Learning Disabilities Source...   ...rcebook

Leukemia Sourcebook   Wom...'s ...

Liver Disorders Sourcebook   E...

Lung Disorders Sourcebook   Workplace Health & Safety Sourcebook

Medical Tests Sourcebook, 3rd Edition   Worldwide Health Sourcebook

Men's Health Concerns Sourcebook, 2nd
    Edition

Mental Health Disorders Sourcebook, 4th
    Edition

Mental Retardation Sourcebook

Movement Disorders Sourcebook, 2nd Edition

Multiple Sclerosis Sourcebook

Muscular Dystrophy Sourcebook

Obesity Sourcebook

Osteoporosis Sourcebook

Pain Sourcebook, 3rd Edition

Pediatric Cancer Sourcebook

Physical & Mental Issues in Aging Sourcebook

Podiatry Sourcebook, 2nd Edition

Pregnancy & Birth Sourcebook, 2nd Edition

Prostate Cancer Sourcebook

Prostate & Urological Disorders Sourcebook

Reconstructive & Cosmetic Surgery
    Sourcebook

Rehabilitation Sourcebook

Respiratory Disorders Sourcebook, 2nd
    Edition

Sexually Transmitted Diseases Sourcebook,
    3rd Edition

Sleep Disorders Sourcebook, 2nd Edition

Smoking Concerns Sourcebook

Sports Injuries Sourcebook, 3rd Edition

Stress-Related Disorders Sourcebook, 2nd
    Edition

Stroke Sourcebook, 2nd Edition

Surgery Sourcebook, 2nd Edition

Thyroid Disorders Sourcebook

Transplantation Sourcebook

Traveler's Health Sourcebook

Urinary Tract & Kidney Diseases & Disorders
    Sourcebook, 2nd Edition

Teen Health Series

Abuse & Violence Information for
    Teens

Accident & Safety Information for Teens

Alcohol Information for Teens, 2nd
    Edition

Allergy Information for Teens

Asthma Information for Teens

Body Information for Teens

Cancer Information for Teens

Complementary & Alternative
    Medicine Information for Teens

Diabetes Information for Teens

Diet Information for Teens, 2nd Edition

Drug Information for Teens, 2nd Edition

Eating Disorders Information for Teens,
    2nd Edition

Fitness Information for Teens, 2nd
    Edition

Learning Disabilities Information for
    Teens

Mental Health Information for Teens,
    2nd Edition

Pregnancy Information for Teens

Sexual Health Information for Teens,
    2nd Edition

Skin Health Information for Teens, 2nd
    Edition

Sleep Information for Teens

Sports Injuries Information for Teens,
    2nd Edition

Stress Information for Teens

Suicide Information for Teens

Tobacco Information for Teens

Arthritis
SOURCEBOOK
Third Edition

Health Reference Series

Third Edition

Arthritis
SOURCEBOOK

Basic Consumer Health Information about the Risk Factors, Symptoms, Diagnosis, and Treatment of Osteoarthritis, Rheumatoid Arthritis, Juvenile Arthritis, Gout, Infectious Arthritis, and Auto-immune Disorders Associated with Arthritis

Along with Facts about Medications, Surgeries, and Self-Care Techniques to Manage Pain and Disability, Tips on Living with Arthritis, a Glossary of Related Terms, and Resources for Additional Help and Information

Edited by
Amy L. Sutton

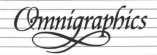

Omnigraphics

P.O. Box 31-1640, Detroit, MI 48231

Bibliographic Note
Because this page cannot legibly accommodate all the copyright notices, the Bibliographic
Note portion of the Preface constitutes an extension of the copyright notice.

Edited by Amy L. Sutton

Health Reference Series

Karen Bellenir, *Managing Editor*
David A. Cooke, MD, FACP, *Medical Consultant*
Elizabeth Collins, *Research and Permissions Coordinator*
Cherry Edwards, *Permissions Assistant*
EdIndex, Services for Publishers, *Indexers*

* * *

Omnigraphics, Inc.
Matthew P. Barbour, *Senior Vice President*
Kevin M. Hayes, *Operations Manager*

* * *

Peter E. Ruffner, *Publisher*

Copyright © 2010 Omnigraphics, Inc.
ISBN 978-0-7808-1077-8

Library of Congress Cataloging-in-Publication Data

Arthritis sourcebook : basic consumer health information about the risk
factors, symptoms, diagnosis, and treatment of osteoarthritis, rheumatoid
arthritis, juvenile arthritis, gout, infectious ... / edited by Amy L.
Sutton. -- 3rd ed.
    p. cm. -- (Health reference series)
  Includes bibliographical references and index.
  Summary: "Provides basic consumer health information about symptoms,
diagnosis, and treatment for major forms of arthritis, along with self-care
tips and coping strategies. Includes index, glossary of related terms, and
other resources"--Provided by publisher.
  ISBN 978-0-7808-1077-8 (hardcover : alk. paper) 1. Arthritis--Popular
works. I. Sutton, Amy L.
  RC933.A665257 2010
  616.7'22--dc22
                                                              2009044768

Table of Contents

Visit www.healthreferenceseries.com to view *A Contents Guide to the Health Reference Series*, a listing of more than 15,000 topics and the volumes in which they are covered.

Part II: Types of Arthritis, Related Rheumatic Diseases, and Other Associated Medical Conditions

ix

Part V: Living with Arthritis

Part VI: Additional Help and Information

Preface

About This Book

About 46 million adults in the United States experience joint pain, stiffness, and inflammation associated with arthritis and related rheumatic diseases. These physical symptoms can interfere with activities of daily life, school, and employment, whereas the fatigue and emotional consequences of the disease can negatively impact relationships and mental well-being. The good news is that medications, surgery, appropriate physical exercise, proper nutrition, and complementary and alternative therapies often offer pain and symptom relief. Although a cure remains elusive, these types of care strategies enable many people to experience significant improvements in daily functioning and overall quality of life.

Arthritis Sourcebook, Third Edition provides updated information about diagnosing, treating, and managing degenerative, inflammatory, and other specific forms of arthritis. It also explains the symptoms and treatments of related diseases that affect the joints, tendons, ligaments, bones, and muscles. Details about currently used medical, surgical, and self-care management strategies are included along with tips for reducing joint pain and inflammation and managing arthritis-related disability. The book concludes with a glossary of terms and directory of resources for additional help and information.

How to Use This Book

This book is divided into parts and chapters. Parts focus on broad areas of interest. Chapters are devoted to single topics within a part.

Part I: Introduction to Arthritis provides general information about the types, prevalence, risk factors, and causes of arthritis and related rheumatic diseases. Information about how arthritis affects specific joints in different parts of the body—the shoulder, wrist, hip, knee, ankle, and foot—is also included.

Part II: Types of Arthritis, Related Rheumatic Diseases, and Other Associated Medical Conditions discusses the symptoms, diagnosis, and treatments for common forms of arthritis, including osteoarthritis, rheumatoid arthritis, and juvenile arthritis. Separate individual chapters focus on rheumatic diseases caused by or related to arthritis. These disorders, such as ankylosing spondylitis, fibromyalgia, gout, lupus, psoriasis, and scleroderma, may also cause chronic joint pain, stiffness, and inflammation.

Part III: Medical and Surgical Treatments for Arthritis begins with information about how arthritis patients can find and communicate with appropriate health care providers. It describes corticosteroid and botulinum toxin injections, which are often used for pain relief, and it provides information about over-the-counter and prescription medications used for arthritis-related pain and inflammation. Surgical procedures, including arthroscopic, bone fusion, and joint replacement surgery, are also described.

Part IV: Arthritis Self-Management: Strategies to Reduce Pain and Inflammation highlights various ways arthritis patients can cope with pain, sleep deprivation, and other symptoms that may accompany arthritis. Weight management tips, exercise programs, and nutrition-related strategies are discussed, and facts about the use of herbs, dietary supplements, and other complementary and alternative therapies are provided.

Part V: Living with Arthritis describes some of the emotional concerns and daily challenges encountered by people who are coping with the effects and limitations of joint disease. These include handling depression, managing stress, maintaining independence, and preserving healthy relationships. Tips are also provided for arthritis patients who have questions about starting a family or handling disability-related financial, legal, and employment issues.

Part VI: Additional Help and Information offers a glossary of important terms related to arthritis and rheumatic diseases. A directory of resources contains a list of organizations able to help people with arthritis, and it includes facts about programs that assist with the cost of medications.

Bibliographic Note

This volume contains documents and excerpts from publications issued by the following U.S. government agencies: Agency for Healthcare Research and Quality (AHRQ); Centers for Disease Control and Prevention (CDC); National Center for Complementary and Alternative Medicine (NCCAM); National Guideline Clearinghouse (NGC); National Highway Traffic Safety Administration (NHTSA); National Institute of Arthritis and Musculoskeletal and Skin Diseases (NIAMS); National Institute of Diabetes and Digestive and Kidney Diseases (NIDDK); National Institute of Neurological Disorders and Stroke (NINDS); National Institute on Aging (NIA); National Institutes of Health (NIH); National Library of Medicine (NLM); Office of Women's Health (OWH); and the U.S. Food and Drug Administration (FDA).

In addition, this volume contains copyrighted documents from the following organizations and publications: A.D.A.M., Inc.; American Academy of Orthopaedic Surgeons; American College of Rheumatology; American College of Sports Medicine; American Geriatrics Society Foundation for Health in Aging; *Atlanta Journal Constitution*; Biological Sciences Curriculum Study; Center for Effective Parenting—Arkansas State Parent Information and Resource Center; DePuy Orthopaedics, Inc.; eMedicine.com; Gillette Children's Specialty Healthcare; Hospital for Special Surgery; International Still's Disease Foundation; Johns Hopkins Medicine Office of Corporate Communications; MediZine LLC; Missouri Arthritis Rehabilitation Research and Training Center; National Fibromyalgia Association; National Pain Foundation; National Psoriasis Foundation; The Nemours Foundation; Rehabilitation Institute of Chicago; Spondylitis Association of America; Vancouver Coastal Health; and Wake Forest University Baptist Medical Center.

Full citation information is provided on the first page of each chapter or section. Every effort has been made to secure all necessary rights to reprint the copyrighted material. If any omissions have been made, please contact Omnigraphics to make corrections for future editions.

Acknowledgements

Thanks go to the many organizations, agencies, and individuals who have contributed materials for this *Sourcebook* and to medical consultant Dr. David Cooke and document engineer Bruce Bellenir. Special thanks go to managing editor Karen Bellenir and research and permissions coordinator Liz Collins for their help and support.

About the Health Reference Series

The *Health Reference Series* is designed to provide basic medical information for patients, families, caregivers, and the general public. Each volume takes a particular topic and provides comprehensive coverage. This is especially important for people who may be dealing with a newly diagnosed disease or a chronic disorder in themselves or in a family member. People looking for preventive guidance, information about disease warning signs, medical statistics, and risk factors for health problems will also find answers to their questions in the *Health Reference Series*. The *Series*, however, is not intended to serve as a tool for diagnosing illness, in prescribing treatments, or as a substitute for the physician/patient relationship. All people concerned about medical symptoms or the possibility of disease are encouraged to seek professional care from an appropriate health care provider.

A Note about Spelling and Style

Health Reference Series editors use *Stedman's Medical Dictionary* as an authority for questions related to the spelling of medical terms and the *Chicago Manual of Style* for questions related to grammatical structures, punctuation, and other editorial concerns. Consistent adherence is not always possible, however, because the individual volumes within the *Series* include many documents from a wide variety of different producers and copyright holders, and the editor's primary goal is to present material from each source as accurately as is possible following the terms specified by each document's producer. This sometimes means that information in different chapters or sections may follow other guidelines and alternate spelling authorities. For example, occasionally a copyright holder may require that eponymous terms be shown in possessive forms (Crohn's disease *vs.* Crohn disease) or that British spelling norms be retained (leukaemia *vs.* leukemia).

Locating Information within the Health Reference Series

The *Health Reference Series* contains a wealth of information about a wide variety of medical topics. Ensuring easy access to all the fact sheets, research reports, in-depth discussions, and other material contained within the individual books of the *Series* remains one of our highest priorities. As the *Series* continues to grow in size and scope, however, locating the precise information needed by a reader may become more challenging.

A Contents Guide to the Health Reference Series was developed to direct readers to the specific volumes that address their concerns. It presents an extensive list of diseases, treatments, and other topics of general interest compiled from the Tables of Contents and major index headings. To access *A Contents Guide to the Health Reference Series*, visit www.healthreferenceseries.com.

Medical Consultant

Medical consultation services are provided to the *Health Reference Series* editors by David A. Cooke, MD, FACP. Dr. Cooke is a graduate of Brandeis University, and he received his M.D. degree from the University of Michigan. He completed residency training at the University of Wisconsin Hospital and Clinics. He is board-certified in Internal Medicine. Dr. Cooke currently works as part of the University of Michigan Health System and practices in Ann Arbor, MI. In his free time, he enjoys writing, science fiction, and spending time with his family.

Our Advisory Board

We would like to thank the following board members for providing guidance to the development of this *Series*:

- Dr. Lynda Baker, Associate Professor of Library and Information Science, Wayne State University, Detroit, MI

- Nancy Bulgarelli, William Beaumont Hospital Library, Royal Oak, MI

- Karen Imarisio, Bloomfield Township Public Library, Bloomfield Township, MI

- Karen Morgan, Mardigian Library, University of Michigan-Dearborn, Dearborn, MI

- Rosemary Orlando, St. Clair Shores Public Library, St. Clair Shores, MI

Health Reference Series *Update Policy*

The inaugural book in the *Health Reference Series* was the first edition of *Cancer Sourcebook* published in 1989. Since then, the *Series* has been enthusiastically received by librarians and in the medical community. In order to maintain the standard of providing high-quality health information for the layperson the editorial staff at Omnigraphics felt it was necessary to implement a policy of updating volumes when warranted.

Medical researchers have been making tremendous strides, and it is the purpose of the *Health Reference Series* to stay current with the most recent advances. Each decision to update a volume is made on an individual basis. Some of the considerations include how much new information is available and the feedback we receive from people who use the books. If there is a topic you would like to see added to the update list, or an area of medical concern you feel has not been adequately addressed, please write to:

Editor
Health Reference Series
Omnigraphics, Inc.
P.O. Box 31-1640
Detroit, MI 48231
E-mail: editorial@omnigraphics.com

Part One

Introduction to Arthritis

Chapter 1

Understanding the Bones, Muscles, and Joints

Characteristics of Bone, Muscle, and Skin

Human development is a complex process that begins with a fertilized egg cell and eventually gives rise to an adult human composed of over 100 trillion cells. As development proceeds, cells begin to take on specialized roles that remain stable throughout the life of the individual. Cells with the same function may group together in specific ways to form a colony of cells called a tissue. An adult human makes use of over 200 different tissues. One or more tissues may work together to form one of the body's organs. As the number of cells in the developing human increases, the fate of the individual cells becomes ever more restricted. This process by which a cell becomes committed to a specific function is called differentiation.

Just as the human body has different organs that carry out specific functions, the human cell has different organelles that have specialized functions. All human cells share certain characteristics. They:

- possess a plasma membrane that separates their inside contents from the outside environment;

- enclose their genetic material inside a membrane-bound organelle called a nucleus;

- generate usable energy within organelles called mitochondria; and

- synthesize proteins using ribosomes.

Despite these similarities, differentiation produces cells that differ in significant ways from one another. The shapes of different cells relate to their functions within the body. For example, nerve cells have many long branches that enable them to communicate with each other and with other cells. Even the presence or absence of a critical organelle, such as the nucleus, can vary by cell type. A mature red blood cell has no nucleus, while a mature skeletal muscle cell has many nuclei derived from cells that have fused together. We shall learn in the following information how the cells of the musculoskeletal and skin systems have characteristic shapes that relate to their functions and how they combine to form specialized tissues.

Bone

Bones serve many important functions. They allow us to do things we take for granted, such as stand and sit, walk and run. They do this in concert with muscles, which attach to bones via tendons. Our bones provide structural support for the body and help determine our shape. Bones also protect internal organs (the skull protects the brain, and the ribs protect the heart and lungs), and the bone marrow produces red blood cells and the white blood cells of the immune system. Bones are lightweight yet very strong, static in appearance yet very dynamic. How does the structure of bones determine how they function in the body?

Bones have a unique structure. The human skeleton has 206 bones of different sizes and shapes. Bones such as those in the arms and legs are called long bones. Others, such as those in the skull, are called flat bones. Other categories include the short bones (for instance, the carpal bones of the wrist) and the irregular bones (for instance, vertebrae). In general, adult human bones are composed of about 70 percent minerals and 30 percent organic matter. The minerals are primarily a crystalline complex of calcium and phosphate called hydroxyapatite, while 90 to 95 percent of the organic matter is the protein collagen. The remainder of the organic matter consists of a gelatinous medium called ground substance, which contains extracellular fluid and specialized proteins called proteoglycans.

Looking at a cross section of a long bone, one sees an inner cavity surrounded by an outer fibrous matrix. The inner cavity contains bone marrow, which consists of fatty tissue and cells that give rise to the red and white blood cells that circulate in the body. The bone matrix contains hydroxyapatite and calcium salts deposited in a network of collagen fibers. On the outside of the bone is a fibrous layer called the periosteum.

A closer look reveals more details. There are two forms of bone—compact (hard) bone, the solid, hard outside part of bone that is optimized to handle compressive and bending forces, and spongy (cancellous) bone, which is found inside the compact bone and near the ends of the bone. Blood vessels are also present and allow nutrients to be brought to bone cells and waste products to be carried away. Blood vessels and nerves pass through narrow openings, or canals, that run parallel to the surface and along the long axis of the bone.

Bone contains three specialized cell types. The name of each begins with osteo, since this is the Greek word for bone. Osteoblasts are cells that form new bone. They are found on the surface of new bone and they have a single nucleus. They are derived from stem cells in the bone marrow. Osteoblasts produce collagen found in bone and the proteoglycans found in ground substance. They are rich in alkaline phosphatase, a phosphate-splitting enzyme required for bone mineralization, a process that osteoblasts control. When osteoblasts have completed making new bone, the cells take on a flattened appearance and line the surface of the bone. Now in a more mature, less active state, the cells are called bone-lining cells. They still serve important functions, however. For instance, bone-lining cells respond to specific hormones and produce proteins that activate another type of bone cell called the osteoclast.

Osteoclasts are large, multinucleated cells that are capable of movement. They are formed by the fusion of mononuclear cells derived from stem cells in the bone marrow. Unlike osteoblasts, osteoclasts lie in depressions where their function is to dissolve (resorb) bone and help shape it. They begin by attacking the mineral portion of bone and then they degrade the bone proteins.

Osteocytes are cells that reside inside bone. They are derived from osteoblasts as new bone is being formed and then become surrounded by the new bone. However, rather than being isolated, osteocytes communicate through long branches that connect these cells to one another. These cells regulate the response of bone to its mechanical environment. Osteocytes sense pressures or cracks in bone and help direct osteoclasts to locations where bone will be remodeled.

Bone formation involves an organic matrix. To understand how bone is formed and why its properties confer such strength, imagine that you have steel rods and cement that you will use to construct a wall or a bridge. Pouring cement around steel rods placed in a suitable frame produces a material (reinforced concrete) that is stronger and more capable of withstanding movement than either steel rods or cement alone. Bone has a similar organization. The steel rods are chains of collagen, which confer resiliency, and the cement is hydroxyapatite, which confers strength.

Bone formation begins with synthesis of the organic matrix by osteoblasts. The matrix can be likened to a protein scaffolding. Next, through a mechanism not yet understood, osteoblasts deposit mineral crystals in the spaces between the protein scaffolding. The mineral consists primarily of calcium and phosphorus. Finally, osteoclasts work with osteocytes to shape or remodel the bone by breaking down the proteins and resorbing the minerals. Bone formation is not a strictly linear process, however. Bones are constantly being formed, broken down, and reformed. Bone is a very dynamic, continually changing tissue. Osteoblasts, osteoclasts, and osteocytes function to maintain a balance between bone deposition and bone resorption that allows bones to grow, repair themselves, and remain strong.

The activity of osteoblasts and osteoclasts is influenced by a number of factors. Vitamin D helps the intestine absorb calcium from foods into the bloodstream after digestion. It is also important in regulating phosphate in the body. Additionally, when blood-calcium levels are low, the parathyroid glands release parathyroid hormone into the blood. Parathyroid hormone activates the osteoclasts, thereby increasing the rate of bone breakdown. Other factors that regulate the dynamic balance between bone deposition and bone breakdown include growth factors and hormones. Importantly, exercise is an important factor in normal bone growth and development. Also, the composition of bone mineral is not fixed. Other ions, if present, can be incorporated into new or remodeled bone. Fluoride, for example, can be incorporated into bone mineral to form fluorapatite, which is harder, less soluble, and more resistant to resorption than is hydroxyapatite.

Bones grow as we grow. This is no surprise. In fact, more bone is formed during the first 20 to 30 years of life than is resorbed, resulting in an increase in bone mass. However, contrary to what some might think, long bones do not grow (or elongate) from the middle, a region called the diaphysis. Rather, the bones grow from their ends, regions called the epiphyses (singular is epiphysis).

Cartilage is a connective tissue specialized to handle mechanical stress without becoming distorted permanently. It is found in areas where shock-absorbing properties are needed or where smooth movement between bones (that is, at a joint) is required. As bones grow, additional cartilage is deposited at the epiphyseal, or growth, plate. This cartilage is the framework on which bone matrix is deposited. Bone growth continues as long as the growth plates are able to produce chondrocytes (cartilage-producing cells). The growth plate determines the length and shape of the mature bone and is the weakest part of the growing skeleton. The growth plate can be injured (fractured) during an acute incident, such as a fall, or from overuse, such as during intense sports training. If untreated, some growth plate fractures can lead to permanent damage and can cause bone growth to stop prematurely.

Hormones are responsible for the cessation of growth. At the end of puberty, high levels of estrogen or testosterone cause the chondrocytes to die, and they are replaced by bone. It is during late adolescence that humans achieve their peak bone mass. Over the next 30 or more years, the human adult skeleton is maintained by precisely balanced bone formation and bone resorption. Sometime after humans reach their 60s, bone mass begins to decrease because new bone formation can no longer keep pace with bone resorption.

Muscle

Muscle is the most abundant tissue in most animals. In vertebrates, such as humans, there are different types of muscle, and each has a unique cellular structure and function. Skeletal muscle enables us to walk, run, lift, or do other physical movements. It enables people to maintain their body posture. Skeletal muscle is also referred to as striated muscle because the arrangement of muscle fibers has a striped (striated) appearance when viewed under a microscope. Smooth muscle is found in the walls of the stomach and intestines, the urinary bladder, the bronchi of the lungs, and the arterial blood vessels. It functions to propel substances along their tracts within the body. Smooth muscle lacks striations and is composed of cells that are spindle shaped. A third type of muscle, cardiac muscle, makes up the heart and pumps blood throughout the body. As the name implies, skeletal muscle is intimately associated with the skeletal system, and for this reason, this information focuses on skeletal muscle and does not discuss cardiac and smooth muscle. Unless otherwise noted, the term muscle refers to skeletal muscle from this point on.

During human development, the differentiation of the muscle system is essentially complete just 8 weeks after fertilization. The first cells committed to form muscle in the developing embryo are called myoblasts. Some myoblasts divide rapidly, while others migrate to areas where muscle tissue needs to form, such as the developing limb buds. Once myoblasts arrive at their needed location, they stop cell division and begin to fuse together with adjoining myoblasts. The results of this cell fusion create a larger cell with many nuclei that share the same cytoplasm. These multinucleated cells continue to differentiate into a myotube, which is the basic structural cell of muscle tissue.

The most essential feature of muscle cells is their ability to generate force by contracting, or shortening—a function unlike that of other types of cells. In skeletal muscle, numerous myotubes bundle together to form a muscle. Within each myotube are thin and thick filaments. Under the microscope, the regular arrangement of these filaments accounts for the alternating light and dark bands seen in the tissue. The functional unit of the muscle is called the sarcomere. Each sarcomere has a dark Z line at each end. By examining the structure of the sarcomere, we can begin to appreciate how a muscle cell is able to contract and exert force on the skeletal system.

When researchers observed muscle contraction under the microscope, they noticed that the sarcomere shortened, that is, the Z lines moved closer together. This observation suggested that muscle contraction proceeds by having thin and thick filaments slide past each other, shortening the sarcomere.

This process is described by the sliding filament model of muscle contraction. According to this model, the lengths of the thin and thick filaments do not change. Rather, the extent to which they overlap changes. As the amount of overlap between the thin and thick filaments increases, the length of the sarcomere decreases. Thin filaments are made of a protein called actin, and thick filaments are made of a protein called myosin. The myosin molecule has a long "tail" region with a protruding "head" at one end. The myosin head provides the energy needed to move the filaments past each other by breaking down the high-energy molecule ATP [adenosine triphosphate] into ADP [adenosine diphosphate] and inorganic phosphate.

Muscle contraction is controlled by the nervous system. Nerves that interact with a muscle cell release a neurotransmitter, known as acetylcholine. This triggers electrical changes within the muscle cell that lead to the release of calcium ions from the sarcoplasmic reticulum (a specialized form of the endoplasmic reticulum). The calcium ions release an inhibitory mechanism and allow the actin and myosin filaments to slide past each other. The muscle fibers themselves are not all identical. They can be classified as slow-twitch fibers or fast-twitch fibers. At Thanksgiving dinner, we refer to these different types of turkey muscle as dark meat and light meat. The dark meat is composed of muscle that has a large proportion of slow-twitch fibers. The slow-twitch fibers are made of muscle cells that have more mitochondria and therefore more red-colored cytochromes than cells from fast-twitch fibers. Slow-twitch fibers have less sarcoplasmic reticulum as compared with fast twitch fibers. Slow-twitch fibers contract at a rate about five times longer than fast-twitch fibers. Fast-twitch fibers are specialized for generating rapid, forceful contractions for short term activities such as jumping or sprinting over a period of a few seconds to about a minute. Some of our muscles, such as those controlling eye movements, are made almost exclusively from fast-twitch fibers. Slow-twitch fibers are specialized for prolonged activity over a period of minutes or hours. The soleus muscle in the lower leg is made up of slow-twitch fibers.

Most of our muscles are composed of a mixture of slow-twitch and fast-twitch fibers, and this mix varies among individuals. The ratio of slow-twitch to fast-twitch fibers for a given muscle is largely genetically determined, though some studies have shown that rigorous training can alter the ratio. This partly explains why some individuals excel at running sprints while others excel at running long distances.

This means that in order to move a limb either up and down or back and forth, a pair of muscles must be involved. Indeed, skeletal muscles work in antagonistic pairs. For example, when a person bends his or her arm, the biceps contract (shorten) and the triceps relax (lengthen). When the arm straightens, the biceps relax and the triceps contract. Contraction is called the concentric phase, whereas the relaxation of the muscle is the eccentric phase. In general, most people think of muscles generating force only as they contract and get shorter. In the case of eccentric contractions, however, the muscles exert force even as they are lengthening. For example, to descend stairs in a controlled way, the quadriceps, or thigh muscle, must contract even as the movement of the knee joint tends to stretch it. Scientists are now recognizing that understanding more about eccentric contractions is important because they are common physiologically, are often associated with muscle soreness and injuries, and may be important in muscle-strengthening activities.

Scientists continue to learn more about the value of regular exercise for maintaining or improving health. Exercise reduces the risk of certain medical conditions including heart disease and obesity and can help reduce complications in other diseases such as diabetes. Exercise is important for children and adolescents as well as for adults. Although in the past, weight (or resistance) training was not recommended for children, the American College of Sports Medicine recently advised that resistance training using nonmaximal weights and the supervision of a trained instructor is safe. In addition to helping build optimal bone mass and reducing the risk of obesity, youth resistance training may decrease the incidence of some sports injuries. The increase in muscular strength that occurs when an adolescent participates in resistance training appears to be a result of increased neuromuscular activation and coordination rather than muscle growth.

Skin

Skin is the largest organ of the human body. Skin is in constant contact with the environment and plays several important roles in maintaining our health and well-being. It serves many purposes, including:

- providing a barrier to microorganisms and toxins;
- preventing us from drying out;
- helping us to maintain temperature control;
- helping us sense pressure and temperature; and
- providing aesthetic and beauty qualities.

Skin is composed of distinct layers. In humans, a functional skin barrier is acquired by about 8.5 months of prenatal development. Babies born prematurely do not have an effective skin barrier and must be kept alive in sterile incubators until they develop the requisite protection. Skin has three layers—the epidermis, the dermis, and the subcutaneous fat layer. The thickness of the epidermis and dermis is different for skin with or without hair. Glabrous skin (skin without hair) has an epidermal layer that is about 1.5 millimeters (mm) thick and a dermal layer that is about 3 mm thick. Hairy skin has an epidermal layer that is 0.07 mm thick and a dermal layer that is 1 to 2 mm thick. The thickness of the subcutaneous fat layer varies throughout the body and from one individual to another.

10

The outermost layer of skin, which we can see, is called the epidermis. The epidermis itself also has multiple layers. The outer layer of the epidermis consists largely of dead skin cells, which are being continuously sloughed off. In fact, most of the house dust that you see is actually composed of dead skin cells. This layer of skin does not feel pain because it lacks blood vessels and nerves. The living, multiplying skin cells are found at the bottom of the epidermis, the basal layer.

Beneath the epidermis is the dermis, which provides a strong, resilient, and flexible infrastructure for the skin. The main component of the dermis is collagen, which accounts for nearly 70 to 75 percent of the skin's dry weight. Collagen is a versatile protein that provides strength. It is necessary for healing wounds, but overproduction during healing leads to scars. Stretch marks are caused by collagen fibers that have been stretched to the point of tearing. Another important component of the dermis is elastin, which gives skin its elasticity. Collagen and elastin degenerate with age, causing wrinkles and sagging.

The dermis is supplied with nutrients and oxygen by blood vessels. A recent study suggests that blood vessels are not the only way skin cells get oxygen, however. According to Markus Stücker of Ruhr University, the atmosphere, thought to be unimportant, actually supplies the top 0.25 to 0.40 mm of skin with oxygen. This corresponds to the entire epidermis and a portion of the dermis below. This finding has implications for doctors treating skin diseases. Healthy skin that is cut off from the air can compensate by obtaining oxygen from the blood, while diseased skin appears unable to do this.

The blood vessels in the dermis hold as much as 25 percent of the body's blood supply at one time. Transdermal drugs take advantage of this vast network of blood vessels. Any substance that penetrates the epidermis and reaches the dermis can enter the bloodstream.

The dermis is also rich in nerves. Sensations transmitted by nerves in the skin include touch, temperature, pain, itching, and pressure. Free nerve endings are scattered throughout the skin and are grouped around the bases of hair. They can register pain and pressure.

The dermis contains hair follicles, sebaceous glands, and sweat glands. (Hair grows from the bulb at the hair follicle's base, which is in the subcutaneous fat layer.) On one side of the follicle is a sebaceous gland that produces an oily substance that lubricates the hair and epidermis. On the other side of the follicle is the erector pili muscle used to erect the hairs.

There are two types of sweat glands. The eccrine glands are located all over the skin surface. They produce a salty liquid that functions as a cooling mechanism when it evaporates from the skin surface. This liquid is somewhat acidic, which helps retard the growth of bacteria that live on the skin. The apocrine glands are thought to produce odors that serve as sexual messages. They are located under the armpits and on the genitals. Starting at puberty, these glands begin secreting a mixture of protein and fat. Bacteria can thrive in these environments and are responsible for body odor.

The bottom layer of the skin is the subcutaneous fat layer. This layer consists primarily of fat cells separated by bands of fibrous connective tissue. It provides a reservoir of energy as well as insulation and gives us our shape. The subcutaneous fat layer may best be known because of cellulite. Cellulite is the puckered appearance of skin thought to be caused by fibrous bands dividing lobules of fat.

Skin cells come in several types. The epidermis is formed by multiple layers of keratinocytes. These cells make keratin, which is a type of protein that provides the skin with its structural integrity. Keratinocytes make up 90 to 95 percent of the cells in the epidermis. The keratinocytes in the outer layer are dead, whereas the keratinocytes in the bottom layer are alive and produce the keratinocytes, which eventually make their way up to the surface of the skin. Keratinocytes also produce hair and nails.

The epidermis also contains melanocytes. There is about one melanocyte for every keratinocyte in the skin. Melanocytes are cells that produce a pigment called melanin. Melanin is transferred to the cells of the epidermis and hair, giving skin and hair their color. The number of melanocytes in the epidermis is the same for all races, but the amount of melanin produced varies. Melanin absorbs ultraviolet light and protects us from sun damage. The melanin shields the DNA of the nucleus in keratinocytes from the mutating effects of the sun.

Other skin cells include Merkel's cells, Langerhans cells, and fibroblast cells. Merkel's cells are sensory receptors that respond to sensations of pressure and are more numerous in the palms and soles of the feet. Langerhans cells are found in the epidermis and dermis as well as other parts of the body. They monitor immune reactions in the skin and play an important role in reactions to poison ivy and other skin irritants. Fibroblast cells, which produce collagen, are the primary cell type in the dermis.

Skin can reflect an individual's general state of health. Skin can suggest that a person is tired or ill. A skin problem also can reflect the onset of another disease. For example, skin itches may be harbingers of diabetes and kidney disease. Clear skin is an important aspect of sexual attraction in virtually all cultures. From an evolutionary point of view, the association between good health (and fertility) and unblemished skin may be responsible for our attraction to those with clear skin.

Since skin is important to sexual attraction, it is not surprising that some people modify the appearance of their skin to enhance their attractiveness. The most common methods include tanning, piercing, and tattoos. Unfortunately, all of these practices can have negative and potentially serious health consequences. A recent survey of 454 university students revealed that more than half had a body piercing and about one-quarter had a tattoo. Nearly one-fifth reported that they had a medical complication due to the procedure itself or how they cared for the piercing or tattoo afterward.

Research into the science of skin is leading to new understandings about how the skin performs its vital functions. For example, studies are shedding light on how skin senses heat, interacts with the immune system in wound repair, and elicits responses to antigens presented at the skin surface. Other studies are concerned with developing new ways for treating people whose skin has been damaged by accident or disease. Each year, there are about 13,000 hospitalizations in the United States that require extensive skin grafting. Unfortunately, the existing skin graft technology has limitations. One company called Stratatech has discovered a rare mutation in a culture of skin cells that allows the cells to grow indefinitely. Tests using animals have shown that skin from this culture can be used successfully to treat wounds. It is hoped that this culture will develop into an off-the-shelf product used by doctors performing skin grafts. Researchers looking at skin stem cells taken from mice have found that they can develop into other types of cells such as nerve, muscle, and fat cells. Their intention is to coax human skin cells to form other cell types that could be used to treat patients with a variety of disorders.

The skin is also being exploited in drug-delivery techniques. Such techniques involve widening the skin's pores using ultrasound waves or an electric shock, or even using a grid of microscopic needles. These approaches offer a number of advantages over traditional means of drug delivery. They can ensure the steady release of a drug over long periods of time and bypass the rapid breakdown that occurs in the digestive system. They are also painless and convenient.

Interactions

As discussed in previous text, bone, muscle, and skin are living systems and are active metabolically. They are connected, as are all other organs, by the body's cardiovascular system. This allows bone, muscle, and skin to respond to hormones and growth factors produced by other tissues. As a result, growth and other metabolic activities in bone, muscle, and skin occur in a coordinated manner. The nervous system also allows interactions between bone, muscle, and skin. Consider what occurs when nerves in the skin of fingers contact a hot object—the muscles of the arm quickly contract, and the arm is moved away from the heat.

In this text, we consider two examples of how bone, muscle, and skin interact. First, we consider joints, which involve interactions between bones and muscles, and then we look at interactions among all three systems related to vitamin D.

Joints

A joint is the place where two bones meet. Because bones are hard, tough structures that resist movement individually, joints form new structures that can move. By joining, or articulating, all the bones of the body, a skeleton of defined shape that is capable of movement is formed.

Joints can be classified in several ways, but for our purposes, joints will be classified by the type of movement they allow. Accordingly, joints can be separated into three main groups: fixed or immovable, slightly movable, and freely movable. Fixed or immovable joints are found between the bones of the skull. The individual bones are joined by dense, fibrous connective tissue, which is why these joints are also called fibrous joints. Fixed joints serve a protective function, although they do allow growth to occur. Teeth are attached to the jaws by fixed joints.

Slightly movable joints are found, for example, between individual vertebra of the vertebral, or spinal, column and where ribs join to the breastbone. In slightly movable joints, the bones are attached to one another by pads or disks of the connective tissue, or cartilage.

Most joints in the human body are freely movable and are characterized by a cavity that contains a fluid, called synovial fluid, that provides lubrication. The ends of adjacent bones have complementary shapes, which further reduces friction, and are covered with a layer of smooth, hard cartilage. These joints are completely enclosed by a bag-like ligament that holds the joint together and prevents the synovial fluid from leaking out.

There are six basic categories of freely movable joints:

- Ball-and-socket joints allow more freedom of movement than any other joint. One bone of the joint has a rounded head that fits into the socket of the other bone. Ball-and-socket joints are found at the hips and shoulders.

- Gliding joints are composed of bones that are almost flat and slide over one another. They offer flexibility in movement direction, although they do not allow great range in movement. The bones of the wrist are connected through gliding joints.

- Hinge joints allow movement up and down, although they do not allow twisting or sliding. One bone, the humerus (bone of the upper arm), for example, fits into the rounded part of another bone, the ulna (the fixed bone of the forearm), thus forming a hinge joint (the elbow).

- Pivot joints allow bones to spin around one another. They are formed when one bone fits into the ring shape of another bone. A pivot joint allows the twisting motion of the elbow (as opposed to the up-and-down motion of the hinge joint). Additionally, a pivot joint is found between the first two vertebrae in the neck, allowing us to provide a negative response by rotating our head left and right.

- Condyloid joints allow movement in many directions, although they do not allow rotation. One bone of the joint is concave while the other is convex. The lower jaw is attached to the skull through a condyloid joint.

- Saddle joints allow side-to-side movement and limited rotation. The bones of a saddle joint have odd shapes but are completely complementary to one another. The lower finger bones are connected to the bones of the hand through saddle joints.

Chapter 2

Overview of Arthritis and Rheumatic Diseases

What is arthritis and what are rheumatic diseases?

Arthritis literally means joint inflammation. Although joint inflammation describes a symptom or sign rather than a specific diagnosis, the term "arthritis" is often used to refer to any disorder that affects the joints. These disorders fall within the broader category of rheumatic diseases. These are diseases characterized by inflammation (signs include redness or heat, swelling, and symptoms such as pain) and loss of function of one or more connecting or supporting structures of the body. These diseases especially affect joints, tendons, ligaments, bones, and muscles. Common signs and symptoms are pain, swelling, and stiffness. Some rheumatic diseases also can involve internal organs.

There are more than 100 rheumatic diseases. Some are described as connective tissue diseases because they affect the supporting framework of the body and its internal organs. Others are known as autoimmune diseases because they occur when the immune system, which normally protects the body from infection and disease, harms the body's own healthy tissues. Throughout this text, the terms "arthritis" and "rheumatic diseases" are used interchangeably.

The burden of arthritis in the United States is enormous. More than 46 million people in the United States have arthritis or other

Excerpted from "Questions and Answers about Arthritis and Rheumatic Diseases," by the National Institute of Arthritis and Musculoskeletal and Skin Diseases (NIAMS, www.niams.nih.gov), part of the National Institutes of Health, October 2008.

rheumatic conditions. Adults with arthritis and other rheumatic conditions incurred mean medical care expenditures of $6,978 in 2003, of which $1,635 was for prescriptions. Expenditures for adults with arthritis and other rheumatic conditions totaled $321.8 billion in 2003. Persons age 18 to 64 with arthritis and other rheumatic conditions earned $3,613 less than other persons. Of this amount, $1,590 in lost wages was attributable to arthritis and other rheumatic conditions.

What are some examples of rheumatic diseases?

Osteoarthritis: This is the most common type of arthritis, affecting an estimated 27 million adults in the United States. Osteoarthritis affects both the cartilage, which is the tissue that cushions the ends of bones within the joint, as well as the underlying bone. In osteoarthritis, there is damage to the cartilage, which begins to fray and may wear away entirely. There is also damage to the bond stock of the joint. Osteoarthritis can cause joint pain and stiffness. Disability results most often when the disease affects the spine and the weight-bearing joints (the knees and hips).

Rheumatoid arthritis: This inflammatory disease of the immune system targets first the synovium, or lining of the joint, resulting in pain, stiffness, swelling, joint damage, and loss of function of the joints. Inflammation most often affects joints of the hands and feet and tends to be symmetrical (occurring equally on both sides of the body). This symmetry helps distinguish rheumatoid arthritis from other forms of the disease. About 0.6 percent of the U.S. population (about 1.3 million people) has rheumatoid arthritis.

Juvenile idiopathic arthritis: This disease is the most common form of arthritis in childhood, causing pain, stiffness, swelling, and loss of function of the joints. This condition may be associated with rashes or fevers and may affect various parts of the body.

Fibromyalgia: Fibromyalgia is a chronic disorder that causes pain throughout the tissues that support and move the bones and joints. Pain, stiffness, and localized tender points occur in the muscles and tendons, particularly those of the neck, spine, shoulders, and hips. Patients also may experience fatigue and sleep disturbances. Fibromyalgia affects millions of adults in the United States.

Systemic lupus erythematosus: Systemic lupus erythematosus (also known as lupus or SLE) is an autoimmune disease in which the immune system harms the body's own healthy cells and tissues. This can result in inflammation of and damage to the joints, skin, kidneys, heart, lungs, blood vessels, and brain. By conservative estimates, lupus affects about 150,000 people.

Scleroderma: Also known as systemic sclerosis, scleroderma means literally "hard skin." The disease affects the skin, blood vessels, and joints. It may also affect internal organs, such as the lungs and kidneys. In scleroderma, there is an abnormal and excessive production of collagen (a fiber-like protein) in the skin and internal organs.

Spondyloarthropathies: This group of rheumatic diseases principally affects the spine. One common form—ankylosing spondylitis—also may affect the hips, shoulders, and knees. The tendons and ligaments around the bones and joints become inflamed, resulting in pain and stiffness. Ankylosing spondylitis tends to affect people in late adolescence or early adulthood. Reactive arthritis, sometimes called Reiter syndrome, is another spondyloarthropathy. It develops after an infection involving the lower urinary tract, bowel, or other organ. It is commonly associated with eye problems, skin rashes, and mouth sores.

Infectious arthritis: This is a general term used to describe forms of arthritis that are caused by infectious agents, such as bacteria or viruses. Parvovirus arthritis and gonococcal arthritis are examples of infectious arthritis. Arthritis symptoms also may occur in Lyme disease, which is caused by a bacterial infection following the bite of certain ticks. In those cases of arthritis caused by bacteria, early diagnosis and treatment with antibiotics are crucial to removing the infection and minimizing damage to the joints.

Gout: This type of arthritis results from deposits of needle-like crystals of uric acid in the joints. The crystals cause episodic inflammation, swelling, and pain in the affected joint, which is often the big toe. An estimated 2.1 million Americans have gout.

Polymyalgia rheumatica: Because this disease involves tendons, muscles, ligaments, and tissues around the joint, symptoms often include pain, aching, and morning stiffness in the shoulders, hips, neck, and lower back. It is sometimes the first sign of giant cell arteritis, a disease of the arteries characterized by headaches, inflammation, weakness, weight loss, and fever.

Polymyositis: This rheumatic disease causes inflammation and weakness in the muscles. The disease may affect the whole body and cause disability.

Psoriatic arthritis: This form of arthritis occurs in some patients with psoriasis, a scaling skin disorder. Psoriatic arthritis often affects the joints at the ends of the fingers and toes and is accompanied by changes in the fingernails and toenails. Back pain may occur if the spine is involved.

Bursitis: This condition involves inflammation of the bursae, small, fluid-filled sacs that help reduce friction between bones and other moving structures in the joints. The inflammation may result from arthritis in the joint or injury or infection of the bursae. Bursitis produces pain and tenderness and may limit the movement of nearby joints.

Tendonitis: This condition refers to inflammation of tendons (tough cords of tissue that connect muscle to bone) caused by overuse, injury, or a rheumatic condition. Tendonitis produces pain and tenderness and may restrict movement of nearby joints.

What causes rheumatic diseases?

Rheumatic diseases are generally believed to be caused by a combination of genetic and environmental factors. In other words, you may be born with a susceptibility to a disease, but it may take something in your environment to get the disease started.

Some of these factors have been identified. For example, in osteoarthritis, inherited cartilage weakness or excessive stress on the joint from repeated injury may play a role. In rheumatoid arthritis, juvenile idiopathic arthritis, and lupus, patients may have a variation in a gene that codes for an enzyme called protein tyrosine phosphatase nonreceptor 22 (PTPN22).

Certain viruses may trigger disease in genetically susceptible people. For example, scientists have found a connection between Epstein-Barr virus and lupus. There are likely many genes and combinations of genes that predispose people to rheumatic diseases, and many different environmental factors that trigger them.

Gender is another factor in some rheumatic diseases. Lupus, rheumatoid arthritis, scleroderma, and fibromyalgia are more common among women. This indicates that hormones or other male-female differences may play a role in the development of these conditions.

Who is affected by rheumatic diseases?

An estimated 43 million people in the United States have arthritis or other rheumatic conditions. By the year 2020, this number is expected to reach 60 million. Rheumatic diseases are a more frequent cause of activity limitation than heart disease, cancer, or diabetes.

Rheumatic diseases affect people of all races and ages. Some rheumatic conditions are more common among certain populations.

- Rheumatoid arthritis occurs two to three times more often in women than in men.

- Scleroderma is more common in women than in men.

- Nine out of 10 people who have lupus are women.

- Nine out of 10 people who have fibromyalgia are women.

- Gout is more common in men than in women. After menopause, the incidence of gout for women begins to rise.

- Systemic lupus erythematosus is more common in women than in men, and it occurs more often in African Americans and Hispanics than in Caucasians.

What are the signs and symptoms of arthritis and rheumatic diseases?

Different types of arthritis and rheumatic diseases have different signs and symptoms. In general, people who have arthritis feel pain and stiffness in the joints. Early diagnosis and treatment help decrease further joint damage and help control symptoms of arthritis and many other rheumatic diseases.

What research is being done on arthritis and rheumatic diseases?

Biomarkers: Recent scientific breakthroughs in basic research have provided new information about what happens to the body's cells and other structures as rheumatic diseases progress. Biomarkers (laboratory and imaging signposts that detect disease) help researchers determine both the likelihood that a person will develop a specific disease as well as its possible severity and outcome.

Biomarkers have the potential to lead to novel and more effective ways of predicting and monitoring both disease activity and responses to treatment. NIAMS supports research on biomarkers for rheumatic and skin diseases, including initiatives to identify and validate biomarkers for osteoarthritis and lupus.

PROMIS: NIAMS has responsibility for managing an NIH [National Institutes of Health]-wide initiative known as PROMIS (Patient-Reported Outcomes Measurement Information System). The goal of this initiative is to develop ways to measure patient-reported symptoms such as pain and fatigue as well as other aspects of health-related quality-of-life across a wide variety of chronic diseases and conditions. Arthritis and many other diseases that compromise daily life involve pain, fatigue, and other quality-of-life outcomes that are hard to measure. A means of measuring changes in these symptoms could enhance clinical research and practice, providing a significant benefit to patients and their health care providers.

Fibromyalgia: In recent years, NIAMS has supported an increasing amount of research into this condition, which is not well understood. Scientists are using imaging studies of the central nervous system to better understand the overresponsiveness to painful stimuli in people with this disorder. They are studying the role of sex hormones, stress, and other factors on fibromyalgia. They are also examining the effectiveness of behavior therapy, exercise, medications, micronutrients, acupuncture, and other alternative approaches for dealing with pain, fatigue, and loss of sleep.

Osteoarthritis: NIAMS has embarked on several innovative efforts to understand the causes and identify effective treatment and prevention methods for osteoarthritis. Through a public/private partnership, researchers are identifying biomarkers for osteoarthritis that will help develop and test new drugs. Imaging studies designed to better identify joint disorders and assess their progression are taking place as well.

NIH's National Center for Complementary and Alternative Medicine and NIAMS funded a major, 16-center study on the usefulness of the dietary supplements glucosamine and chondroitin sulfate, which previous studies have suggested may be useful for osteoarthritis.

Some genetic and behavioral studies are focusing on factors that may cause osteoarthritis to develop. Among behavioral risk factors, excessive weight and lack of exercise have been identified as contributing to knee and hip disability.

Researchers are working to understand the role certain enzymes play in the breakdown of joint cartilage in osteoarthritis. They also are testing drugs that block the action of these enzymes and looking at new ways to administer drugs.

Studies show that young adults who have had a previous joint injury are more likely to develop osteoarthritis. These studies underscore the need for increased education about joint injury prevention and use of proper sports equipment. They are also prompting scientists to look for ways to prevent joint cartilage breakdown after injury.

Rheumatoid arthritis: Researchers are trying to identify the cause of rheumatoid arthritis so they can develop better and more specific treatments. They are examining the roles that the endocrine (hormonal), nervous, and immune systems play, and the ways in which these systems interact with environmental and genetic factors in the development of rheumatoid arthritis. Some scientists are trying to determine whether an infectious agent triggers rheumatoid arthritis. Others are studying the role of certain enzymes (specialized proteins in the body that spark biochemical reactions) in breaking down cartilage. Researchers are also trying to identify the genetic factors that place some people at higher risk than others for developing rheumatoid arthritis.

Moreover, scientists are looking at new ways to treat rheumatoid arthritis. They are experimenting with new drugs, genetic therapies, and biologic agents that selectively block certain immune system activities associated with inflammation.

In recent years, several biologic agents have been approved. These include etanercept (Enbrel) and infliximab (Remicade), which block a cytokine, or chemical messenger, called tumor necrosis factor (TNF); anakinra (Kineret), which blocks the cytokine interleukin-1 (IL-1); and abatacept (Orencia), which interferes with function of some cells such as T-lymphocytes. These cells are important in rheumatoid arthritis. Followup studies of biologics have shown that they not only relieve signs and symptoms of rheumatoid arthritis, but also block the joint destruction it causes. Studies for additional new drugs targeting other cytokines and inflammation pathways continue.

Recently, scientists discovered that the presence of proteins called anti-citrulline antibodies can help identify people with early rheumatoid arthritis who are likely to have aggressive disease. This enables doctors to begin aggressive treatment early and help prevent damage. Researchers continue to search for biomarkers that identify people at risk of aggressive disease as well as those most likely to respond to a particular treatment.

Researchers are also studying non-medication treatments for rheumatoid arthritis, such as green tea, fish oil, borage seed oil, and relaxation techniques.

Scleroderma: Current studies on scleroderma are focusing on overproduction of collagen, blood vessel injury, and abnormal immune system activity. Researchers hope to discover how these three elements interact to cause and promote scleroderma. In a number of studies, researchers have found evidence of fetal cells within the blood and skin lesions of women who had been pregnant years before developing scleroderma.

These studies suggest that fetal cells may somehow play a role in scleroderma. Scientists are continuing to study the implications of this finding. Scientists are also trying to better understand the organ complications that can occur in people with scleroderma and to find factors that predict who is at greatest risk for these complications.

Treatment studies are under way as well. One study in particular has looked at the effectiveness of ultraviolet light in softening the thickened skin of people with scleroderma, and others have shown that drugs affecting the circulation can improve symptoms of scleroderma.

Spondyloarthropathies: Researchers are working to understand the genetic and environmental causes of spondyloarthropathies, which include ankylosing spondylitis, psoriatic arthritis, reactive arthritis, and arthritis associated with inflammatory bowel disease. They are also looking at genetic determinants of disease severity, the development of associated eye problems, and potential new treatments for the diseases and their complications.

Systemic lupus erythematosus: Researchers are looking at how genetic, environmental, and hormonal factors influence the development of systemic lupus erythematosus. They are trying to find out why lupus is more common or more severe in certain populations, and they have made progress in identifying the genes that may be responsible for lupus. Researchers also continue to study the cellular and molecular basis of autoimmune disorders such as lupus. Promising areas of research on treatment include biologic agents; newer, more selective drugs that suppress the immune system; and bone marrow transplants to correct immune abnormalities. Contrary to the widely held belief that estrogens can make the disease worse, a major NIAMS-supported study has shown that it may be safe to use estrogens for hormone replacement therapy and birth control in women with lupus.

Chapter 3

Statistics on Arthritis in the United States

Based on 2003–2005 data from the National Health Interview Survey (NHIS), an estimated 46 million (22%) of adults have self-reported doctor-diagnosed arthritis. Nineteen million (9% of all adults) have arthritis and arthritis-attributable activity limitation.

Based on 2003 NHIS data an estimated 67 million (25%) adults aged 18 years and older will have doctor-diagnosed arthritis by the year 2030. An estimated 25 million adults (37%) of those with arthritis will report arthritis-attributable activity limitations.

The best source for national arthritis prevalence estimates is the National Health Interview Survey (NHIS), an annual survey conducted by the National Center for Health Statistics. Each year, the NHIS samples U.S. households and gathers information on select adult and child members living in each household. Estimates of health conditions and behaviors from the NHIS are representative of the U.S. civilian, non-institutionalized population.

Prevalence of Arthritis

- An estimated 46 million adults in the United States reported being told by a doctor that they have some form of arthritis, rheumatoid arthritis, gout, lupus, or fibromyalgia.

Excerpted from "Arthritis: Data and Statistics," by the Centers for Disease Control and Prevention (CDC, www.cdc.gov), National Center for Chronic Disease Prevention and Health Promotion, October 15, 2008. For complete references, see www.cdc.gov/arthritis/data_statistics/index.htm.

- One in five (22+%) adults in the United States report having doctor-diagnosed arthritis.

- In 2003–2005, 50% of adults 65 years or older reported an arthritis diagnosis.

- By 2030, an estimated 67 million Americans ages 18 years or older are projected to have doctor-diagnosed arthritis.

- An estimated 294,000 children under age 18 have some form of arthritis or rheumatic condition; this represents approximately 1 in every 250 children.

Prevalence of Specific Types of Arthritis

- The most common form of arthritis is osteoarthritis. Other common rheumatic conditions include gout, fibromyalgia, and rheumatoid arthritis.

- An estimated 27 million adults had osteoarthritis in 2005.

- An estimated 1.3 million adults were affected by rheumatoid arthritis in 2005.

- An estimated 3.0 million adults had gout in 2005, and 6.1 million adults have ever had gout.

- An estimated 5.0 million adults had fibromyalgia in 2005.

Prevalence of Arthritis by Age/Race/Gender

- Of persons aged 18–44, 7.9% (8.7 million) report doctor-diagnosed arthritis. Of persons aged 45–64, 29.3% (20.5 million) report doctor-diagnosed arthritis. Of persons aged 65+, 50.0% (17.2 million) report doctor-diagnosed arthritis.

- 28.3 million women and 18.1 million men report doctor-diagnosed arthritis.

- 3.1 million Hispanic adults report doctor-diagnosed arthritis.

- 4.6 million non-Hispanic Blacks report doctor-diagnosed arthritis.

- An estimated 294,000 children under age 18 have some form of arthritis or rheumatic condition; this represents approximately 1 in every 250 children.

Overweight/Obesity and Arthritis

People who are overweight or obese report more doctor-diagnosed arthritis than people with a lower body mass index (BMI).

- 16% of under/normal weight adults report doctor-diagnosed arthritis.

- 21.7% of overweight and 30.6% obese Americans report doctor-diagnosed arthritis.

- 66% of adults with doctor-diagnosed arthritis are overweight or obese (compared with 53% of adults without doctor-diagnosed arthritis).

- Weight loss of as little as 11 pounds reduces the risk of developing knee osteoarthritis among women by 50%.

Physical Activity and Arthritis

- Almost 44% of adults with doctor-diagnosed arthritis report no leisure time physical activity, compared with 36% of adults without arthritis.

- Among older adults with knee osteoarthritis, engaging in moderate physical activity at least three times per week can reduce the risk of arthritis-related disability by 47%.

Disability/Limitations and Arthritis

- State-specific prevalence estimates of arthritis-attributable work limitation show a high impact of arthritis in working-age (18–64 years) adults in all U.S. states, ranging from a low of 3.4% to a high of 15% of adults in this age group.

- Approximately 5% of all U.S. adults between the ages of 18 and 64 have arthritis and are affected by arthritis-attributable work limitation.

- Approximately 1 in 3 people with arthritis in this age group report arthritis-attributable work limitation.

- Arthritis and other rheumatic conditions are the most common cause of disability in the United States.

- Among all civilian, non-institutionalized U.S. adults 8.8% (19 million) report both doctor-diagnosed and arthritis-attributable activity limitations.

- Nearly 41% of adults with doctor-diagnosed arthritis report arthritis-attributable activity limitations.

- Among adults with doctor-diagnosed arthritis, many report significant limitations in vital activities such as the following:

  - Walking 1/4 mile—6 million

  - Stooping/bending/kneeling—7.8 million

  - Climbing stairs—4.8 million

  - Social activities such as church and family gatherings—2.1 million

- Among all civilian, non-institutionalized U.S. adults aged 18–64, 4.8% (8.2 million) report both doctor-diagnosed arthritis and arthritis-attributable work limitations.

- 30.6% of adults aged 18–64 with doctor-diagnosed arthritis report an arthritis-attributable work limitation.

Health Related Quality of Life (HRQOL) and Arthritis

Persons with doctor-diagnosed arthritis have significantly worse HRQOL than those without arthritis. People with doctor-diagnosed report more than twice as many unhealthy days and three times as many days with activity limitations in the past month than those without arthritis.

Arthritis Healthcare Utilization

- **Hospitalizations:** In 1997, there were an estimated 744,000 hospitalizations with a principal diagnosis of arthritis (3% of all hospitalizations).

- **Outpatient care:** There were 36.5 million ambulatory care visits for arthritis and other rheumatic conditions in 1997, or nearly 4% of all ambulatory care visits that year.

Arthritis-Related Mortality

- From 1979–1998, the annual number of arthritis and other related rheumatic conditions (AORC) deaths rose from 5,537 to 9,367.

- Three categories of AORC account for almost 80% of deaths: diffuse connective tissue diseases (34%), other specified rheumatic conditions (23%), and rheumatoid arthritis (22%).

- In 1979, the crude death rate from AORC was 2.46 per 100,000 population. In 1998, it was 3.48 per 100,000 population; rates age-standardized to the year 2000 population were 2.75 and 3.51, respectively.

Arthritis Costs

- In 2003, the total cost attributed to arthritis and other rheumatic conditions in the United States was 128 billion dollars, up from 86.2 billion dollars in 1997.

- Medical expenditures (direct costs) for arthritis and other rheumatic conditions in 2003 were 80.8 billion dollars, up from 51.1 billion in 1997.

- Earnings losses (indirect costs) for arthritis and other rheumatic conditions in 2003 were 47 billion dollars, up from 35.1 billion in 1997.

Mental/Emotional Health and Arthritis

Arthritis is strongly associated with major depression (attributable risk of 18.1%), probably through its role in creating functional limitation.

Total Joint Replacements in Arthritis

- In 2004, there were 454,652 total knee replacements performed, primarily for arthritis.

- In 2004, there were 232,857 total hip replacements, 41,934 shoulder, and 12, 055 other joint replacements.

Chapter 4

Risk Factors for Arthritis

Chapter Contents

Section 4.1

Genetic Risk Factor for Arthritis Identified

From "Study Identifies Genetic Risk Factor for Rheumatoid Arthritis, Lupus," by the National Institutes of Health (NIH, www.nih.gov), September 6, 2007.

A genetic variation has been identified that increases the risk of two chronic, autoimmune inflammatory diseases: rheumatoid arthritis (RA) and systemic lupus erythematosus (lupus). These research findings result from a long-time collaboration between the Intramural Research Program (IRP) of the National Institute of Arthritis and Musculoskeletal and Skin Diseases (NIAMS) and other organizations. NIAMS is part of the National Institutes of Health.

These results appear in the Sept. 6 [2007] issue of the *New England Journal of Medicine*.

"Although both diseases are believed to have a strong genetic component, identifying the relevant genes has been extremely difficult," says study coauthor Elaine Remmers, PhD, of the Genetics and Genomics Branch of the Intramural Research Program at the National Institute of Arthritis and Musculoskeletal and Skin Diseases. Dr. Remmers and her colleagues tested variants within 13 candidate genes located in a region of chromosome 2, which they had previously linked with RA, for association with disease in large collections of RA and lupus patients and controls. Among the variants were several disease-associated single nucleotide polymorphisms (SNPs)—small differences in DNA sequence that represent the most common genetic variations between individuals—in a large segment of the STAT4 gene. The STAT4 gene encodes a protein that plays an important role in the regulation and activation of certain cells of the immune system.

"It may be too early to predict the impact of identifying the STAT4 gene as a susceptibility locus for rheumatoid arthritis—whether the presence of the variant and others will serve as a predictor of disease, disease outcome or response to therapy," says coauthor and NARAC principal investigator Peter K. Gregersen, MD, of The Feinstein

Institute for Medical Research, part of the North Shore Long Island Jewish Health System, in Manhasset, NY. "It also remains to be found whether the STAT4 pathway plays such a crucial role in RA and lupus that new therapies targeting this pathway would be effective in these and perhaps other autoimmune diseases."

One variant form of the gene was present at a significantly higher frequency in RA patient samples from the North American Rheumatoid Arthritis Consortium (NARAC) as compared with controls. The scientists replicated that result in two independent collections of RA cases and controls.

The researchers also found that the same variant of the STAT4 gene was even more strongly linked with lupus in three independent collections of patients and controls. Frequency data on the genetic profiles of the patients and controls suggest that individuals who carry two copies of the disease-risk variant form of the STAT4 gene have a 60 percent increased risk for RA and more than double the risk for lupus compared with people who carry no copies of the variant form. The research also suggests a shared disease pathway for RA and lupus.

"For this complex disease, rheumatoid arthritis, this is the first instance of a genetic linkage study leading to a chromosomal location, which then, in a genetic association study, identified a disease susceptibility gene," says Dr. Gregersen.

The study's success, according to NIAMS Director Stephen I. Katz, MD, PhD, can be attributed in part to the uncommon and longstanding collaboration between NIAMS intramural researchers and other scientists the Institute supports around the country. "This work required the collection and genotyping of thousands of RA and lupus cases and controls, a task that would have been difficult to accomplish without the strong partnerships we forged," he says. NARAC was established 10 years ago by Dr. Gregersen, NIAMS Clinical Director and Genetics and Genomics Branch Chief Daniel Kastner, MD, PhD, and investigators at several academic health centers to facilitate the collection and analysis of RA genetic samples.

Adds Dr. Remmers, "Although we do not yet know precisely how the disease-associated variant of the STAT4 gene increases the risk for developing RA or lupus, it is very exciting to know that this gene plays a fundamental role in these important autoimmune diseases."

Both RA and lupus are considered autoimmune diseases, or diseases in which the body's immune system attacks healthy tissue. In RA, the immune system attacks the linings of the joints and sometimes other organs. In lupus, it attacks the internal organs, joints, and skin. If not well controlled, both diseases can lead to significant disability.

Reference: Remmers E, et al. STAT4 and the risk of rheumatoid arthritis and systemic lupus erythematosus. *NEJM* 2007;357(10):13–22.

Section 4.2

Veterans' Orthopedic Injuries Contribute to Arthritis

From "One-third of U.S. veterans suffer from arthritis, perhaps due to orthopedic injuries sustained in the military," by the Agency for Healthcare Research and Quality (AHRQ, www.ahrq.gov), February 2006.

About one-third of U.S. veterans suffer from arthritis, according to a new study. For some, the arthritis may have resulted from orthopedic injuries they sustained while in the military. Military training and service often involve situations that place personnel at greater risk for orthopedic injuries. For example, soldiers deployed to the Persian Gulf during Operation Desert Storm often wore Kevlar helmets and heavy battle gear while riding in trucks over desert terrain. These soldiers commonly reported extreme posterior neck pain. Screening individuals entering military service for predisposing factors for orthopedic injury, such as skeletal malalignment, may help reduce these injuries. Use of foot orthotics, supportive shoes, bracing, and individualized stretching and strengthening programs may also reduce the risk of injury to veterans, suggest the Duke University Medical Center investigators.

They found that 32 percent of veterans surveyed in 36 states had been diagnosed with arthritis, compared with 22 percent of nonveterans. Also, 43 percent of veterans using the Veterans Affairs (VA) health care system (who tend to have more disabilities and poorer health) had been diagnosed with arthritis compared with 30 percent of veterans who did not use VA health care.

Veterans were twice as likely as nonveterans to report chronic joint symptoms and activity limitations, as were veteran users of VA health compared with veterans who did not use VA health care. The findings were based on responses from 123,395 veterans and nonveterans to the arthritis survey of the 2000 Behavioral Risk Factor Surveillance System. The study was supported in part by the Agency for Healthcare Research and Quality.

Reference: See "Arthritis prevalence and symptoms among U.S. non-veterans, veterans, and veterans receiving Department of Veterans Affairs healthcare," by Kelli L. Dominick, PhD, Yvonne M. Golightly, PT, MS, and George L. Jackson, PhD, in the February 2006 *Journal of Rheumatology* 33(2), pp. 348–354.

Section 4.3

Weight and Joint Pain

"Osteoarthritis Another Health Detriment of Obesity,"
News release, May 28, 2008. Reprinted with permission of the
American College of Sports Medicine (www.acsm.org).

The escalating obesity epidemic in the United States has focused attention on obesity as a risk factor for coronary artery disease, type 2 diabetes, and hypertension. But being overweight is also a risk factor for osteoarthritis (OA), the degeneration of the cartilage at the ends of bones, which results in painful and restricted movement, said an expert at the 55th Annual Meeting of the American College of Sports Medicine.

Stephen P. Messier, PhD, FACSM, presented a lecture on *The Burden of Obesity: A Biomechanical Perspective*. Messier has been involved in research on understanding and treating OA for more than 25 years. His current work looks at the biomechanics of obesity among adults aged 55 and older.

He says extra weight also puts added stress on joints, impacts movement, affects gait (how a person walks), increases foot pressure, and decreases strength.

Messier notes that people who are overweight or obese have a higher risk of OA and the progression of the disease is greater. Every excess pound of body weight puts an additional four-pound stress on the knee, he explains, adding, "A weight gain of about 11 pounds over a 10-year period causes a 50 percent increase in the likelihood of developing OA."

Messier points out that OA is the leading cause of disability among older adults. It affects about 27 million older adults in the United States.

In looking at the biomechanics of walking, Messier comments that being overweight can change an individual's gait, thus causing or exacerbating joint pain. In addition, obesity creates more pressure on the feet. This pressure can contribute to plantar fasciitis, a painful inflammatory condition caused by excessive wear to the connective tissue that supports the arch of the foot. Obese individuals—those with a body mass index (BMI) greater than 30—are five to six times more likely to have plantar fasciitis than individuals with a normal BMI (18.5 to 25).

In addition to joint and foot pain, obesity lessens a person's physical strength, which can impact activities of daily living.

"At first consideration, one might think obese individuals are stronger than normal-weight individuals," said Messier. "However, when you consider strength relative to body weight, obese people tend to be much weaker." He says this is because excessive fat in obese individuals infiltrates and weakens muscle tissue. Fat cells also release cytokines, chemicals that increase inflammation. Cytokines can also get into the joints and degrade cartilage.

The pain and disability suffered due to OA, plantar fasciitis, and loss of strength can cause a vicious cycle. When physical activity is painful, people tend to become more sedentary, and that inactive behavior can result in even more weight gain.

But there is good news. In his work, Messier found that weight loss and exercise can improve function and reduce the pain from OA. His research shows that a five percent drop in body weight, combined with a moderate exercise program, results in a 24-percent increase in function, and a 30-percent decrease in pain over an 18-month period. For a 250-pound individual, this translates to a weight loss of 12.5 pounds with moderate physical activity, such as walking 30 minutes a day, five days a week.

The American College of Sports Medicine is the largest sports medicine and exercise science organization in the world. More than 20,000 international, national, and regional members are dedicated to advancing and integrating scientific research to provide educational and practical applications of exercise science and sports medicine.

Chapter 5

Joints Affected by Arthritis

Chapter Contents

Section 5.1

Arthritis of the Shoulder

Excerpted from "Questions and Answers about Shoulder Problems," by the National Institute of Arthritis and Musculoskeletal and Skin Diseases (NIAMS, www.niams.nih.gov), part of the National Institutes of Health, March 2006.

What are the most common shoulder problems?

The most movable joint in the body, the shoulder is also one of the most potentially unstable joints. As a result, it is the site of many common problems. They include sprains, strains, dislocations, separations, tendonitis, bursitis, torn rotator cuffs, frozen shoulder, fractures, and arthritis.

How common are shoulder problems?

According to the Centers for Disease Control and Prevention, about 13.7 million people in the United States sought medical care in 2003 for shoulder problems.

What are the structures of the shoulder and how does it function?

To better understand shoulder problems and how they occur, it helps to begin with an explanation of the shoulder's structure and how it functions.

The shoulder joint is composed of three bones: the clavicle (collarbone), the scapula (shoulder blade), and the humerus (upper arm bone). Two joints facilitate shoulder movement. The acromioclavicular (AC) joint is located between the acromion (part of the scapula that forms the highest point of the shoulder) and the clavicle. The glenohumeral joint, commonly called the shoulder joint, is a ball-and-socket-type joint that helps move the shoulder forward and backward and allows the arm to rotate in a circular fashion or hinge out and up away from the body. (The "ball," or humerus, is the top, rounded portion of the upper arm bone; the "socket," or glenoid, is a dish-shaped part of the outer edge of the scapula into which the ball fits.) The capsule is a soft tissue envelope that encircles the glenohumeral joint. It is lined by a thin, smooth synovial membrane.

In contrast to the hip joint, which more closely approximates a true ball-and-socket joint, the shoulder joint can be compared to a golf ball and tee, in which the ball can easily slip off the flat tee. Because the bones provide little inherent stability to the shoulder joint, it is highly dependent on surrounding soft tissues such as capsule ligaments and the muscles surrounding the rotator cuff to hold the ball in place. Whereas the hip joint is inherently quite stable because of the encircling bony anatomy, it also is relatively immobile. The shoulder, on the other hand, is relatively unstable but highly mobile, allowing an individual to place the hand in numerous positions. It is in fact, one of the most mobile joints in the human body.

The bones of the shoulder are held in place by muscles, tendons, and ligaments. Tendons are tough cords of tissue that attach the shoulder muscles to bone and assist the muscles in moving the shoulder. Ligaments attach shoulder bones to each other, providing stability. For example, the front of the joint capsule is anchored by three glenohumeral ligaments. The rotator cuff is a structure composed of tendons that work along with associated muscles to hold the ball at the top of the humerus in the glenoid socket and provide mobility and strength to the shoulder joint. Two filmy sac-like structures called bursae permit smooth gliding between bones, muscles, and tendons. They cushion and protect the rotator cuff from the bony arch of the acromion.

What are the origins and causes of shoulder problems?

The shoulder is easily injured because the ball of the upper arm is larger than the shoulder socket that holds it. To remain stable, the shoulder must be anchored by its muscles, tendons, and ligaments.

Although the shoulder is easily injured during sporting activities and manual labor, the primary source of shoulder problems appears to be the natural age-related degeneration of the surrounding soft tissues such as those found in the rotator cuff. The incidence of rotator cuff problems rises dramatically as a function of age and is generally seen among individuals who are more than 60 years old. Often, the dominant and nondominant arm will be affected to a similar degree. Overuse of the shoulder can lead to more rapid age-related deterioration.

Shoulder pain may be localized or may be felt in areas around the shoulder or down the arm. Disease within the body (such as gallbladder, liver, or heart disease, or disease of the cervical spine of the neck) also may generate pain that travels along nerves to the shoulder.

How are shoulder problems diagnosed?

As with any medical issue, a shoulder problem is generally diagnosed using a three-part process:

- **Medical history:** The patient tells the doctor about any injury or other condition that might be causing the pain.

- **Physical examination:** The doctor examines the patient to feel for injury and to discover the limits of movement, location of pain, and extent of joint instability.

- **Tests:** The doctor may order one or more of the tests listed in the following text to make a specific diagnosis. These tests may include the following:

  - **Standard x-ray:** A familiar procedure in which low-level radiation is passed through the body to produce a picture called a radiograph. An x-ray is useful for diagnosing fractures or other problems of the bones. Soft tissues, such as muscles and tendons, do not show up on x-rays.

  - **Arthrogram:** A diagnostic record that can be seen on an x-ray after injection of a contrast fluid into the shoulder joint to outline structures such as the rotator cuff. In disease or injury, this contrast fluid may either leak into an area where it does not belong, indicating a tear or opening, or be blocked from entering an area where there normally is an opening.

  - **Ultrasound:** A noninvasive, patient-friendly procedure in which a small, handheld scanner is placed on the skin of the shoulder. Just as ultrasound waves can be used to visualize the fetus during pregnancy, they can also be reflected off the rotator cuff and other structures to form a high quality image of them. The accuracy of ultrasound for the rotator cuff is particularly high.

  - **MRI (magnetic resonance imaging):** A noninvasive procedure in which a machine with a strong magnet passes a force through the body to produce a series of cross-sectional images of the shoulder.

What should I know about specific shoulder problems, including their symptoms and treatment?

The symptoms of shoulder problems, as well as their diagnosis and treatment, vary widely, depending on the specific problem. The following is important information to know about some of the most common shoulder problems.

Rotator cuff disease (tendonitis and bursitis): These conditions are closely related and may occur alone or in combination.

Tendonitis is inflammation (redness, soreness, and swelling) of a tendon. In tendonitis of the shoulder, the rotator cuff and/or biceps tendon become inflamed, usually as a result of being pinched by surrounding structures. The injury may vary from mild inflammation to involvement of most of the rotator cuff. When the rotator cuff tendon becomes inflamed and thickened, it may get trapped under the acromion. Squeezing of the rotator cuff is called impingement syndrome.

Bursitis, or inflammation of the bursa sacs that protect the shoulder, may accompany tendonitis and impingement syndrome. Inflammation caused by a disease such as rheumatoid arthritis may cause rotator cuff tendonitis and bursitis. Sports involving overuse of the shoulder and occupations requiring frequent overhead reaching are other potential causes of irritation to the rotator cuff or bursa and may lead to inflammation and impingement.

If the rotator cuff and bursa are irritated, inflamed, and swollen, they may become squeezed between the head of the humerus and the acromion. Repeated motion involving the arms, or the effects of the aging process on shoulder movement over many years, may also irritate and wear down the tendons, muscles, and surrounding structures.

Signs of these conditions include the slow onset of discomfort and pain in the upper shoulder or upper third of the arm and/or difficulty sleeping on the shoulder. Tendonitis and bursitis also cause pain when the arm is lifted away from the body or overhead. If tendonitis involves the biceps tendon (the tendon located in front of the shoulder that helps bend the elbow and turn the forearm), pain will occur in the front or side of the shoulder and may travel down to the elbow and forearm. Pain may also occur when the arm is forcefully pushed upward overhead.

Diagnosis of tendonitis and bursitis begins with a medical history and physical examination. X-rays do not show tendons or the bursae, but may be helpful in ruling out bony abnormalities or arthritis. The doctor may remove and test fluid from the inflamed area to rule out infection. Impingement syndrome may be confirmed when injection of a small amount of anesthetic (lidocaine hydrochloride) into the space under the acromion relieves pain.

The first step in treating these conditions is to reduce pain and inflammation with rest, ice, and anti-inflammatory medicines such as aspirin and ibuprofen (Advil, Motrin). In some cases, the doctor or therapist will use ultrasound (gentle sound-wave vibrations) to warm deep tissues and improve blood flow. Gentle stretching and strengthening exercises are added gradually.

These may be preceded or followed by use of an ice pack. If there is no improvement, the doctor may inject a corticosteroid medicine into the space under the acromion. Although steroid injections are a common treatment, they must be used with caution because they may lead to tendon rupture. If there is still no improvement after 6 to 12 months, the doctor may recommend either arthroscopic or open surgery to repair damage and relieve pressure on the tendons and bursae.

Frozen shoulder (adhesive capsulitis): As the name implies, movement of the shoulder is severely restricted in people with a "frozen shoulder." This condition, which doctors call adhesive capsulitis, is frequently caused by injury that leads to lack of use due to pain. Rheumatic disease progression and recent shoulder surgery can also cause frozen shoulder. Intermittent periods of use may cause inflammation. Adhesions (abnormal bands of tissue) grow between the joint surfaces, restricting motion. There is also a lack of synovial fluid, which normally lubricates the gap between the arm bone and socket to help the shoulder joint move. It is this restricted space between the capsule and ball of the humerus that distinguishes adhesive capsulitis from a less complicated painful, stiff shoulder. People with diabetes, stroke, lung disease, rheumatoid arthritis, and heart disease, or those who have been in an accident, are at a higher risk for frozen shoulder. Frozen shoulder is more common among women than men. People between the ages of 40 and 70 are most likely to experience it.

With a frozen shoulder, the joint becomes so tight and stiff that it is nearly impossible to carry out simple movements, such as raising the arm. Stiffness and discomfort may worsen at night.

A doctor may suspect a frozen shoulder if a physical examination reveals limited shoulder movement. X-rays usually appear normal.

Treatment of this disorder focuses on restoring joint movement and reducing shoulder pain. Usually, treatment begins with nonsteroidal anti-inflammatory drugs and the application of heat, followed by gentle stretching exercises. These stretching exercises, which may be performed in the home with the help of a therapist, are the treatment of choice. In some cases, transcutaneous electrical nerve stimulation (TENS) with a small battery-operated unit may be used to reduce pain by blocking nerve impulses. If these measures are unsuccessful, an intraarticular injection of steroids into the glenoid humeral joint can result in marked improvement of the frozen shoulder in a large percentage of cases. In those rare people who do not improve from nonoperative measures, manipulation of the shoulder under general anesthesia and an arthroscopic procedure to cut the remaining adhesions can be highly effective in most cases.

Arthritis of the shoulder: Arthritis is a degenerative disease caused by either wear and tear of the cartilage (osteoarthritis) or an inflammation (rheumatoid arthritis) of one or more joints. Arthritis not only affects joints, but may also affect supporting structures such as muscles, tendons, and ligaments.

The usual signs of arthritis of the shoulder are pain, particularly over the acromioclavicular joint, and a decrease in shoulder motion.

A doctor may suspect the patient has arthritis when there is both pain and swelling in the joint. The diagnosis may be confirmed by a physical examination and x-rays. Blood tests may be helpful for diagnosing rheumatoid arthritis, but other tests may be needed as well. Analysis of synovial fluid from the shoulder joint may be helpful in diagnosing some kinds of arthritis. Although arthroscopy permits direct visualization of damage to cartilage, tendons, and ligaments, and may confirm a diagnosis, it is usually done only if a repair procedure is to be performed.

Treatment of shoulder arthritis depends in part on the type of arthritis. Osteoarthritis of the shoulder is usually treated with nonsteroidal anti-inflammatory drugs, such as aspirin and ibuprofen. Rheumatoid arthritis may require physical therapy and additional medications such as corticosteroids.

When nonoperative treatment of arthritis of the shoulder fails to relieve pain or improve function, or when there is severe wear and tear of the joint causing parts to loosen and move out of place, shoulder joint replacement (arthroplasty) may provide better results. In this operation, a surgeon replaces the shoulder joint with an artificial ball for the top of the humerus and a cap (glenoid) for the scapula. Passive shoulder exercises (where someone else moves the arm to rotate the shoulder joint) are started soon after surgery. Patients begin exercising on their own about three to six weeks after surgery. Eventually, stretching and strengthening exercises become a major part of the rehabilitation program. The success of the operation often depends on the condition of rotator cuff muscles prior to surgery and the degree to which the patient follows the exercise program.

Section 5.2

Arthritis of the Wrist

"Arthritis of the Wrist." Reproduced with permission from Your Orthopaedic Connection. Rosemont, IL, American Academy of Orthopaedic Surgeons, © 2009.

Arthritis affects millions of people in the United States. A significant number of people suffer from arthritis in their wrists and hands, which makes it difficult for them to perform the activities of daily living.

Cause

Although there are hundreds of kinds of arthritis, most wrist pain is caused by just two types:

Osteoarthritis

Osteoarthritis (OA) is a progressive condition that destroys the smooth joint cartilage covering the ends of bones. The bare bones rub against each other, resulting in pain, stiffness, and weakness.

Osteoarthritis can develop due to normal "wear-and-tear" in the wrist, particularly in people who have a hereditary tendency. It may also develop as a result of a traumatic injury to the wrist bones or ligaments.

Rheumatoid Arthritis

Rheumatoid arthritis (RA) is a systemic inflammatory disease that affects the joint linings and destroys bones, tissues, and joints. Rheumatoid arthritis often starts in smaller joints, like those found in the hand and wrist. It is symmetrical, meaning that it usually affects the same joint on both sides of the body.

Symptoms

OA of the wrist joint manifests with swelling, pain, limited motion, and weakness. These symptoms are usually limited to the wrist joint itself.

RA of the wrist joint also manifests with swelling, pain, limited motion, and weakness. However, in contrast to OA, wrist symptoms will usually be accompanied by pain, swelling, and stiffness in the knuckle joints of the hand.

Doctor Examination

Your physician will use a combination of physical examination, patient history, and blood tests to diagnose arthritis of the wrist.

X-rays can help distinguish among various forms of arthritis. Blood tests sometimes help to diagnose rheumatoid arthritis. Osteoarthritis is never associated with blood abnormalities.

Treatment

Nonsurgical Treatment

In general, early treatment is nonsurgical and designed to help relieve pain and swelling. Several therapies can be used to treat arthritis, including:

- modifying your activities;
- immobilizing the wrist for a short time in a splint;
- taking anti-inflammatory medications such as aspirin or ibuprofen;
- following a prescribed exercise program;
- getting a steroid injection into the joint.

When rheumatoid arthritis symptoms are not adequately controlled by the above therapies, additional medications with varying risks and benefits may be prescribed by your doctor.

Surgical Treatment

When nonsurgical treatments are no longer effective, resulting in progressive loss of hand and wrist function, surgery is an option. The goal of surgery is to relieve pain and to preserve or improve function.

Surgical options include:

- removing the arthritic bones;
- joint fusion (making the joint solid and preventing any movement at the wrist);
- joint replacement.

You and your physician should discuss the options and select the one that is best for you.

Section 5.3

Arthritis of the Hip

Excerpted from "Questions and Answers about Hip Replacement," by the National Institute of Arthritis and Musculoskeletal and Skin Diseases (NIAMS, www.niams.nih.gov), part of the National Institutes of Health, May 2006.

What types of arthritis cause hip pain and damage?

Osteoarthritis is the most common cause of hip joint damage that causes pain and interferes with daily activities despite treatment. However, other conditions, such as rheumatoid arthritis (a chronic inflammatory disease that causes joint pain, stiffness, and swelling), osteonecrosis (or avascular necrosis, which is the death of bone caused by insufficient blood supply), injury, and bone tumors also may lead to breakdown of the hip joint and the need for hip replacement surgery.

What are treatments for arthritis of the hip?

Before considering a total hip replacement, the doctor may try other methods of treatment, such as exercise, walking aids, and medication. An exercise program can strengthen the muscles around the hip joint. Walking aids such as canes and walkers may alleviate some of the stress from painful, damaged hips and help you to avoid or delay surgery.

For hip pain without inflammation, doctors usually recommend the analgesic medication acetaminophen (Tylenol).

For hip pain with inflammation, treatment usually consists of nonsteroidal anti-inflammatory drugs, or NSAIDs. Some common NSAIDs are aspirin and ibuprofen (Motrin, Advil). If you need to take NSAIDs on a long-term basis or at doses that are higher than those obtainable over the counter, you should do so only under a doctor's supervision. When neither NSAIDs nor analgesics are sufficient to relieve pain, doctors sometimes recommend combining the two. Again, this should be done only under a doctor's supervision.

In some cases, a stronger analgesic medication such as tramadol or a product containing both acetaminophen and a narcotic analgesic such as codeine may be necessary to control pain.

Topical analgesic products such as capsaicin and methyl salicylate may provide additional relief. Some people find that the nutritional supplement combination of glucosamine and chondroitin helps ease pain. People taking nutritional supplements, herbs, and other complementary and alternative medicines should inform their doctors to avoid harmful drug interactions.

In a small number of cases, doctors may prescribe corticosteroid medications, such as prednisone or cortisone, if NSAIDs do not relieve pain. Corticosteroids reduce joint inflammation and are frequently used to treat rheumatic diseases such as rheumatoid arthritis. The downside of corticosteroids is that they can cause further damage to the bones in the joint. Also, they carry the risk of side effects such as increased appetite, weight gain, and lower resistance to infections. A doctor must prescribe and monitor corticosteroid treatment. Because corticosteroids alter the body's natural hormone production, which is essential for the body to function, you should not stop taking them suddenly, and you should follow the doctor's instructions for discontinuing treatment.

Sometimes, corticosteroids are injected into the hip joint. A joint lubricant such as Hyaluronan may also be injected into the hip joint to relieve pain.

If exercise and medication do not relieve pain and improve joint function, the doctor may suggest a less complex corrective surgery before proceeding to hip replacement. One common alternative to hip replacement is an osteotomy. This procedure involves cutting and realigning bone, to shift the weight from a damaged and painful bone surface to a healthier one. Recovery from an osteotomy takes 6 to 12 months. Afterward, the function of the hip joint may continue to worsen and additional treatment may be needed. The length of time before another surgery is needed varies greatly and depends on the condition of the joint before the procedure.

Section 5.4

Arthritis of the Knee

Excerpted from "Questions and Answers about Knee Problems," by the National Institute of Arthritis and Musculoskeletal and Skin Diseases (NIAMS, www.niams.nih.gov), part of the National Institutes of Health, May 2006.

What do the knees do? How do they work?

The knee is the joint where the bones of the upper leg meet the bones of the lower leg, allowing hinge-like movement while providing stability and strength to support the weight of the body. Flexibility, strength, and stability are needed for standing and for motions like walking, running, crouching, jumping, and turning.

Several kinds of supporting and moving parts, including bones, cartilage, muscles, ligaments, and tendons, help the knees do their job. Each of these structures is subject to disease and injury. When a knee problem affects your ability to do things, it can have a big impact on your life. Knee problems can interfere with many things, from participation in sports to simply getting up from a chair and walking.

What are the parts of the knee?

The point at which two or more bones are connected is called a joint. In all joints, the bones are kept from grinding against each other by lining called cartilage. Bones are joined to bones by strong, elastic bands of tissue called ligaments. Muscles are connected to bones by tough cords of tissue called tendons. Muscles pull on tendons to move joints. Although muscles are not technically part of a joint, they're important because strong muscles help support and protect joints.

What causes knee problems?

Knee problems can be the result of disease or injury.

Disease: A number of diseases can affect the knee. The most common is arthritis. Although arthritis technically means "joint inflammation," the term is used loosely to describe many different diseases that can affect the joints.

Injury: Knee injuries can occur as the result of a direct blow or sudden movements that strain the knee beyond its normal range of motion. Sometimes knees are injured slowly over time. Problems with the hips or feet, for example, can cause you to walk awkwardly, which throws off the alignment of the knees and leads to damage.

Knee problems can also be the result of a lifetime of normal wear and tear. Much like the treads on a tire, the joint simply wears out over time.

How does arthritis affect the knee?

There are some 100 different forms of arthritis, rheumatic diseases, and related conditions. Virtually all of them have the potential to affect the knees in some way; however, the following are the most common.

Osteoarthritis: Most people with knee problems have a form of arthritis called osteoarthritis. In this disease, the cartilage gradually wears away and changes occur in the adjacent bone. Osteoarthritis may be caused by joint injury or being overweight. It is associated with aging and most typically begins in people age 50 or older. A young person who develops osteoarthritis typically has had an injury to the knee or may have an inherited form of the disease.

Rheumatoid arthritis: Rheumatoid arthritis, which generally affects people at a younger age than does osteoarthritis, is an autoimmune disease. This means it occurs as a result of the immune system attacking components of the body.

In rheumatoid arthritis, the primary site of the immune system's attack is the synovium, the membrane that lines the joint. This attack causes inflammation of the joint. It can lead to destruction of the cartilage and bone and, in some cases, muscles, tendons, and ligaments as well.

Other rheumatic diseases: These include the following:

- Gout: An acute and intensely painful form of arthritis that occurs when crystals of the bodily waste product uric acid are deposited in the joints

- Lupus: An autoimmune disease characterized by destructive inflammation of the skin, internal organs, and other body systems as well as the joints

- Ankylosing spondylitis: An inflammatory form of arthritis that primarily affects the spine, leading to stiffening and in some cases fusing into a stooped position

- Psoriatic arthritis: A condition in which inflamed joints produce symptoms of arthritis for patients who have or will develop psoriasis

- Infectious arthritis: A term describing forms of arthritis that are caused by infectious agents, such as bacteria or viruses. Prompt medical attention is essential to treat the infection and minimize damage to joints, particularly if fever is present.

What are symptoms of arthritis of the knee?

The symptoms are different for the different forms of arthritis. For example, people with rheumatoid arthritis, gout, or other inflammatory conditions may find the knee swollen, red, and even hot to the touch. Any form of arthritis can cause the knee to be painful and stiff.

How is arthritis of the knee diagnosed?

The doctor may confirm the diagnosis by conducting a careful history and physical examination. Blood tests may be helpful for diagnosing rheumatoid arthritis, but other tests may also be needed. Analyzing fluid from the knee joint, for example, may be helpful in diagnosing gout. X-rays may be taken to determine loss or damage to cartilage or bone.

How is arthritis of the knee treated?

Like the symptoms, treatment varies depending on the form of arthritis affecting the knee. For osteoarthritis, treatment is targeted at relieving symptoms and may include pain-reducing medicines such as aspirin or acetaminophen (Tylenol); nonsteroidal anti-inflammatory drugs (NSAIDs) such as ibuprofen (Motrin, Nuprin, Advil); or, in some cases, injections of corticosteroid medications directly into the knee joint. Other treatments for the pain of knee osteoarthritis include injections of hyaluronic acid substitutes and the nutritional supplements glucosamine and chondroitin sulfate.

People with diseases such as rheumatoid arthritis, ankylosing spondylitis, or psoriatic arthritis often require disease-modifying antirheumatic drugs (DMARDs) or biologic response modifiers (biologics) to control the underlying disease that is the source of their knee problems. These drugs are typically prescribed after less potent treatments, such as NSAIDs or intra-articular injections, are deemed ineffective.

DMARDs are a family of medicines that may be able to slow or stop the immune system from attacking the joints. This in turn prevents pain and swelling. DMARDs typically require regular blood tests to monitor side effects. In addition to relieving signs and symptoms, these drugs may help to retard or even stop joint damage from progressing. However, DMARDs cannot fix joint damage that has already occurred. Some of the most commonly prescribed DMARDs are methotrexate, hydroxychloroquine, sulfasalazine, and leflunomide.

Biologic response modifiers, or biologics, are a new family of genetically engineered drugs that block specific molecular pathways of the immune system that are involved in the inflammatory process. They are often prescribed in combination with DMARDs such as methotrexate. Because biologics work by suppressing the immune system, they could be problematic for patients who are prone to frequent infection. They are typically administered by injection at home or by an intravenous infusion at a clinic. Some commonly prescribed biologics include etanercept, adalimumab, infliximab, and anakinra.

People with any type of arthritis may benefit from exercises to strengthen the muscles that support the knee and from weight loss, if needed, to relieve excess stress on the joints.

If arthritis causes serious damage to a knee or there is incapacitating pain or loss of use of the knee from arthritis, joint surgery may be considered. Traditionally, this has been done with what is known as a total knee replacement. However, newer surgical procedures are continuously being developed that include resurfacing or replacing only the damaged cartilage surfaces while leaving the rest of the joint intact.

What kinds of doctors evaluate and treat knee problems?

After an examination by your primary care doctor, he or she may refer you to a rheumatologist, an orthopedic surgeon, or both. A rheumatologist specializes in nonsurgical treatment of arthritis and other rheumatic diseases. An orthopedic surgeon, or orthopedist, specializes in nonsurgical and surgical treatment of bones, joints, and soft tissues such as ligaments, tendons, and muscles.

You may also be referred to a physiatrist. Specializing in physical medicine and rehabilitation, physiatrists seek to restore optimal function to people with injuries to the muscles, bones, tissues, and nervous system.

Minor injuries or arthritis may be treated by an internist (a doctor trained to diagnose and treat nonsurgical diseases) or your primary care doctor.

What is total knee replacement?

Joint replacement is becoming more common, and hips and knees are the most commonly replaced joints. In 2003, more than 638,000 hip or knee replacement surgeries were performed.

The new joint, called a prosthesis, can be made of plastic, metal, or both. It may be cemented into place or uncemented. An uncemented prosthesis is designed so that bones will grow into it.

First made available in the late 1950s, early total knee replacements did a poor job of mimicking the natural motion of the knee. For that reason, these procedures resulted in high failure and complication rates. Advances in total knee replacement technology in the past 10 to 15 years have enhanced the design and fit of knee implants.

Total knee replacement is often the answer for people when x-rays and other tests show joint damage; when moderate-to-severe, persistent pain does not improve adequately with nonsurgical treatment; and when the limited range of motion in their knee joint diminishes their quality of life.

In the past, patients between 60 and 75 years of age were considered to be the best candidates for total knee replacement. Over the past two decades, however, that age range has broadened to include more patients older than 75, who are likely to have other health issues, and patients younger than 60, who are generally more physically active and whose implants will probably be exposed to greater mechanical stress.

About 90 percent of patients appear to experience rapid and substantial reduction in pain, feel better in general, and enjoy improved joint function. Although most total knee replacement surgeries are successful, failure does occur and revision is sometimes necessary. Risk factors include being younger than 55 years old, being male, being obese, and having osteoarthritis or other illnesses.

How can people prevent knee problems?

Some knee problems, such as those resulting from an accident, cannot be foreseen or prevented. However, people can prevent many knee problems by following these suggestions.

- Before exercising or participating in sports, warm up by walking or riding a stationary bicycle, then do stretches. Stretching the muscles in the front of the thigh (quadriceps) and back of the thigh (hamstrings) reduces tension on the tendons and relieves pressure on the knee during activity.

- Strengthen the leg muscles by doing specific exercises (for example, by walking up stairs or hills or by riding a stationary bicycle). A supervised workout with weights is another way to strengthen the leg muscles that support the knee.

- Avoid sudden changes in the intensity of exercise. Increase the force or duration of activity gradually.

- Wear shoes that fit properly and are in good condition. This will help maintain balance and leg alignment when walking or running. Flat feet or overpronated feet (feet that roll inward) can cause knee problems. People can often reduce some of these problems by wearing special shoe inserts (orthotics).

- Maintain a healthy weight to reduce stress on the knee. Obesity increases the risk of osteoarthritis of the knee.

Section 5.5

Arthritis of the Foot and Ankle

Arthritis is the leading cause of disability in the United States. It can occur at any age, and literally means "pain within a joint." As a result, arthritis is a term used broadly to refer to a number of different conditions.

Although there is no cure for arthritis, there are many treatment options available. It is important to seek help early so that treatment can begin as soon as possible. With treatment, people with arthritis are able to manage pain, stay active, and live fulfilling lives, often without surgery.

Description

There are three types of arthritis that may affect your foot and ankle.

Osteoarthritis

Osteoarthritis, also known as degenerative or "wear and tear" arthritis, is a common problem for many people after they reach middle age. Over the years, the smooth, gliding surface covering the ends of bones (cartilage) becomes worn and frayed. This results in inflammation, swelling, and pain in the joint.

Osteoarthritis progresses slowly and the pain and stiffness it causes worsens over time.

Rheumatoid Arthritis

Unlike osteoarthritis which follows a predictable pattern in certain joints, rheumatoid arthritis is a system-wide disease. It is an inflammatory disease where the patient's own immune system attacks and destroys cartilage.

Post-Traumatic Arthritis

Post-traumatic arthritis can develop after an injury to the foot or ankle. This type of arthritis is similar to osteoarthritis and may develop years after a fracture, severe sprain, or ligament injury.

Cause

Osteoarthritis

Many factors increase your risk for developing osteoarthritis. Because the ability of cartilage to heal itself decreases as we age, older people are more likely to develop the disease. Other risk factors include obesity and family history of the disease.

Rheumatoid Arthritis

The exact cause of rheumatoid arthritis is not known. Although it is not an inherited disease, researchers believe that some people have genes that make them more susceptible. There is usually a trigger, such as an infection or environmental factor, which activates the genes. When the body is exposed to this trigger, the immune system begins to produce substances that attack the joint. This is what may lead to the development of rheumatoid arthritis.

Post-Traumatic Arthritis

Fractures—particularly those that damage the joint surface—and dislocations are the most common injuries that lead to this type of arthritis. An injured joint is about seven times more likely to become arthritic, even if the injury is properly treated. In fact, following injury, your body can secrete hormones that stimulate the death of your cartilage cells.

Anatomy

There are 28 bones and more than 30 joints in the foot. Tough bands of tissue, called ligaments, keep the bones and joints in place. If arthritis develops in one or more of these joints, balance and walking may be affected.

The joints most commonly affected by arthritis in the lower extremity include:

- The ankle (tibiotalar joint). The ankle is where the shinbone (tibia) rests on the uppermost bone of the foot (the talus).

- The three joints of the hindfoot. These three joints include:
    - the subtalar or talocalcaneal joint, where the bottom of the talus connects to the heel bone (calcaneus);
    - the talonavicular joint, where the talus connects to the inner midfoot bone (navicular); and
    - the calcaneocuboid joint, where the heel bone connects to the outer midfoot bone (cuboid).
- The midfoot (metatarsocuneiform joint). This is where one of the forefoot bones (metatarsals) connects to the smaller midfoot bones (cuneiforms).
- The great toe (first metatarsophalangeal joint). This is where the first metatarsal connects to the great toe bone (phalange). This is also the area where bunions usually develop.

Symptoms

Signs and symptoms of arthritis of the foot vary, depending on which joint is affected. Common symptoms include:

- pain or tenderness;
- stiffness or reduced motion;
- swelling;
- difficulty walking due to any of the above.

Diagnosis

Your doctor will base a diagnosis using your medical history, symptoms, a physical examination, and additional tests.

Medical History and Examination

A medical history is important to understand more about the problem. Your doctor will want to know when the pain started and when it occurs. Is it worse at night? Does it get worse when walking or running? Is it continuous, or does it come and go?

He or she will want to know if there was a past injury to the foot or ankle. If so, your doctor will discuss your injury, when it occurred, and how it was treated.

Your doctor will want to know if the pain is in both feet or only in one foot, and where it is located exactly. Footwear will be examined, and any medications will be noted.

Additional Tests

One of the tests performed during the physical examination is the gait analysis. This shows how the bones in the leg and foot line up with walking, measures stride, and tests the strength of the ankles and feet.

X-rays can show changes in the spacing between bones or in the shape of the bones themselves. Weight-bearing x-rays are the most valuable additional test in diagnosing the severity of arthritis.

A bone scan, computed tomographic (CT) scan, or magnetic resonance image (MRI) may also be used in the evaluation.

Treatment

Depending on the type, location, and severity of the arthritis, there are many types of treatment available.

Nonsurgical Treatment

Nonsurgical treatment options include:

- pain relievers and anti-inflammatory medications to reduce swelling;
- shoe inserts (orthotics), such as pads or arch supports;
- custom-made shoe, such as a stiff-soled shoe with a rocker bottom;
- an ankle-foot orthosis (AFO);
- a brace or a cane;
- physical therapy and exercises;
- weight control or nutritional supplements;
- medications, such as a steroid medication injected into the joint.

Surgical Treatment

If arthritis doesn't respond to nonsurgical treatment, surgical treatment might be considered. The choice of surgery will depend on the type of arthritis, the impact of the disease on the joints, and the location of the arthritis. Sometimes more than one type of surgery will be needed.

Surgery performed for arthritis of the foot and ankle include arthroscopic debridement, arthrodesis (or fusion of the joints), and arthroplasty (replacement of the affected joint).

Arthroscopic debridement: Arthroscopic surgery may be helpful in the early stages of arthritis.

A flexible, fiberoptic pencil-sized instrument (arthroscope) is inserted into the joint through a series of small incisions through the skin.

The arthroscope is fitted with a small camera and lighting system, as well as various instruments. The camera projects images of the joint on a television monitor. This enables the surgeon to look directly inside the joint and identify the problem areas.

Small instruments at the end of the arthroscope, such as probes, forceps, knives, and shavers, are used to clean the joint area of foreign tissue, inflamed tissue that lines the joint, and bony outgrowths (spurs).

Arthrodesis or fusion: Arthrodesis fuses the bones of the joint completely, making one continuous bone.

The surgeon uses pins, plates and screws, or rods to hold the bones in the proper position while the joint(s) fuse. If the joints do not fuse (nonunion), this hardware may break.

A bone graft is sometimes needed if there is bone loss. The surgeon may use a graft (a piece of bone, taken from one of the lower leg bones or the wing of the pelvis) to replace the missing bone.

This surgery is typically quite successful. A very small percentage of patients have problems with wound healing. These problems can be addressed by bracing or additional surgery.

The biggest long-term problem with fusion is the development of arthritis at the joints adjacent to those fused. This occurs from increased stresses applied to the adjacent joints.

Arthroplasty or joint replacement: In arthroplasty, the damaged ankle joint is replaced with an artificial implant (prosthesis).

Although not as common as total hip or knee joint replacement, advances in implant design have made ankle replacement a feasible option for many people.

In addition to providing pain relief from arthritis, ankle replacements offer patients better mobility and movement compared to fusion. By allowing motion at the formerly arthritic joint, less stress is transferred to the adjacent joints. Less stress results in reduced occurrence of adjacent joint arthritis.

Ankle replacement is most often recommended for patients with:

• advanced arthritis of the ankle;

- destroyed ankle joint surfaces;
- an ankle condition that interferes with daily activities.

As in any joint replacement surgery, the ankle implant may loosen over the years or fail. If the implant failure is severe, revision surgery may be necessary.

Surgical recovery: Foot and ankle surgery can be painful. Pain relievers in the hospital and for a time period after being released from the hospital may help.

It is important to keep your foot elevated above the level of your heart for one to two weeks following surgery.

Your doctor may recommend physical therapy for several months to help you regain strength in your foot or ankle and to restore range of motion. Ordinary daily activities usually can be resumed in three to four months. You may need special shoes or braces.

In most cases, surgery relieves pain and makes it easier to perform daily activities. Full recovery takes four to nine months, depending on the severity of your condition before surgery, and the complexity of your procedure.

Part Two

Types of Arthritis, Related Rheumatic Diseases, and Other Associated Medical Conditions

Chapter 6

Osteoarthritis (OA)

Chapter Contents

Section 6.1

Understanding Osteoarthritis

This section includes text excerpted from "Handout on Health: Osteoarthritis," by the National Institute of Arthritis and Musculoskeletal and Skin Diseases (NIAMS, www.niams.nih.gov), part of the National Institutes of Health, May 2006. The section also includes text from "SMURFs May Cause Osteoarthritis," December 2007, and "NIAMS Researchers Develop Potential Non-Invasive Test for OA," November 2008, NIAMS.

Handout on Health: Osteoarthritis

What is osteoarthritis?

Osteoarthritis is the most common type of arthritis, and is seen especially among older people. Sometimes it is called degenerative joint disease or osteoarthrosis.

Osteoarthritis mostly affects cartilage, the hard but slippery tissue that covers the ends of bones where they meet to form a joint. Healthy cartilage allows bones to glide over one another. It also absorbs energy from the shock of physical movement. In osteoarthritis, the surface layer of cartilage breaks down and wears away. This allows bones under the cartilage to rub together, causing pain, swelling, and loss of motion of the joint. Over time, the joint may lose its normal shape. Also, small deposits of bone—called osteophytes or bone spurs—may grow on the edges of the joint. Bits of bone or cartilage can break off and float inside the joint space. This causes more pain and damage.

People with osteoarthritis usually have joint pain and some movement limitations. Unlike some other forms of arthritis, such as rheumatoid arthritis, osteoarthritis affects only joint function and does not affect skin tissue, the lungs, the eyes, or the blood vessels.

In rheumatoid arthritis, the second most common form of arthritis, the immune system attacks the tissues of the joints, leading to pain, inflammation, and eventually joint damage and malformation. It typically begins at a younger age than osteoarthritis, causes swelling and redness in joints, and may make people feel sick, tired, and uncommonly feverish.

Who has osteoarthritis?

Osteoarthritis is by far the most common type of arthritis, and the percentage of people who have it grows higher with age. An estimated 27 million Americans age 25 and older have osteoarthritis.

Although osteoarthritis is more common in older people, younger people can develop it—usually as the result of a joint injury, a joint malformation, or a genetic defect in joint cartilage. Both men and women have the disease. Before age 45, more men than women have osteoarthritis; after age 45, it is more common in women. It is also more likely to occur in people who are overweight and in those with jobs that stress particular joints.

As the population ages, the number of people with osteoarthritis will only grow. By 2030, 20 percent of Americans—about 72 million people—will have passed their 65th birthday and will be at high risk for the disease.

What areas does osteoarthritis affect?

Osteoarthritis most often occurs in the hands (at the ends of the fingers and thumbs), spine (neck and lower back), knees, and hips.

How does osteoarthritis affect people?

People with osteoarthritis usually experience joint pain and stiffness. The most commonly affected joints are those at the ends of the fingers (closest to the nail), thumbs, neck, lower back, knees, and hips.

Osteoarthritis affects different people differently. Although in some people it progresses quickly, in most individuals joint damage develops gradually over years. In some people, osteoarthritis is relatively mild and interferes little with day-to-day-life; in others, it causes significant pain and disability.

While osteoarthritis is a disease of the joints, its effects are not just physical. In many people with osteoarthritis, lifestyle and finances also decline.

Lifestyle effects include the following:

- Depression
- Anxiety
- Feelings of helplessness
- Limitations on daily activities
- Job limitations

- Difficulty participating in everyday personal and family joys and responsibilities

Financial effects include the following:

- The cost of treatment
- Wages lost because of disability

Fortunately, most people with osteoarthritis live active, productive lives despite these limitations. They do so by using treatment strategies such rest and exercise, pain relief medications, education and support programs, learning self-care, and having a "good attitude."

What are the parts of a joint?

A joint is the point where two or more bones are connected. With a few exceptions (in the skull and pelvis, for example), joints are designed to allow movement between the bones and to absorb shock from movements like walking or repetitive motions. These movable joints are made up of the following parts:

- **Cartilage:** A hard but slippery coating on the end of each bone. Cartilage, which breaks down and wears away in osteoarthritis, is described in more detail on the next page.

- **Joint capsule:** A tough membrane sac that encloses all the bones and other joint parts.

- **Synovium:** A thin membrane inside the joint capsule that secretes synovial fluid.

- **Synovial fluid:** A fluid that lubricates the joint and keeps the cartilage smooth and healthy.

Ligaments, tendons, and muscles are tissues that surround the bones and joints, and allow the joints to bend and move. Ligaments are tough, cord-like tissues that connect one bone to another. Tendons are tough, fibrous cords that connect muscles to bones. Muscles are bundles of specialized cells that, when stimulated by nerves, either relax or contract to produce movement.

How do you know if you have osteoarthritis?

Usually, osteoarthritis comes on slowly. Early in the disease, your joints may ache after physical work or exercise. Later on, joint pain

A Healthy Joint

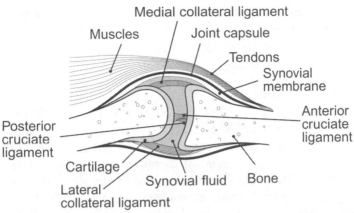

Figure 6.1. *In a healthy joint, the ends of bones are encased in smooth cartilage. Together, they are protected by a joint capsule lined with a synovial membrane that produces synovial fluid. The capsule and fluid protect the cartilage, muscles, and connective tissues.*

A Joint With Severe Osteoarthritis

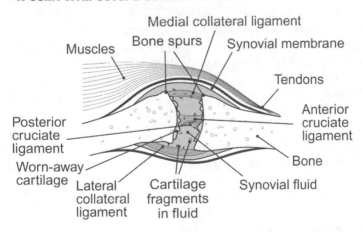

Figure 6.2. *With osteoarthritis, the cartilage becomes worn away. Spurs grow out from the edge of the bone, and synovial fluid increases. Altogether, the joint feels stiff and sore.*

may become more persistent. You may also experience joint stiffness, particularly when you first wake up in the morning or have been in one position for a long time.

Although osteoarthritis can occur in any joint, most often it affects the hands, knees, hips, and spine (either at the neck or lower back). Different characteristics of the disease can depend on the specific joint(s) affected.

Hands: Osteoarthritis of the hands seems to have some hereditary characteristics; that is, it runs in families. If your mother or grand-mother has or had osteoarthritis in their hands, you're at greater-than-average risk of having it, too. Women are more likely than men to have hand involvement and, for most, it develops after menopause.

When osteoarthritis involves the hands, small, bony knobs may appear on the end joints (those closest to the nails) of the fingers. They are called Heberden's nodes. Similar knobs, called Bouchard's nodes, can appear on the middle joints of the fingers. Fingers can become enlarged and gnarled, and they may ache or be stiff and numb. The base of the thumb joint also is commonly affected by osteoarthritis.

Knees: The knees are among the joints most commonly affected by osteoarthritis. Symptoms of knee osteoarthritis include stiffness, swell-ing, and pain, which make it hard to walk, climb, and get in and out of chairs and bathtubs. Osteoarthritis in the knees can lead to disability.

Hips: The hips are also common sites of osteoarthritis. As with knee osteoarthritis, symptoms of hip osteoarthritis include pain and stiffness of the joint itself. But sometimes pain is felt in the groin, inner thigh, buttocks, or even the knees. Osteoarthritis of the hip may limit mov-ing and bending, making daily activities such as dressing and putting on shoes a challenge.

Spine: Osteoarthritis of the spine may show up as stiffness and pain in the neck or lower back. In some cases, arthritis-related changes in the spine can cause pressure on the nerves where they exit the spinal column, resulting in weakness or numbness of the arms and legs.

How do doctors diagnose osteoarthritis?

No single test can diagnose osteoarthritis. Most doctors use a com-bination of the following methods to diagnose the disease and rule out other conditions.

Clinical history: The doctor begins by asking the patient to describe the symptoms, and when and how the condition started, as well as how the symptoms have changed over time. The doctor will also ask about any other medical problems the patient and close family members have and about any medications the patient is taking. Accurate answers to these questions can help the doctor make a diagnosis and understand the impact the disease has on your life.

Physical examination: The doctor will check the patient's reflexes and general health, including muscle strength. The doctor will also examine bothersome joints and observe the patient's ability to walk, bend, and carry out activities of daily living.

X-rays: Doctors take x-rays to see how much joint damage has been done. X-rays of the affected joint can show such things as cartilage loss, bone damage, and bone spurs. But there often is a big difference between the severity of osteoarthritis as shown by the x-ray and the degree of pain and disability felt by the patient. Also, x-rays may not show early osteoarthritis damage before much cartilage loss has taken place.

Magnetic resonance imaging: Also known as an MRI, magnetic resonance imaging provides high-resolution computerized images of internal body tissues. This procedure uses a strong magnet that passes a force through the body to create these images. Doctors often use MRI tests if there is pain; if x-ray findings are minimal; and if the findings suggest damage to other joint tissues such as a ligament, or the pad of connective tissue in the knee known as the meniscus.

Other tests: The doctor may order blood tests to rule out other causes of symptoms. He or she may also order a joint aspiration, which involves drawing fluid from the joint through a needle and examining the fluid under a microscope.

It usually is not difficult to tell if a patient has osteoarthritis. It is more difficult to tell if the disease is causing the patient's symptoms. Osteoarthritis is so common—especially in older people—that symptoms seemingly caused by the disease actually may be due to other medical conditions. The doctor will try to find out what is causing the symptoms by ruling out other disorders and identifying conditions that may make the symptoms worse. The severity of symptoms in osteoarthritis can be influenced greatly by the patient's attitude, anxiety, depression, and daily activity level.

How is osteoarthritis treated?

Most successful treatment programs involve a combination of treatments tailored to the patient's needs, lifestyle, and health. Most programs include ways to manage pain and improve function. These can involve exercise, weight control, rest and relief from stress on joints, pain relief techniques, medications, surgery, and complementary and alternative therapies.

Exercise: Research shows that exercise is one of the best treatments for osteoarthritis. Exercise can improve mood and outlook, decrease pain, increase flexibility, strengthen the heart and improve blood flow, maintain weight, and promote general physical fitness. Exercise is also inexpensive and, if done correctly, has few negative side effects. The amount and form of exercise prescribed will depend on which joints are involved, how stable the joints are, and whether a joint replacement has already been done. Walking, swimming, and water aerobics are a few popular types of exercise for people with osteoarthritis. Your doctor and/or physical therapist can recommend specific types of exercise depending on your particular situation.

Weight control: Osteoarthritis patients who are overweight or obese should try to lose weight. Weight loss can reduce stress on weight-bearing joints, limit further injury, and increase mobility. A dietitian can help you develop healthy eating habits. A healthy diet and regular exercise help reduce weight.

Rest and relief from stress on joints: Treatment plans include regularly scheduled rest. Patients must learn to recognize the body's signals, and know when to stop or slow down. This will prevent the pain caused by overexertion. Although pain can make it difficult to sleep, getting proper sleep is important for managing arthritis pain. If you have trouble sleeping, you may find that relaxation techniques, stress reduction, and biofeedback can help, as can timing medications to provide maximum pain relief through the night.

Some people use canes to take pressure off painful joints. They may use splints or braces to provide extra support for joints and/or keep them in proper position during sleep or activity. Splints should be used only for limited periods of time because joints and muscles need to be exercised to prevent stiffness and weakness. If you need a splint, an occupational therapist or a doctor can help you get a properly fitted one.

If joint pain interferes with your ability to sleep or rest, consult your doctor.

Nondrug pain relief: People with osteoarthritis may find many nondrug ways to relieve pain. Below are some examples:

- Heat and cold: Heat or cold (or a combination of the two) can be useful for joint pain. Heat can be applied in a number of different ways—with warm towels, hot packs, or a warm bath or shower—to increase blood flow and ease pain and stiffness. In some cases, cold packs (bags of ice or frozen vegetables wrapped in a towel), which reduce inflammation, can relieve pain or numb the sore area. (Check with a doctor or physical therapist to find out if heat or cold is the best treatment.)

- Transcutaneous electrical nerve stimulation (TENS): TENS is a technique that uses a small electronic device to direct mild electric pulses to nerve endings that lie beneath the skin in the painful area. TENS may relieve some arthritis pain. It seems to work by blocking pain messages to the brain and by modifying pain perception.

- Massage: In this pain-relief approach, a massage therapist will lightly stroke and/or knead the painful muscles. This may increase blood flow and bring warmth to a stressed area. However, arthritis-stressed joints are sensitive, so the therapist must be familiar with the problems of the disease.

Medications to control pain: Doctors prescribe medicines to eliminate or reduce pain and to improve functioning. Doctors consider a number of factors when choosing medicines for their patients with osteoarthritis. These include the intensity of pain, potential side effects of the medication, your medical history (other health problems you have or are at risk for), and other medications you are taking.

Because some medications can interact with one another and certain health conditions put you at increased risk of drug side effects, it's important to discuss your medication, and health history with your doctor before you start taking any new medication, and to see your doctor regularly while you are taking medication. By working together, you and your doctor can find the medication that best relieves your pain with the least risk of side effects.

The following types of medicines are commonly used in treating osteoarthritis:

- Acetaminophen: A medication commonly used to relieve pain, acetaminophen (for example, Tylenol) is available without a prescription. It is often the first medication doctors recommend for osteoarthritis patients because of its safety relative to some other drugs and its effectiveness against pain.

- NSAIDs (nonsteroidal anti-inflammatory drugs): A large class of medications useful against both pain and inflammation, (NSAIDs) 2 are staples in arthritis treatment. Aspirin, ibuprofen, naproxen, and naproxen sodium are examples of NSAIDs. They are often the first type of medication used. All NSAIDs work similarly: by blocking substances called prostaglandins that contribute to inflammation and pain. However, each NSAID is a different chemical, and each has a slightly different effect on the body. Some NSAIDs are available over the counter, while more than a dozen others, including a subclass called COX-2 inhibitors, are available only with a prescription.

  All NSAIDs can have significant side effects, and for unknown reasons, some people seem to respond better to one NSAID than another. Any person taking NSAIDs regularly should be monitored by a doctor. (Warning: NSAIDs can cause stomach irritation or, less often, they can affect kidney function. The longer a person uses NSAIDs, the more likely he or she is to have side effects, ranging from mild to serious. Many other drugs cannot be taken when a patient is being treated with NSAIDs because NSAIDs alter the way the body uses or eliminates these other drugs. Check with your health care provider or pharmacist before you take NSAIDs. Also, NSAIDs sometimes are associated with serious gastrointestinal problems, including ulcers, bleeding, and perforation of the stomach or intestine. People over age 65 and those with any history of ulcers or gastrointestinal bleeding should use NSAIDs with caution.)

- Other medications: Doctors may prescribe several other medicines for osteoarthritis. They include the following:
  - Topical pain-relieving creams, rubs, and sprays: These products, which are applied directly to the skin over painful joints, contain ingredients that work in one of three different ways: by stimulating the nerve endings to distract the brain's attention from the joint pain; by depleting the amount of a neurotransmitter called substance P that sends pain messages to the brain; or by blocking chemicals called prostaglandins

that cause pain and inflammation. Examples of topical medications are Zostrix, Icy Hot, Therapeutic Mineral Ice, Aspercreme, and Ben Gay.

- Tramadol (Ultram): A prescription pain reliever that is sometimes prescribed when over-the-counter medications don't provide sufficient relief. It carries risks that don't exist with acetaminophen and NSAIDs, including the potential for addiction.

- Mild narcotic painkillers: Medications containing narcotic analgesics such as codeine or hydrocodone are often effective against osteoarthritis pain. But because of concerns about the potential for physical and psychological dependence on these drugs, doctors generally reserve them for short-term use.

- Corticosteroids: Corticosteroids are powerful anti-inflammatory hormones made naturally in the body or manmade for use as medicine. They may be injected into the affected joints to temporarily relieve pain. This is a short-term measure, generally not recommended for more than two to four treatments per year. Oral corticosteroids are not routinely used to treat osteoarthritis. They are occasionally used for inflammatory flares.

- Hyaluronic acid substitutes: Sometimes called viscosupplements, these products are designed to replace a normal component of the joint involved in joint lubrication and nutrition. Depending on the particular product your doctor prescribes, it will be given in a series of three to five injections. These products are approved only for osteoarthritis of the knee.

Because most medicines used to treat osteoarthritis have side effects, it's important to learn as much as possible about the medications you take, even the ones available without a prescription. Certain health problems and lifestyle habits can increase the risk of side effects from NSAIDs. These include a history of peptic ulcers or digestive tract bleeding, use of oral corticosteroids or anticoagulants (blood thinners), smoking, and alcohol use.

There are measures you can take to help reduce the risk of side effects associated with NSAIDs. These include taking medications with food and avoiding stomach irritants such as alcohol, tobacco, and caffeine. In some cases, it may help to take another medication along with an NSAID to coat the stomach or block stomach acids. While these measures may help, they are not always completely effective.

Surgery: For many people, surgery helps relieve the pain and disability of osteoarthritis. Surgery may be performed to achieve one or more of the following:

- Removal of loose pieces of bone and cartilage from the joint if they are causing symptoms of buckling or locking

- Repositioning of bones

- Resurfacing (smoothing out) of bones

Surgeons may replace affected joints with artificial joints called prostheses. These joints can be made from metal alloys, high-density plastic, and ceramic material. Some prostheses are joined to bone surfaces with special cements. Others have porous surfaces and rely on the growth of bone into that surface (a process called biologic fixation) to hold them in place. Artificial joints can last 10 to 15 years or longer. Surgeons choose the design and components of prostheses according to their patient's weight, sex, age, activity level, and other medical conditions.

The decision to use surgery depends on several factors, including the patient's age, occupation, level of disability, pain intensity, and the degree to which arthritis interferes with his or her lifestyle. After surgery and rehabilitation, the patient usually feels less pain and swelling, and can move more easily.

Complementary and alternative therapies: When conventional medical treatment doesn't provide sufficient pain relief, people are more likely to try complementary and alternative therapies. The following are some alternative therapies used to treat osteoarthritis.

- Acupuncture: Some people have found pain relief using acupuncture, a practice in which fine needles are inserted by a licensed acupuncture therapist at specific points on the skin. Preliminary research shows that acupuncture may be a useful component in an osteoarthritis treatment plan for some patients. Scientists think the needles stimulate the release of natural, pain-relieving chemicals produced by the nervous system.

- Folk remedies: These include wearing copper bracelets, drinking herbal teas, taking mud baths, and rubbing WD-40 on joints to "lubricate" them. While these practices may or may not be harmful, no scientific research to date shows that they are helpful in treating osteoarthritis. They can also be expensive, and using them may cause people to delay or even abandon useful medical treatment.

- Nutritional supplements: Nutrients such as glucosamine and chondroitin sulfate have been reported to improve the symptoms of people with osteoarthritis, as have certain vitamins. Additional studies have been carried out to further evaluate these claims.

Who treats osteoarthritis?

Treating arthritis often requires a multidisciplinary or team approach. Many types of health professionals care for people with arthritis. You may choose a few or more of the following professionals to be part of your health care team:

- **Primary care physicians:** Doctors who treat patients before they are referred to other specialists in the health care system.

- **Rheumatologists:** Doctors who specialize in treating arthritis and related conditions that affect joints, muscles, and bones.

- **Orthopedists:** Surgeons who specialize in the treatment of, and surgery for, bone and joint diseases.

- **Physical therapists:** Health professionals who work with patients to improve joint function.

- **Occupational therapists:** Health professionals who teach ways to protect joints, minimize pain, perform activities of daily living, and conserve energy.

- **Dietitians:** Health professionals who teach ways to use a good diet to improve health and maintain a healthy weight.

- **Nurse educators:** Nurses who specialize in helping patients understand their overall condition and implement their treatment plans.

- **Physiatrists (rehabilitation specialists):** Medical doctors who help patients make the most of their physical potential.

- **Licensed acupuncture therapists:** Health professionals who reduce pain and improve physical functioning by inserting fine needles into the skin at specific points on the body.

- **Psychologists:** Health professionals who seek to help patients cope with difficulties in the home and workplace resulting from their medical conditions.

- **Social workers:** Professionals who assist patients with social challenges caused by disability, unemployment, financial hardships, home health care, and other needs resulting from their medical conditions.

SMURFs May Cause Osteoarthritis

If you grew up in the 1980s—or had children who did—you probably know Smurfs as the friendly blue cartoon characters who showed up everywhere from Saturday morning television to lunch boxes and ice shows. But for NIAMS-supported osteoarthritis (OA) researchers, "Smurfs" are neither blue nor necessarily friendly; they're a potentially harmful type of enzyme (full name: Smad Ubiquitination Regulatory Factors), which controls the response of cells to growth factors. Researchers believe a particular form of the enzyme, Smurf2, may hold important clues to the development of OA and quite possibly its prevention.

Smurf2 controls whether a cartilage cell matures and calcifies into hard bone, which is a good thing when it's turned on in areas of the body where we are supposed to have hard bone, says Randy Rosier, MD, PhD, director of the Center of Research Translation in Orthopaedics and senior associate dean for clinical research at the University of Rochester. But when Smurf2 is active in joint cartilage—perhaps as the result of a cartilage injury—it may set off a chain reaction that leads to the steady deterioration of the cartilage that normally comprises the joint surface. When this happens, cartilage breaks down, resulting in damage to the weight-bearing surface of a joint—in other words, OA.

Dr. Rosier believes Smurf2 may be the reason as many as half of people who suffer joint injuries later develop OA in the injured joint. To test his suspicion, he has teamed up with University of Rochester sports medicine surgeon Michael Maloney, MD, to examine tissue samples from healthy patients without arthritis who have sustained an injury to the meniscus (the crescent-shaped piece of cartilage that cushions the knee joint) to determine the level of Smurf2 in their cartilage at the beginning of the trial.

In addition, the researchers will use magnetic resonance imaging (MRI) to measure the cartilage at the time of injury and again three years later. If MRI results confirm the team's earlier findings, the MRIs of patients with high Smurf2 expression will show the beginning signs of OA as measured by hardening of the cartilage and bone loss.

"Our ultimate goal is to create a simple diagnostic test to determine whether a person with a knee injury has a high level of Smurf2 enzyme in their cartilage," says Dr. Rosier, whose work is being supported by one of a special type of NIAMS grant called a Center of Research Translation (CORT) grant. CORT grants require centers to encompass at least three projects, including one clinical and one basic research study. The grants are awarded to research programs that show promise of quickly translating basic science discoveries into patient treatments.

People found to have high levels of Smurf2 could be advised to stop high-intensity, wear-and-tear activity to slow the onset of arthritis and lessen its intensity, says Dr. Rosier. Eventually, the researchers hope to create an injection that will stop Smurf2's ability to turn on the calcification and degeneration process in cartilage that leads to osteoarthritis.

NIAMS Researchers Develop Potential Non-Invasive Test for OA

Researchers funded by the National Institute of Arthritis and Musculoskeletal and Skin Diseases (NIAMS) have identified a new method to diagnose and monitor cartilage changes in people with osteoarthritis (OA). Their discovery, which was reported in the *Proceedings of the National Academy of Sciences*, holds promise for interventions to preserve joint function in individuals identified at early stages of the disease.

Osteoarthritis is caused by the breakdown of cartilage, the tissue that covers the ends of bones where they meet to form a joint. People with OA often experience pain and loss of movement in their joints. Treatment approaches focus on reducing pain, improving mobility, and slowing the progression of the disease.

Although radiographs (x-rays) have traditionally been used as the diagnostic tool for OA, these tests do not show damage from the disease until significant cartilage loss has taken place. Newer imaging techniques also have limitations, including their reliance on contrast dye injections, which can be problematic for older people and those with kidney disease. In light of these issues, Ravinder Regatte, Ph.D., and researchers from New York and Tel Aviv Universities have developed a new method to detect early and progressive changes in cartilage tissue.

Regatte's work focused on proteoglycans, molecules that serve as building blocks for cartilage. "The loss of proteoglycans from cartilage appears to be the initiating event in OA," says Regatte. He and his team adapted an established magnetic resonance imaging (MRI) technique to separately visualize proteoglycans from water molecules in tissue samples of knee cartilage and intravertebral discs. Through a series of experiments, they demonstrated that their method provided accurate measurements of proteoglycans that were as reliable as measurements from more sophisticated and invasive technologies. And, unlike other imaging methods, Regatte's approach did not involve the use of a contrast agent, making it a safer diagnostic tool.

Although further research and refinements are needed, Regatte is hopeful that this non-invasive approach could one day play an important role in the management of people with OA. "Early detection is the key to preventing damage and disability from osteoarthritis, and could allow clinicians the opportunity to monitor the impact of therapeutic interventions very early in the disease process. Such an approach could result in a significant reduction in health care costs from joint replacement surgery."

Ling W, Regatte RR, Navon G, Jerschow A. Assessment of glycosaminoglycan concentration in vivo by chemical exchange-dependent saturation transfer (gagCEST). *Proc Natl Acad Sci* USA. 2008 Feb 19;105(7):2266–70.

Section 6.2

Spinal Stenosis Can Be Caused by OA

Excerpted from "Fast Facts About Spinal Stenosis," by the National Institute of Arthritis and Musculoskeletal and Skin Diseases (NIAMS, www.niams.nih.gov), part of the National Institutes of Health, June 2009.

Who gets spinal stenosis?

Spinal stenosis is most common in men and women over 50 years old. Younger people who were born with a narrow spinal canal or who hurt their spines may also get spinal stenosis.

What causes spinal stenosis?

Aging: Changes that occur in the spine as people get older are the most common cause of spinal stenosis. As people get older, the following changes occur:

- The bands of tissue that support the spine may get thick and hard.
- Bones and joints may get bigger.
- Surfaces of the bones may bulge out (these are called bone spurs).

Arthritis: In some cases arthritis, a degenerative (gets worse over time) condition can cause spinal stenosis. Two forms of arthritis may affect the spine: osteoarthritis and rheumatoid arthritis.
Osteoarthritis:

- is the most common form of arthritis;
- most often occurs in middle-aged and older people;
- doesn't go away;
- may involve many joints in the body;
- wears away the tough tissue (cartilage) that keeps the joints in place;
- causes bone spurs and problems with joints.

79

Rheumatoid arthritis:

- affects most people at a younger age than osteoarthritis;
- causes the soft tissues of the joints to swell and can affect the internal organs and systems;
- is not a common cause of spinal stenosis;
- can cause severe damage, especially to joints.

Inherited conditions: Some people are born with conditions that cause spinal stenosis. For instance, some people are born with a small spinal canal. Others are born with a curved spine (scoliosis).

Other causes: Other causes of spinal stenosis include the following:

- Tumors of the spine
- Injuries
- Paget disease (a disease that affects the bones)
- Too much fluoride in the body
- Calcium deposits on the ligaments that run along the spine

What are the symptoms of spinal stenosis?

There may be no symptoms of spinal stenosis, or symptoms may appear slowly and get worse over time. Signs of spinal stenosis include the following:

- Pain in the neck or back
- Numbness, weakness, cramping, or pain in the arms or legs
- Pain going down the leg
- Foot problems

One type of spinal stenosis, cauda equine syndrome, is very serious. This type occurs when there is pressure on nerves in the lower back. Symptoms may include the following:

- Loss of control of the bowel or bladder
- Problems having sex
- Pain, weakness, or loss of feeling in one or both legs

If you have any of these symptoms, you should call your doctor right away.

How is spinal stenosis diagnosed?

To diagnose spinal stenosis, your doctor will ask about your medical history and conduct a physical exam. Your doctor may also order one or more tests, such as the following:

- X-rays
- Magnetic resonance imaging (MRI): A test that uses radio waves to look at your spine
- Computerized axial tomography (CAT): A series of x-rays that give your doctor a detailed image of your spine
- Myelogram: A test in which the doctor injects liquid dye into your spinal column
- Bone scan: A test in which you are given a shot of radioactive substance that shows where bone is breaking down or being formed

Who treats spinal stenosis?

Because spinal stenosis has many causes and symptoms, you may require treatment from doctors who specialize in certain aspects of the condition. Based on your symptoms, your doctor may refer you to one of the following:

- Rheumatologists (doctors who treat arthritis and related disorders)
- Neurologists and neurosurgeons (doctors who treat diseases of the nervous system)
- Orthopedic surgeons (doctors who treat problems with the bones, joints, and ligaments)
- Physical therapists

What are some nonsurgical treatments for spinal stenosis?

There are many nonsurgical treatments for spinal stenosis. Your doctor may prescribe one or more of the following:

- Medicines to reduce swelling

- Medicines to relieve pain
- Limits on your activity
- Exercises and/or physical therapy
- A brace for your lower back

When should surgery be considered?

Your doctor will likely suggest nonsurgical treatment first unless you have one of the following:

- Symptoms that get in the way of walking
- Problems with bowel or bladder function
- Problems with your nervous system

Your doctor will take many factors into account in deciding if surgery is right for you.

- The success of nonsurgical treatments
- The extent of the pain
- Your preferences

What are some alternative treatments for spinal stenosis?

Alternative treatments are those that are not part of standard treatment. For spinal stenosis, such treatments include chiropractic treatment and acupuncture.

More research is needed on the value of these treatments. Your doctor may suggest alternative treatments in addition to standard treatments.

Chapter 7

Rheumatoid Arthritis (RA)

Chapter Contents

Section 7.1

All about RA

Excerpted from "Handout on Health: Rheumatoid Arthritis," by the National Institute of Arthritis and Musculoskeletal and Skin Diseases (NIAMS, www.niams.nih.gov), part of the National Institutes of Health, May 2004. Reviewed and revised by David A. Cooke, MD, FACP, June 29, 2009. Brand names included in this section are provided as examples only, and their inclusion does not mean that these products are endorsed by the National Institutes of Health or any other government agency. Also, if a particular band name is not mentioned, this does not mean or imply that the product is unsatisfactory.

Features of Rheumatoid Arthritis

Rheumatoid arthritis is an inflammatory disease that causes pain, swelling, stiffness, and loss of function in the joints. It has several special features that make it different from other kinds of arthritis. For example, rheumatoid arthritis generally occurs in a symmetrical pattern, meaning that if one knee or hand is involved, the other one also is. The disease often affects the wrist joints and the finger joints closest to the hand. It can also affect other parts of the body besides the joints. In addition, people with rheumatoid arthritis may have fatigue, occasional fevers, and a general sense of not feeling well.

Rheumatoid arthritis affects people differently. For some people, it lasts only a few months or a year or two and goes away without causing any noticeable damage. Other people have mild or moderate forms of the disease, with periods of worsening symptoms, called flares, and periods in which they feel better, called remissions. Still others have a severe form of the disease that is active most of the time, lasts for many years or a lifetime, and leads to serious joint damage and disability.

Although rheumatoid arthritis can have serious effects on a person's life and well-being, current treatment strategies—including pain-relieving drugs and medications that slow joint damage, a balance between rest and exercise, and patient education and support programs—allow most people with the disease to lead active and productive lives. In recent years, research has led to a new understanding of rheumatoid arthritis and has increased the likelihood that, in time, researchers will find even better ways to treat the disease.

Normal Joint

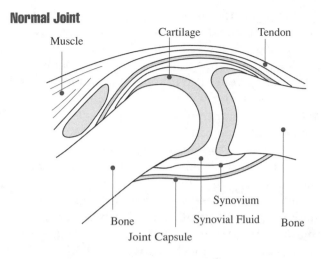

Joint Affected by Rheumatoid Arthritis

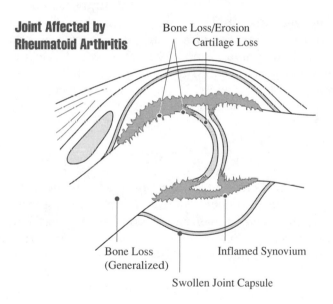

Figure 7.1. How a joint is affected by rheumatoid arthritis.

How Rheumatoid Arthritis Develops and Progresses

The Joints

A joint is a place where two bones meet. The ends of the bones are covered by cartilage, which allows for easy movement of the two bones.

85

The joint is surrounded by a capsule that protects and supports it. The joint capsule is lined with a type of tissue called synovium, which produces synovial fluid, a clear substance that lubricates and nourishes the cartilage and bones inside the joint capsule.

Like many other rheumatic diseases, rheumatoid arthritis is an autoimmune disease (auto means self), so-called because a person's immune system, which normally helps protect the body from infection and disease, attacks joint tissues for unknown reasons. White blood cells, the agents of the immune system, travel to the synovium and cause inflammation (synovitis), characterized by warmth, redness, swelling, and pain—typical symptoms of rheumatoid arthritis. During the inflammation process, the normally thin synovium becomes thick and makes the joint swollen and puffy to the touch.

As rheumatoid arthritis progresses, the inflamed synovium invades and destroys the cartilage and bone within the joint. The surrounding muscles, ligaments, and tendons that support and stabilize the joint become weak and unable to work normally. These effects lead to the pain and joint damage often seen in rheumatoid arthritis. Researchers studying rheumatoid arthritis now believe that it begins to damage bones during the first year or two that a person has the disease, one reason why early diagnosis and treatment are so important.

Other Parts of the Body

Some people with rheumatoid arthritis also have symptoms in places other than their joints. Many people with rheumatoid arthritis develop anemia, or a decrease in the production of red blood cells. Other effects that occur less often include neck pain and dry eyes and mouth. Very rarely, people may have inflammation of the blood vessels, the lining of the lungs, or the sac enclosing the heart.

Occurrence and Impact of Rheumatoid Arthritis

Scientists estimate that about 1.3 million people, or about 0.6 percent of the U.S. adult population, have rheumatoid arthritis. Interestingly, some recent studies have suggested that although the number of new cases of rheumatoid arthritis for older people is increasing, the overall number of new cases may actually be going down. (According to the National Arthritis Data Workgroup, the actual number of new cases of rheumatoid arthritis is lower than previous estimates due to changes in the classification for the condition, as cited in "Estimates of the Prevalence of Arthritis and Other Rheumatic Conditions in the United States," *Arthritis and Rheumatism*, 58(1):15–25, January 2008.)

Rheumatoid arthritis occurs in all races and ethnic groups. Although the disease often begins in middle age and occurs with increased frequency in older people, children and young adults also develop it. Like some other forms of arthritis, rheumatoid arthritis occurs much more frequently in women than in men. About two to three times as many women as men have the disease.

By all measures, the financial and social impact of all types of arthritis, including rheumatoid arthritis, is substantial, both for the nation and for individuals. From an economic standpoint, the medical and surgical treatment for rheumatoid arthritis and the wages lost because of disability caused by the disease add up to billions of dollars annually. Daily joint pain is an inevitable consequence of the disease, and most patients also experience some degree of depression, anxiety, and feelings of helplessness. For some people, rheumatoid arthritis can interfere with normal daily activities, limit job opportunities, or disrupt the joys and responsibilities of family life. However, there are arthritis self-management programs that help people cope with the pain and other effects of the disease and help them lead independent and productive lives.

Searching for the Causes of Rheumatoid Arthritis

Scientists still do not know exactly what causes the immune system to turn against itself in rheumatoid arthritis, but research over the last few years has begun to piece together the factors involved.

Genetic (inherited) factors: Scientists have discovered that certain genes known to play a role in the immune system are associated with a tendency to develop rheumatoid arthritis. Some people with rheumatoid arthritis do not have these particular genes; still others have these genes but never develop the disease. These somewhat contradictory data suggest that a person's genetic makeup plays an important role in determining if he or she will develop rheumatoid arthritis, but it is not the only factor. What is clear, however, is that more than one gene is involved in determining whether a person develops rheumatoid arthritis and how severe the disease will become.

Environmental factors: Many scientists think that something must occur to trigger the disease process in people whose genetic makeup makes them susceptible to rheumatoid arthritis. A viral or bacterial infection appears likely, but the exact agent is not yet known. This does not mean that rheumatoid arthritis is contagious: a person cannot catch it from someone else.

Other factors: Some scientists also think that a variety of hormonal factors may be involved. Women are more likely to develop rheumatoid arthritis than men, pregnancy may improve the disease, and the disease may flare after a pregnancy. Breastfeeding may also aggravate the disease. Contraceptive use may alter a person's likelihood of developing rheumatoid arthritis. Scientists think that levels of the immune system molecules interleukin 12 (IL-12) and tumor necrosis factor-alpha (TNF-α;) may change along with the changing hormone levels seen in pregnant women. This change may contribute to the swelling and tissue destruction seen in rheumatoid arthritis. These hormones, or possibly deficiencies or changes in certain hormones, may promote the development of rheumatoid arthritis in a genetically susceptible person who has been exposed to a triggering agent from the environment.

Even though all the answers are not known, one thing is certain: Rheumatoid arthritis develops as a result of an interaction of many factors. Researchers are trying to understand these factors and how they work together.

Diagnosing and Treating Rheumatoid Arthritis

Diagnosing and treating rheumatoid arthritis requires a team effort involving the patient and several types of health care professionals. A person can go to his or her family doctor or internist or to a rheumatologist. A rheumatologist is a doctor who specializes in arthritis and other diseases of the joints, bones, and muscles. As treatment progresses, other professionals often help. These may include nurses, physical or occupational therapists, orthopedic surgeons, psychologists, and social workers.

Studies have shown that patients who are well informed and participate actively in their own care have less pain and make fewer visits to the doctor than do other patients with rheumatoid arthritis.

Patient education and arthritis self-management programs, as well as support groups, help people to become better informed and to participate in their own care. An example of a self-management program is the Arthritis Self-Help Course offered by the Arthritis Foundation and developed at a NIAMS-supported Multipurpose Arthritis and

Musculoskeletal Diseases Center. Self-management programs teach about rheumatoid arthritis and its treatments, exercise and relaxation approaches, communication between patients and health care providers, and problem solving. Research on these programs has shown that they help people do the following:

- Understand the disease
- Reduce their pain while remaining active
- Cope physically, emotionally, and mentally
- Feel greater control over the disease and build a sense of confidence in the ability to function and lead full, active, and independent lives

Diagnosis

Rheumatoid arthritis can be difficult to diagnose in its early stages for several reasons. First, there is no single test for the disease. In addition, symptoms differ from person to person and can be more severe in some people than in others. Also, symptoms can be similar to those of other types of arthritis and joint conditions, and it may take some time for other conditions to be ruled out. Finally, the full range of symptoms develops over time, and only a few symptoms may be present in the early stages. As a result, doctors use a variety of the following tools to diagnose the disease and to rule out other conditions:

Medical history: This is the patient's description of symptoms and when and how they began. Good communication between patient and doctor is especially important here. For example, the patient's description of pain, stiffness, and joint function and how these change over time is critical to the doctor's initial assessment of the disease and how it changes over time.

Physical examination: This includes the doctor's examination of the joints, skin, reflexes, and muscle strength.

Laboratory tests: One common test is for rheumatoid factor, an antibody that is present eventually in the blood of most people with rheumatoid arthritis. (An antibody is a special protein made by the immune system that normally helps fight foreign substances in the body.) Not all people with rheumatoid arthritis test positive for rheumatoid factor, however, especially early in the disease. Also, some people test positive for rheumatoid factor, yet never develop the disease. A newer blood test, anti-cyclic citrullinated peptide antibodies (anti-CCP), appears to be more accurate that the rheumatoid factor test, and is increasingly being used for diagnosis. Other common laboratory tests include a white blood cell count, a blood test for anemia, and a test of the erythrocyte sedimentation rate (often called the sed rate), which measures inflammation in the body. C-reactive protein is another common test that measures disease activity.

X-rays: X-rays are used to determine the degree of joint destruction. They are not useful in the early stages of rheumatoid arthritis before bone damage is evident, but they can be used later to monitor the progression of the disease.

Treatment

Doctors use a variety of approaches to treat rheumatoid arthritis. These are used in different combinations and at different times during the course of the disease and are chosen according to the patient's individual situation. No matter what treatment the doctor and patient choose, however, the goals are the same: to relieve pain, reduce inflammation, slow down or stop joint damage, and improve the person's sense of well-being and ability to function.

Good communication between the patient and doctor is necessary for effective treatment. Talking to the doctor can help ensure that exercise and pain management programs are provided as needed, and that drugs are prescribed appropriately. Talking to the doctor can also help people who are making decisions about surgery.

Health behavior changes: Certain activities can help improve a person's ability to function independently and maintain a positive outlook.

- **Rest and exercise:** People with rheumatoid arthritis need a good balance between rest and exercise, with more rest when the disease is active and more exercise when it is not. Rest helps to reduce active joint inflammation and pain and to fight fatigue. The length of time for rest will vary from person to person, but in general, shorter rest breaks every now and then are more helpful than long times spent in bed. Exercise is important for maintaining healthy and strong muscles, preserving joint mobility, and maintaining flexibility. Exercise can also help people sleep well, reduce pain, maintain a positive attitude, and lose weight. Exercise programs should take into account the person's physical abilities, limitations, and changing needs.

- **Joint care:** Some people find using a splint for a short time around a painful joint reduces pain and swelling by supporting the joint and letting it rest. Splints are used mostly on wrists and hands, but also on ankles and feet. A doctor or a physical or occupational therapist can help a person choose a splint and make sure it fits properly. Other ways to reduce stress on joints include self-help devices (for example, zipper pullers, long-handled shoe horns); devices to help with getting on and off chairs, toilet seats, and beds; and changes in the ways that a person carries out daily activities.

- **Stress reduction:** People with rheumatoid arthritis face emotional challenges as well as physical ones. The emotions they feel because of the disease—fear, anger, and frustration—combined with any pain and physical limitations can increase their stress level. Although there is no evidence that stress plays a role in causing rheumatoid arthritis, it can make living with the disease difficult at times. Stress also may affect the amount of pain a person feels. There are a number of successful techniques for coping with stress. Regular rest periods can help, as can relaxation, distraction, or visualization exercises. Exercise programs, participation in support groups, and good communication with the health care team are other ways to reduce stress.

- **Healthful diet:** With the exception of several specific types of oils, there is no scientific evidence that any specific food or nutrient helps or harms people with rheumatoid arthritis. However, an overall nutritious diet with enough—but not an excess of—calories, protein, and calcium is important. Some people may need to be careful about drinking alcoholic beverages because of the medications they take for rheumatoid arthritis. Those taking methotrexate may need to avoid alcohol altogether because one of the most serious long-term side effects of methotrexate is liver damage.

- **Climate:** Some people notice that their arthritis gets worse when there is a sudden change in the weather. However, there is no evidence that a specific climate can prevent or reduce the effects of rheumatoid arthritis. Moving to a new place with a different climate usually does not make a long-term difference in a person's rheumatoid arthritis.

91

Medications: Most people who have rheumatoid arthritis take medications. Some medications are used only for pain relief; others are used to reduce inflammation. Still others, often called disease-modifying antirheumatic drugs (DMARDs), are used to try to slow the course of the disease. The person's general condition, the current and predicted severity of the illness, the length of time he or she will take the drug, and the drug's effectiveness and potential side effects are important considerations in prescribing drugs for rheumatoid arthritis. Table 7.1 shows currently used rheumatoid arthritis medications, along with their uses and effects, side effects, and monitoring requirements.

At present, the first choice drug for most patients with rheumatoid arthritis is methotrexate. This medication was originally developed for cancer treatment, but has been since found to be very useful for conditions such as rheumatoid arthritis. It selectively kills rapidly dividing white blood cells and sharply reduces the degree of joint inflammation. Starting this medication early in the disease can dramatically reduce the progressive joint damage, which had once been considered inevitable.

Biologic response modifiers are new drugs used for the treatment of rheumatoid arthritis. They can help reduce inflammation and structural damage to the joints by blocking the action of cytokines, proteins of the body's immune system that trigger inflammation during normal immune responses. Three of these drugs, etanercept (Enbrel), infliximab (Remicade), and adalimumab (Humira), reduce inflammation by blocking the reaction of TNF α molecules. Another drug, called anakinra (Kineret), works by blocking a protein called interleukin 1 (IL-1) that is seen in excess in patients with rheumatoid arthritis. Still another drug, abatacept (Orencia), blocks several different molecules important in inflammation, TNF α, interleukin 2 (IL-2), and interferon-γ.

For many years, doctors initially prescribed aspirin or other pain-relieving drugs for rheumatoid arthritis, as well as rest and physical therapy. They usually prescribed more powerful drugs later only if the disease worsened.

Today, however, most doctors have changed their approach, especially for patients with severe, rapidly progressing rheumatoid arthritis. Studies show that early treatment with more powerful drugs, and the use of drug combinations instead of one medication alone, is more effective in preventing serious complications. Once the disease improves or is in remission, the doctor may gradually reduce the dosage or prescribe a milder medication.

Surgery: Several types of surgery are available to patients with severe joint damage. The primary purpose of these procedures is to reduce pain, improve the affected joint's function, and improve the patient's ability to perform daily activities. Surgery is not for everyone, however, and the decision should be made only after careful consideration by patient and doctor. Together they should discuss the patient's overall health, the condition of the joint or tendon that will be operated on, and the reason for, as well as the risks and benefits of, the surgical procedure. Cost may be another factor. Commonly performed surgical procedures include joint replacement, tendon reconstruction, and synovectomy.

- **Joint replacement:** This is the most frequently performed surgery for rheumatoid arthritis, and it is done primarily to relieve pain and improve or preserve joint function. Artificial joints are not always permanent and may eventually have to be replaced. This may be an important consideration for young people.

- **Tendon reconstruction:** Rheumatoid arthritis can damage and even rupture tendons, the tissues that attach muscle to bone. This surgery, which is used most frequently on the hands, reconstructs the damaged tendon by attaching an intact tendon to it. This procedure can help to restore hand function, especially if the tendon is completely ruptured.

- **Synovectomy:** In this surgery, the doctor actually removes the inflamed synovial tissue. Synovectomy by itself is seldom performed now because not all of the tissue can be removed, and it eventually grows back. Synovectomy is done as part of reconstructive surgery, especially tendon reconstruction.

Routine monitoring and ongoing care: Regular medical care is important to monitor the course of the disease, determine the effectiveness and any negative effects of medications, and change therapies as needed. Monitoring typically includes regular visits to the doctor. It also may include blood, urine, and other laboratory tests and x-rays.

People with rheumatoid arthritis may want to discuss preventing osteoporosis with their doctors as part of their long-term, ongoing care. Osteoporosis is a condition in which bones become weakened and fragile. Having rheumatoid arthritis increases the risk of developing osteoporosis for both men and women, particularly if a person takes corticosteroids. Such patients may want to discuss with their doctors the potential benefits of calcium and vitamin D supplements, antiresorptive medications, or other treatments for osteoporosis.

Alternative and complementary therapies: Special diets, vitamin supplements, and other alternative approaches have been suggested for treating rheumatoid arthritis. Although many of these approaches may not be harmful in and of themselves, controlled scientific studies either have not been conducted on them or have found no definite benefit to these therapies. Some alternative or complementary approaches may help the patient cope or reduce some of the stress associated with living with a chronic illness. As with any therapy, patients should discuss the benefits and drawbacks with their doctors before beginning an alternative or new type of therapy. If the doctor feels the approach has value and will not be harmful, it can be incorporated into a patient's treatment plan. However, it is important not to neglect regular health care.

Current Research

Over the last several decades, research has greatly increased our understanding of the immune system, genetics, and biology. This research is now showing results in several areas important to rheumatoid arthritis. Scientists are thinking about rheumatoid arthritis in exciting ways that were not possible even 10 years ago.

Scientists are looking at the immune systems of people with rheumatoid arthritis and in some animal models of the disease to understand why and how the disease develops. For example, small studies are looking at the role of T cells, which play an important role in immunity and in the progression of rheumatoid arthritis. Findings from these studies may lead to precise, targeted therapies that could stop the inflammatory process in its earliest stages. They may even lead to a vaccine that could prevent rheumatoid arthritis.

Researchers are studying genetic factors that predispose some people to developing rheumatoid arthritis, as well as factors connected with disease severity. For example, by studying genetically engineered mice, scientists supported by the National Institutes of Health (NIH) discovered that immune cells called mast cells play a key role in the development of rheumatoid arthritis. Findings from these studies should increase our understanding of the disease and will help develop new therapies, as well as guide treatment decisions.

In a major effort aimed at identifying genes involved in rheumatoid arthritis, the NIH and the Arthritis Foundation have joined together

Table 7.1. Medications Used to Treat Rheumatoid Arthritis (continued on next page)

Medication: Analgesics and Nonsteroidal Anti-inflammatory Drugs (NSAIDs)
Uses/Effects: Analgesics relieve pain; NSAIDs are a large class of medications useful against pain and inflammation. A number of NSAIDs are available over the counter. More than a dozen others—including a subclass called COX-2 inhibitors—are available only with a prescription.
Side Effects: NSAIDs can cause stomach irritation or, less often, can affect kidney function. The longer a person uses NSAIDs, the more likely he or she is to have side effects, ranging from mild to serious. Many other drugs cannot be taken when a patient is being treated with NSAIDs because they alter the way the body uses or eliminates these other drugs. NSAIDs sometimes are associated with serious gastrointestinal problems, including ulcers, bleeding, and perforation of the stomach or intestine. People over age 65 and those with any history of ulcers or gastrointestinal bleeding should use NSAIDs with caution.
Monitoring: Check with your health care provider or pharmacist before you take NSAIDs. Before taking traditional NSAIDs, let your provider know if you drink alcohol or use blood thinners or if you have any of the following: sensitivity or allergy to aspirin or similar drugs, kidney or liver disease, heart disease, high blood pressure, asthma, or peptic ulcers.

Medication: Acetaminophen
Uses/Effects: Nonprescription medications used to relieve pain. Examples are aspirin-free Anacin, Excedrin caplets, Panadol, Tylenol, and Tylenol Arthritis.
Side Effects: Usually no side effects when taken as directed.
Monitoring: Not to be taken with alcohol or with other products containing acetaminophen. Not to be used for more than 10 days unless directed by a physician.

Medication: Aspirin (Buffered, Plain)
Uses/Effects: Aspirin is used to reduce pain, swelling, and inflammation, allowing patients to move more easily and carry out normal activities. It is generally part of early and ongoing therapy.
Side Effects: Upset stomach; tendency to bruise easily; ulcers, pain, or discomfort; diarrhea; headache; heartburn or indigestion; nausea or vomiting.
Monitoring: Doctor monitoring is needed.

Medication: Traditional NSAIDs (Ibuprofen, Ketoprofen, Naproxen)
Uses/Effects: NSAIDs help relieve pain within hours of administration in dosages available over-the-counter (available for all three medications). They relieve pain and inflammation in dosages available in prescription form (ibuprofen and ketoprofen). It may take several days to reduce inflammation.
Side Effects: For all traditional NSAIDs: Abdominal or stomach cramps, pain, or discomfort; diarrhea; dizziness; drowsiness or light-headedness; headache; heartburn or indigestion; peptic ulcers; nausea or vomiting; possible kidney and liver damage (rare).
Monitoring: For all traditional NSAIDs: Before taking these drugs, let your doctor know if you drink alcohol or use blood thinners or if you have or have had any of the following: sensitivity or allergy to aspirin or similar drugs, kidney or liver disease, heart disease, high blood pressure, asthma, or peptic ulcers.

Table 7.1. Medications Used to Treat Rheumatoid Arthritis (continued from previous page)

Medication: Corticosteroids
Uses/Effects: These are steroids given by mouth or injection. They are used to relieve inflammation and reduce swelling, redness, itching, and allergic reactions.
Side Effects: Increased appetite, indigestion, nervousness, or restlessness.
Monitoring: For all corticosteroids, let your doctor know if you have one of the following: fungal infection, history of tuberculosis, underactive thyroid, herpes simplex of the eye, high blood pressure, osteoporosis, or stomach ulcer.

Medication: Methylprednisolone/Prednisone
Uses/Effects: These steroids are available in pill form or as an injection into a joint. Improvements are seen in several hours up to 24 hours after administration. There is potential for serious side effects, especially at high doses. They are used for severe flares and when the disease does not respond to NSAIDs and DMARDs.
Side Effects: Osteoporosis, mood changes, fragile skin, easy bruising, fluid retention, weight gain, muscle weakness, onset or worsening of diabetes, cataracts, increased risk of infection, hypertension (high blood pressure).
Monitoring: Doctor monitoring for continued effectiveness of medication and for side effects is needed.

Medication: Disease-modifying antirheumatic drugs (DMARDs)
Uses/Effects: These are common arthritis medications. They relieve painful, swollen joints and slow joint damage, and several DMARDs may be used over the disease course. They take a few weeks or months to have an effect, and may produce significant improvements for many patients. Exactly how they work is still unknown.
Side Effects: Side effects vary with each medicine. DMARDs may increase risk of infection, hair loss, and kidney or liver damage.
Monitoring: Doctor monitoring allows the risk of toxicities to be weighed against the potential benefits of individual medications.

Medication: Azathioprine
Uses/Effects: This drug was first used in higher doses in cancer chemotherapy and organ transplantation. It is used in patients who have not responded to other drugs, and in combination therapy.
Side Effects: Cough or hoarseness, fever or chills, loss of appetite, lower back or side pain, nausea or vomiting, painful or difficult urination, unusual tiredness or weakness.
Monitoring: Before taking this drug, tell your doctor if you use allopurinol or have kidney or liver disease. This drug can reduce your ability to fight infection, so call your doctor immediately if you develop chills, fever, or a cough. Regular blood and liver function tests are needed.

Medication: Cyclosporine
Uses/Effects: This medication was first used in organ transplantation to prevent rejection. It is used in patients who have not responded to other drugs.
Side Effects: Bleeding, tender, or enlarged gums; high blood pressure; increase in hair growth; kidney problems; trembling and shaking of hands.

Table 7.1. Medications Used to Treat Rheumatoid Arthritis (continued on next page)

Medication: Cyclosporine (continued)
Monitoring: Before taking this drug, tell your doctor if you have one of the following: sensitivity to castor oil (if receiving the drug by injection), liver or kidney disease, active infection, or high blood pressure. Using this drug may make you more susceptible to infection and certain cancers. Do not take live vaccines while on this drug.

Medication: Hydroxychloroquine
Uses/Effects: It may take several months to notice the benefits of this drug, which include reducing the signs and symptoms of rheumatoid arthritis.
Side Effects: Diarrhea, eye problems (rare), headache, loss of appetite, nausea or vomiting, stomach cramps, or pain.
Monitoring: Doctor monitoring is important, particularly if you have an allergy to any antimalarial drug or a retinal abnormality.

Medication: Gold sodium thiomalate
Uses/Effects: This was one of the first DMARDs used to treat rheumatoid arthritis.
Side Effects: Redness or soreness of tongue; swelling or bleeding gums; skin rash or itching; ulcers or sores on lips, mouth, or throat; irritation on tongue. Joint pain may occur for one or two days after injection.
Monitoring: Before taking this drug, tell your doctor if you have any of the following: lupus, skin rash, kidney disease, or colitis. Periodic urine and blood tests are needed to check for side effects.

Medication: Leflunomide
Uses/Effects: This drug reduces signs and symptoms and slows structural damage to joints caused by arthritis.
Side Effects: Bloody or cloudy urine; congestion in chest; cough; diarrhea; difficult, burning, or painful urination or breathing; fever; hair loss; headache; heartburn; loss of appetite; nausea and/or vomiting; skin rash; stomach pain; sneezing; and sore throat.
Monitoring: Before taking this medication, let your doctor know if you have one of the following: active infection, liver disease, known immune deficiency, renal insufficiency, or underlying malignancy. You will need regular blood tests, including liver function tests. Leflunomide must not be taken during pregnancy because it may cause birth defects in humans.

Medication: Methotrexate
Uses/Effects: This drug can be taken by mouth or by injection and results in rapid improvement (it usually takes 3–6 weeks to begin working). It is very effective, especially in combination with infliximab or etanercept. In general, it produces more favorable long-term responses compared with other DMARDs such as sulfasalazine, gold sodium thiomalate, and hydroxychloroquine.
Side Effects: Abdominal discomfort, chest pain, chills, nausea, mouth sores, painful urination, sore throat, unusual tiredness or weakness.

Table 7.1. Medications Used to Treat Rheumatoid Arthritis (continued from previous page)

Medication: Methotrexate (continued)
Monitoring: Doctor monitoring is important, particularly if you have an abnormal blood count, liver or lung disease, alcoholism, immune-system deficiency, or active infection. Methotrexate must not be taken during pregnancy because it may cause birth defects in humans.

Medication: Sulfasalazine
Uses/Effects: This drug works to reduce the signs and symptoms of rheumatoid arthritis by suppressing the immune system.
Side Effects: Abdominal pain, aching joints, diarrhea, headache, sensitivity to sunlight, loss of appetite, nausea or vomiting, skin rash.
Monitoring: Doctor monitoring is important, particularly if you are allergic to sulfa drugs or aspirin, or if you have a kidney, liver, or blood disease.

Medication: Biologic Response Modifiers
Uses/Effects: These drugs selectively block parts of the immune system called cytokines. Cytokines play a role in inflammation. Long-term efficacy and safety are uncertain.
Side Effects: Increased risk of infection, especially tuberculosis. Increased risk of pneumonia, and listeriosis (a foodborne illness caused by the bacterium *Listeria monocytogenes*).
Monitoring: It is important to avoid eating undercooked foods (including unpasteurized cheeses, cold cuts, and hot dogs) because undercooked food can cause listeriosis for patients taking biologic response modifiers.

Medication: Tumor Necrosis Factor Inhibitors (Etanercept, Infliximab, Adalimumab)
Uses/Effects: These medications are highly effective for treating patients with an inadequate response to DMARDs. They may be prescribed in combination with some DMARDs, particularly methotrexate. Etanercept requires subcutaneous (beneath the skin) injections two times per week. Infliximab is taken intravenously (IV) during a 2-hour procedure. It is administered with methotrexate. Adalimumab requires injections every 2 weeks. Long-term efficacy and safety are uncertain.
Side Effects: *Etanercept*: Pain or burning in throat; redness, itching, pain, and/or swelling at injection site; runny or stuffy nose. *Infliximab*: Abdominal pain, cough, dizziness, fainting, headache, muscle pain, runny nose, shortness of breath, sore throat, vomiting, wheezing. *Adalimumab*: Redness, rash, swelling, itching, bruising, sinus infection, headache, nausea.
Monitoring: Long-term efficacy and safety are uncertain. Doctor monitoring is important, particularly if you have an active infection, exposure to tuberculosis, or a central nervous system disorder. Evaluation for tuberculosis is necessary before treatment begins.

Medication: Interleukin1 Inhibitor (Anakinra)
Uses/Effects: This medication requires daily injections. Long-term efficacy and safety are uncertain.

Table 7.1. Medications Used to Treat Rheumatoid Arthritis (continued)

Medication: Interleukin1 Inhibitor (Anakinra) (continued)
Side Effects: Redness, swelling, bruising, or pain at the site of injection; headache; upset stomach; diarrhea; runny nose; and stomach pain.
Monitoring: Doctor monitoring is required.

Medication: Abatacept (Orencia)
Uses/Effects: This medication cannot be used in combination with other TNF or IL-1 blocking biologic response modifiers.
Side Effects: Common side effects include headache, sore throat, and nausea. Serious infections and cancers have been reported in patients taking this medication.
Monitoring: Close monitoring by a doctor is very important, and evaluation for tuberculosis or other serious infections must be performed before the start of therapy.

to support the North American Rheumatoid Arthritis Consortium. This group of 10 research centers around the United States is collecting medical information and genetic material from 1,000 families in which two or more siblings have rheumatoid arthritis. It serves as a national resource for genetic studies of this disease.

To help identify the multiple factors that predict disease course and outcomes in rheumatoid arthritis in African Americans, the NIH is supporting the Consortium for the Longitudinal Evaluations of African Americans with Early Rheumatoid Arthritis (CLEAR) Registry at the University of Alabama at Birmingham. This registry aims to collect clinical and x-ray data and DNA [deoxyribonucleic acid] to help scientists analyze genetic and nongenetic factors that predict disease course and outcomes of rheumatoid arthritis.

Scientists are also unearthing the genetic basis of rheumatoid arthritis by studying rats with a condition that resembles rheumatoid arthritis in humans. NIAMS researchers have identified several genetic regions that affect arthritis susceptibility and severity in these animal models of the disease. These genetic regions are important because they can assist scientists in predicting the symptoms and severity of rheumatoid arthritis. Replacing malfunctioning genes with healthy genes (gene transfer) is being tested in mice, and it may eventually be used in humans to treat rheumatoid arthritis.

Researchers are also uncovering the complex relationships between the hormonal, nervous, and immune systems in rheumatoid arthritis. For example, they are exploring whether and how the normal changes in the levels of naturally produced steroid hormones (such as estrogen and testosterone) during a person's lifetime may be related to the development, improvement, or flares of the disease. Scientists also are researching how these systems interact with environmental and genetic factors. The results of this research may suggest new treatment strategies.

Scientists are exploring why so many more women than men develop rheumatoid arthritis. In hopes of finding clues, they are studying female and male hormones and other differences between women and men.

Scientists are examining why rheumatoid arthritis often improves during pregnancy. Results of one study suggest that the explanation may be related to differences in certain special proteins that pass between a mother and her unborn child. These proteins help the immune system distinguish between the body's own cells and foreign cells. Such differences, the scientists speculate, may change the activity of the mother's immune system during pregnancy.

A growing body of evidence indicates that infectious agents, such as viruses and bacteria, may trigger rheumatoid arthritis in people who have an inherited predisposition to the disease. Scientists are trying to discover which infectious agents may be responsible and how they trigger arthritis.

Researchers are searching for new drugs or combinations of drugs that can reduce inflammation and slow or stop the progression of rheumatoid arthritis with few side effects. Already, the new biologic response modifiers infliximab and etanercept are proving to be extremely effective for some people. Studies show that these treatments are more effective at slowing joint damage than methotrexate alone. Combination treatment with etanercept and methotrexate or infliximab and methotrexate has been found even more effective than either of the new treatments alone. (Methotrexate was used for comparison because it is a commonly prescribed "front-line" treatment.) The U.S. Food and Drug Administration has approved adalimumab (Humira), anakinra (Kineret), and abatacept (Orencia) for slowing the progression of structural damage in adults with moderate to severe rheumatoid arthritis who have not responded well to one or more disease modifying antirheumatic drugs.

Investigators have also shown that treatment of rheumatoid arthritis with minocycline, a drug in the tetracycline family, has a modest benefit. Other studies have shown that the omega-3 fatty acids in certain fish or plant seed oils also may reduce rheumatoid arthritis inflammation. However, many people are not able to tolerate the large amounts of oil necessary for any benefit.

Scientists are examining many issues related to quality of life for people with rheumatoid arthritis and the quality, cost, and effectiveness of the health care services they receive. Some new techniques for managing symptoms under investigation include tai chi (a form of movement-based meditation), and cognitive-behavioral therapy (a technique that teaches you to anticipate and prepare yourself for the situations and bodily sensations that may trigger painful symptoms). Scientists have found that even a small improvement in a patient's sense of physical and mental well-being can have an impact on his or her quality of life and use of health care services.

Section 7.2

Heart Disease and RA

"Doctors Urge More Aggressive Cardiac Screening for People with Rheumatoid Arthritis," © 2005 Missouri Arthritis Rehabilitation Research and Training Center (MARRTC). Reprinted with permission. For additional information, visit http://marrtc.missouri.edu.

If you have rheumatoid arthritis, listen to your heart. This is what doctors are urging people who have the disease to do, after two Mayo Clinic studies found that rheumatoid arthritis ups one's risk for heart failure, heart disease, and sudden cardiac death.

About 2 million people in the United States have rheumatoid arthritis, an autoimmune disease that causes inflammation, pain, and damage to the joints.

Researchers are not sure why and how people with rheumatoid arthritis develop heart disease, and there are no recommendations for prevention and treatment at this time. So what is a person with rheumatoid arthritis to do?

"When studies like these come out, they should increase our awareness that we need to look beyond joint pain and stiffness in people with rheumatoid arthritis and start thinking about heart disease," says Michael Lim, MD, assistant professor of cardiology at St. Louis University. Doctors suspect that the inflammation caused by rheumatoid arthritis is the most likely culprit.

"While the exact mechanism remains unknown, there is enough anecdotal evidence to suggest that the inflammation caused by rheumatoid arthritis damages the arteries," Lim says.

In fact, doctors now can measure the level of inflammation in the body by gauging levels of an enzyme called CRP, C-reactive protein. Elevated levels of CRP are associated with increased heart disease risk in everyone, not just people with rheumatoid arthritis. CRP testing, while not used regularly as a screening tool for heart disease, has a reliable predictive power and is beginning to gain more mainstream diagnostic popularity, Lim says.

People with rheumatoid arthritis who have elevated CRP levels and borderline cholesterol levels might benefit from treatment with statins, a class of drugs that lower cholesterol and also have been shown to curb inflammation, Lim says.

Everyone who has been diagnosed with rheumatoid arthritis, regardless of age and the severity of the disease, should have a serious discussion with a primary care physician about screening and testing for heart disease even if they do not have symptoms or traditional risk factors, such as family history, high blood pressure, diabetes, and high cholesterol. Researchers found that people with rheumatoid arthritis can develop heart disease even in the absence of these factors.

"In general, people with rheumatoid arthritis develop heart disease earlier in life, so we should lower the age where we start to think about heart disease," Lim says.

The Mayo Clinic studies found that about one-third of the patients who were studied developed heart failure over a 30-year period. Heart failure is caused by weakened heart muscle, which prevents the heart from pumping blood. Symptoms include fatigue, shortness of breath, persistent cough, swelling of the legs, ankles, and abdomen due to water retention, and sudden weight gain (three or more pounds in one day, five or more pounds in one week). The risk of heart failure increases soon after the onset of rheumatoid arthritis and remains constant throughout the course of the disease, the study found. People with rheumatoid arthritis are also more likely to experience fewer symptoms, silent heart attacks, and sudden cardiac death than people without rheumatoid arthritis, researchers found.

Chapter 8

Childhood Arthritis

Chapter Contents

Section 8.1

Questions and Answers about Childhood Arthritis

Excerpted from "Questions and Answers about Juvenile Arthritis (Juvenile Idiopathic Arthritis, Juvenile Rheumatoid Arthritis, and Other Forms of Arthritis Affecting Children)," by the National Institute of Arthritis and Musculoskeletal and Skin Diseases (NIAMS, www.niams.nih.gov), part of the National Institutes of Health, September 2008.

What is juvenile arthritis?

Arthritis means joint inflammation. This term refers to a group of diseases that cause pain, swelling, stiffness, and loss of motion in the joints.

Arthritis is also used more generally to describe the more than 100 rheumatic diseases that may affect the joints but can also cause pain, swelling, and stiffness in other supporting structures of the body such as muscles, tendons, ligaments, and bones. Some rheumatic diseases can affect other parts of the body, including various internal organs. Juvenile arthritis (JA) is a term often used to describe arthritis in children. Children can develop almost all types of arthritis that affect adults, but the most common type that affects children is juvenile idiopathic arthritis.

Both juvenile idiopathic arthritis (JIA) and juvenile rheumatoid arthritis (JRA) are classification systems for chronic arthritis in children. The JRA classification system was developed about 30 years ago and had three different subtypes. More recently, pediatric rheumatologists throughout the world developed the JIA classification system, which includes more types of chronic arthritis that affect children. This classification system also provides a more accurate separation of the three JRA subtypes.

Prevalence statistics for JA vary, but according to a 2008 report from the National Arthritis Data Workgroup, about 294,000 children age 0 to 17 are affected with arthritis or other rheumatic conditions. [Note: According to the National Arthritis Data Workgroup, the actual number of new cases of JA is higher than previously reported because the statistic includes conditions not previously captured, as cited in Helmick CG, Felson DT, Lawrence RC, Gabriel S, Hirsch R, Kwoh CK, et al.; National Arthritis Data Workgroup. Estimates of the prevalence of arthritis and other rheumatic conditions in the United States. Part I. *Arthritis & Rheumatism*, 58(1):15–25, January 2008.]

What is juvenile idiopathic arthritis?

JIA is currently the most widely accepted term to describe various types of chronic arthritis in children.

In general, the symptoms of JIA include joint pain, swelling, tenderness, warmth, and stiffness that last for more than 6 continuous weeks. It is divided into seven separate subtypes, each with characteristic symptoms.

Systemic arthritis (formerly known as systemic juvenile rheumatoid arthritis): A patient has arthritis with, or preceded by, a fever that has lasted for at least 2 weeks. It must be documented as an intermittent fever, spiking for at least 3 days, and it must be accompanied by at least one or more of the following symptoms:

- Generalized enlargement of the lymph nodes

- Enlargement of the liver or spleen

- Inflammation of the lining of the heart or the lungs (pericarditis or pleuritis)

- The characteristic rheumatoid rash, which is flat, pale, pink, and generally not itchy

The individual spots of the rash are usually the size of a quarter or smaller. They are present for a few minutes to a few hours, and then disappear without any changes in the skin. The rash may move from one part of the body to another.

Oligoarthritis (formerly known as pauciarticular juvenile rheumatoid arthritis): A patient has arthritis affecting one to four joints during the first 6 months of disease. Two subcategories are recognized:

- Persistent oligoarthritis, which means the child never has more than four joints involved throughout the disease course

- Extended oligoarthritis, which means that more than four joints are involved after the first 6 months of the disease

Polyarthritis—rheumatoid factor negative (formerly known as polyarticular rheumatoid arthritis—rheumatoid factor negative): A patient has arthritis in five or more joints during the first 6 months of disease, and all tests for rheumatoid factor are negative.

Polyarthritis—rheumatoid factor positive (formerly known as polyarticular rheumatoid arthritis—rheumatoid factor positive): A patient has arthritis in five or more joints during the first 6 months of the disease. Also, at least two tests for rheumatoid factor, at least 3 months apart, are positive.

Psoriatic arthritis: Patients have both arthritis and psoriasis (a skin rash), or they have arthritis and at least two of the following symptoms:

- Inflammation and swelling of an entire finger or toe (this is called dactylitis)
- Nail pitting or splitting
- A first-degree relative with psoriasis

Enthesitis-related arthritis: The enthesis is the point at which a ligament, tendon, or joint capsule attaches to the bone. If this point becomes inflamed, it can be tender, swollen, and painful with use. The most common locations are around the knee and at the Achilles tendon on the back of the ankle. Patients are diagnosed with this JIA subtype if they have both arthritis and inflammation of an enthesitis site, or if they have either arthritis or enthesitis with at least two of the following symptoms:

- Inflammation of the sacroiliac joints (at the bottom of the back) or pain and stiffness in the lumbosacral area (in the lower back)
- A positive blood test for the human leukocyte antigen (HLA) B27 gene
- Onset of arthritis in males after age 6 years
- A first-degree relative diagnosed with ankylosing spondylitis, enthesitis-related arthritis, inflammation of the sacroiliac joint

in association with inflammatory bowel disease, Reiter syndrome, or acute inflammation of the eye

Undifferentiated arthritis: A child is said to have this subtype of JIA if the arthritis manifestations do not fulfill the criteria for one of the other six categories or if they fulfill the criteria for more than one category.

What causes juvenile arthritis?

Most forms of juvenile arthritis are autoimmune disorders, which means that the body's immune system—which normally helps to fight off bacteria or viruses—mistakenly attacks some of its own healthy cells and tissues. The result is inflammation, marked by redness, heat, pain, and swelling. Inflammation can cause joint damage. Doctors do not know why the immune system attacks healthy tissues in children who develop JA. Scientists suspect that it is a two-step process. First, something in a child's genetic makeup gives him or her a tendency to develop JA; then an environmental factor, such as a virus, triggers the development of the disease.

Not all cases of JA are autoimmune, however. Recent research has demonstrated that some people, such as many with systemic arthritis, have what is more accurately called an autoinflammatory condition. Although the two terms sound somewhat similar, the disease processes behind autoimmune and autoinflammatory disorders are different.

When the immune system is working properly, foreign invaders such as bacteria and viruses provoke the body to produce proteins called antibodies. Antibodies attach to these invaders so that they can be recognized and destroyed. In an autoimmune reaction, the antibodies attach to the body's own healthy tissues by mistake, signaling the body to attack them. Because they target the self, these proteins are called autoantibodies.

Like autoimmune disorders, autoinflammatory conditions also cause inflammation. And like autoimmune disorders, they also involve an overactive immune system. However, autoinflammation is not caused by autoantibodies. Instead, autoinflammation involves a more primitive part of the immune system that in healthy people causes white blood cells to destroy harmful substances. When this system goes awry, it causes inflammation for unknown reasons. In addition to inflammation, autoinflammatory diseases often cause fever and rashes.

What are its symptoms and signs?

The most common symptom of all types of juvenile arthritis is persistent joint swelling, pain, and stiffness that is typically worse in the morning or after a nap. The pain may limit movement of the affected joint, although many children, especially younger ones, will not complain of pain. JA commonly affects the knees and the joints in the hands and feet. One of the earliest signs of JA may be limping in the morning because of an affected knee. Besides joint symptoms, children with systemic JA have a high fever and a skin rash. The rash and fever may appear and disappear very quickly. Systemic arthritis also may cause the lymph nodes located in the neck and other parts of the body to swell. In some cases (fewer than half), internal organs including the heart and (very rarely) the lungs, may be involved.

Eye inflammation is a potentially severe complication that commonly occurs in children with oligoarthritis but can also be seen in other types of JA. All children with JA need to have regular eye exams, including a special exam called a slit lamp exam. Eye diseases such as iritis or uveitis can be present at the beginning of arthritis but often develop some time after a child first develops JA. Very commonly, JA-associated eye inflammation does not cause any symptoms and is found only by performing eye exams.

Typically, there are periods when the symptoms of JA are better or disappear (remissions) and times when symptoms flare, or get worse. JA is different in each child; some may have just one or two flares and never have symptoms again, while others experience many flares or even have symptoms that never go away.

Some children with JA have growth problems. Depending on the severity of the disease and the joints involved, bone growth at the affected joints may be too fast or too slow, causing one leg or arm to be longer than the other. Overall growth also may be slowed. Doctors are exploring the use of growth hormone to treat this problem. JA may also cause joints to grow unevenly.

How is it diagnosed?

Doctors usually suspect JA, along with several other possible conditions, when they see children with persistent joint pain or swelling, unexplained skin rashes, and fever associated with swelling of lymph nodes or inflammation of internal organs. A diagnosis of JA also is considered in children with an unexplained limp or excessive clumsiness.

No single test can be used to diagnose JA. A doctor diagnoses JA by carefully examining the patient and considering his or her medical history and the results of tests that help confirm JA or rule out other conditions. Specific findings or problems that relate to the joints are the main factors that go into making a JA diagnosis.

Symptoms: When diagnosing JA, a doctor must consider not only the symptoms a child has but also the length of time these symptoms have been present. Joint swelling or other objective changes in the joint with arthritis must be present continuously for at least 6 weeks for the doctor to establish a diagnosis of JA. Because this factor is so important, it may be useful to keep a record of the symptoms and changes in the joints, noting when they first appeared and when they are worse or better.

Family history: It is very rare for more than one member of a family to have JA. But children with a family member who has JA are at a small increased risk of developing it. Research shows that JA is also more likely in families with a history of any autoimmune disease. One study showed that families of children with JA are three times more likely to have a member with an autoimmune disease such as rheumatoid arthritis, multiple sclerosis, or thyroid inflammation (Hashimoto thyroiditis) than are families of children without JA. For that reason, having an autoimmune disease in the family may raise the doctor's suspicions that a child's joint symptoms are caused by JA or some other autoimmune disease.

Laboratory tests: Laboratory tests, usually blood tests, cannot alone provide the doctor with a clear diagnosis. But these tests can be used to help rule out other conditions and classify the type of JA that a patient has. Blood samples may be taken to test for anti-CCP antibodies, rheumatoid factor, and antinuclear antibodies, and to determine the erythrocyte sedimentation rate (ESR), described below.

- Anti-cyclic citrullinated peptide (anti-CCP) antibodies: Anti-CCP antibodies may be detected in healthy individuals years before onset of clinical rheumatoid arthritis. They may predict the eventual development of undifferentiated arthritis into rheumatoid arthritis.

- Rheumatoid factor (RF): Rheumatoid factor, an autoantibody that is produced in large amounts in adults with rheumatoid arthritis, also may be detected in children with JA, although it is rare. The RF test helps the doctor differentiate among the different types of JA.

- Antinuclear antibody (ANA): An autoantibody directed against substances in the cells' nuclei, ANA is found in some JA patients. However, the presence of ANA in children generally points to some type of connective tissue disease, helping the doctor to narrow down the diagnosis. A positive test in a child with oligoarthritis markedly increases his or her risk of developing eye disease.

- Erythrocyte sedimentation rate (ESR or sed rate): This blood test, which measures how fast red blood cells fall to the bottom of a test tube, can tell the doctor if inflammation is present. Inflammation is a hallmark of JA and a number of other conditions.

X-rays: X-rays are needed if the doctor suspects injury to the bone or unusual bone development. Early in the disease, some x-rays can show changes in soft tissue. In general, x- rays are more useful later in the disease, when bones may be affected.

Other tests: Because there are many causes of joint pain and swelling, the doctor must rule out other conditions before diagnosing JA. These include physical injury, bacterial or viral infection, Lyme disease, inflammatory bowel disease, lupus, dermatomyositis, and some forms of cancer. The doctor may use additional laboratory tests to help rule out these and other possible conditions.

Who treats it?

Treating juvenile arthritis often requires a team approach, encompassing the child and his or her family and a number of different health professionals. Ideally, the child's care should be managed by a pediatric rheumatologist: a doctor who has been specially trained to treat the rheumatic diseases in children. However, many pediatricians and "adult" rheumatologists also treat children with JA. Because there are relatively few pediatric rheumatologists and they are mainly concentrated at major medical centers in metropolitan areas, children who live in smaller towns and rural areas may benefit from having a doctor in their town coordinate care through a pediatric rheumatologist. Many large centers now conduct outreach clinics, in which doctors and a supporting team travel from large cities to smaller towns for 1 or 2 days to treat local patients.

Other members of your child's health care team may include one or more of the following health professionals:

- **Physical therapist:** This health professional can work with your child to develop a plan of exercises that will improve joint function and strengthen muscles without causing further harm to affected joints.

- **Occupational therapist:** This health professional can teach ways to protect joints, minimize pain, conserve energy, and exercise. Occupational therapists specialize in the upper extremities (hands, wrists, elbows, arms, shoulders, and neck).

- **Counselor or psychologist:** Being a child or adolescent with a chronic disease isn't easy, for the child or his or her family. Some children may benefit from sorting out their feelings with a psychologist or counselor trained to help children in this situation. Members of the child's family may benefit from counseling as well.

- **Ophthalmologist:** If your child's medications or form of arthritis can affect the eyes, catching problems early can help keep them from becoming serious. All children with JA need to have regular exams by an ophthalmologist (eye doctor) to detect eye inflammation.

- **Dentist and orthodontist:** Dental care can be difficult if a child's hands are so affected by arthritis that thorough brushing and flossing of the teeth becomes difficult. In addition, children with involvement of the jaw may have difficulty opening the mouth for proper brushing. Therefore, regular dental exams are important. Because JA can affect the alignment of the jaw, it is important for children with this disease to be evaluated by an orthodontist.

- **Orthopedic surgeon:** For some children, surgery is necessary to help minimize or repair the effects of their disease. Orthopedic surgeons are doctors who perform surgery on the joints and bones.

- **Dietitian:** For children with chronic diseases, good nutrition is particularly important. A dietitian can help design a nutritious diet that will benefit the whole family.

- **Pharmacist:** A pharmacist is a good source of information about medications, including possible side effects and drugs that have the potential to interact with one another. If a child has trouble swallowing large pills or taking other medication, the pharmacist may have suggestions for different ways to take the medication or may be able to formulate or help you get kid-friendly versions of some medications.

- **Social worker:** A social worker can help a child and his or her family deal with life and lifestyle changes caused by arthritis. A social worker also can help you identify helpful resources for your child.

- **Rheumatology nurse:** A rheumatology nurse likely will be intimately involved in a child's care, serving as the main point of contact with the doctor's office concerning appointments, tests, medications, and instructions.

- **School nurse:** For a school-age child, the school nurse also may be considered a member of the treatment team, particularly if the child is required to take medications regularly during school hours.

How is it treated?

The main goals of treatment are to preserve a high level of physical and social functioning and maintain a good quality of life. To achieve these goals, doctors recommend treatments to reduce swelling, maintain full movement in the affected joints, relieve pain, and prevent, identify, and treat complications. Most children with JA need a combination of medication and nonmedication treatments to reach these goals.

What are some treatments with medication?

Nonsteroidal anti-inflammatory drugs (NSAIDs): Aspirin, ibuprofen, naproxen, and naproxen sodium are examples of NSAIDs. They are often the first type of medication used. All NSAIDs work similarly: by blocking substances called prostaglandins that contribute to inflammation and pain. However, each NSAID is a different chemical, and each has a slightly different effect on the body.

Some NSAIDs are available over the counter, while more than a dozen others, including a subclass called COX-2 inhibitors, are available only with a prescription.

All NSAIDs can have significant side effects, so consult a doctor before taking any of these medications. For unknown reasons, some children seem to respond better to one NSAID than another. A doctor should monitor any child taking NSAIDs regularly to control JA symptoms as effectively as possible, at the optimal dose.

Disease-modifying anti-rheumatic drugs (DMARDs): If NSAIDs do not relieve symptoms of JA, the doctor is likely to prescribe this type of medication. DMARDs slow the progression of JA, but because they may take weeks or months to relieve symptoms, they often are taken with an NSAID. Although many different types of DMARDs are available, doctors are most likely to use one particular DMARD, methotrexate, for children with JA.

Researchers have learned that methotrexate is safe and effective for some children with JA whose symptoms are not relieved by other medications. Because only small doses of methotrexate are needed to relieve arthritis symptoms, potentially dangerous side effects rarely occur. The most serious complication is liver damage, but it can be avoided with regular blood screening tests and doctor followup. Careful monitoring for side effects is important for people taking methotrexate. When side effects are noticed early, the doctor can reduce the dose and eliminate the side effects.

Corticosteroids: In children with very severe JA, stronger medicines may be needed to stop serious symptoms such as inflammation of the sac around the heart (pericarditis). Corticosteroids such as prednisone may be added to the treatment plan to control severe symptoms. This medication can be given either intravenously (directly into the vein) or by mouth. Corticosteroids can interfere with a child's normal growth and can cause other side effects, such as a round face, weakened bones, and increased susceptibility to infections.

Once the medication controls severe symptoms, the doctor will reduce the dose gradually and eventually stop it completely. Because it can be dangerous to stop taking corticosteroids suddenly, it is important that the patient carefully follow the doctor's instructions about how to take or reduce the dose. For inflammation in one or just a few joints, injecting a corticosteroid compound into the affected joint or joints can often bring quick relief without the systemic side effects of oral or intravenous medication.

Biologic agents: Children with JA who have received little relief from other drugs may be given one of a newer class of drug treatments called biologic response modifiers, or biologic agents. Five such agents—etanercept, infliximab, adalimumab, abatacept, and anakinra—are

113

helpful for polyarthritis, extended oligoarthritis, and systemic arthritis. Etanercept, infliximab, and adalimumab work by blocking the actions of tumor necrosis factor (TNF), a naturally occurring protein in the body that helps cause inflammation. Anakinra works by blocking a different inflammatory protein called interleukin-1. Abatacept works by blocking the activation of certain inflammatory cells called T cells.

What are some treatments without medication?

Physical therapy: A regular, general exercise program is an important part of a child's treatment plan. It can help to maintain muscle tone and preserve and recover the range of motion of the joints. A physiatrist (rehabilitation specialist) or a physical therapist can design an appropriate exercise program for a person with JA. The specialist also may recommend using splints and other devices to help maintain normal bone and joint growth.

Complementary and alternative therapies: Many adults seek alternative ways of treating arthritis, such as special diets, supplements, acupuncture, massage, or even magnetic jewelry or mattress pads. Research shows that increasing numbers of children are using alternative and complementary therapies as well.

Although there is little research to support many alternative treatments, some people seem to benefit from them. If a child's doctor feels the approach has value and is not harmful, it can be incorporated into the treatment plan. However, it is important not to neglect regular health care or treatment of serious symptoms.

How can the family help a child live well with juvenile arthritis?

Juvenile arthritis affects the entire family, all of whom must cope with the special challenges of this disease. JA can strain a child's participation in social and after-school activities and make schoolwork more difficult. Family members can do several things to help the child physically and emotionally.

- Get the best care possible. Ensure that the child receives appropriate medical care and follows the doctor's instructions. If possible, have a pediatric rheumatologist manage your child's care. If such a specialist is not close by, consider having your child see one yearly or twice a year. A pediatric rheumatologist can devise a treatment plan and consult with your child's doctor, who will help you carry it out and monitor your child's progress.

- Learn as much as you can about your child's disease and its treatment. Many treatment options are available, and because JA is different in each child, what works for one may not work for another. If the medications that the doctor prescribes do not relieve symptoms or if they cause unpleasant side effects, you and your child should discuss other choices with the doctor. A person with JA can be more active when symptoms are controlled.

- Insist that your child take the treatment. Although it can be difficult to give your child a weekly shot or unpleasant-tasting medication, it's important that you do so—for his or her sake. If your child truly has a problem with one form of medication, speak with the doctor. He or she may be able to recommend a different medication or at least suggest ways to make taking the medication a little easier.

- Consider joining a support group. Try to find other parents and kids who face similar experiences. It can help you—and your child—to know you're not alone.

- Treat the child as normally as possible. Don't cut your child too much slack just because he or she has arthritis. Too much coddling can keep your child from being responsible and independent and can cause resentment in siblings.

- Encourage exercise and physical therapy for the child. For many young people, exercise and physical therapy play important roles in managing JA. Parents can arrange for children to participate in activities that the doctor recommends.

- During symptom-free periods, many doctors suggest playing team sports or doing other activities. The goal is to help keep the joints strong and flexible, to provide play time with other children, and to encourage appropriate social development.

- Work closely with your child's school. Help your child's school to develop a suitable lesson plan, and educate your child's teacher and classmates about JA. Some children with JA may be absent from school for prolonged periods and need to have the teacher send assignments home. Some minor changes—such as having an extra set of books or leaving class a few minutes early to get to the next class on time—can be a great help. With proper attention, most children progress normally through school.

- Talk with your child. Explain that getting JA is nobody's fault. Some children believe that JA is a punishment for something they did. Let your child know you are always available to listen, and help him or her in any way you can.

- Work with therapists or social workers. They can help you and your child adapt more easily to the lifestyle changes JA may bring.

Do these children have to limit activities?

Although pain sometimes limits physical activity, exercise is important for reducing the symptoms of juvenile arthritis and maintaining function and range of motion of the joints. Most children with JA can take part fully in physical activities and selected sports when their symptoms are under control. During a disease flare, however, the doctor may advise limiting certain activities, depending on the joints involved. Once the flare is over, the child can start regular activities again. Swimming is particularly useful because it uses many joints and muscles without putting weight on the joints. A doctor or physical therapist can recommend exercises and activities.

Section 8.2

Systemic-Onset Juvenile Rheumatoid Arthritis (Still Disease)

What is Still's disease?

Still's disease is a form of arthritis that is characterized by high spiking fevers and evanescent (transient) salmon-colored rash. Still's disease was first described in children, but it is now known to occur, much less commonly, in adults (in whom it is referred to as adult-onset Still's disease).

What causes Still's disease?

There have been a number of schools of thought. One is that Still's disease is due to infection with a microbe. Another concept is that Still's disease is a hypersensitive or autoimmune disorder. In truth, the cause of Still's disease is still not known.

How does Still's disease fit in with juvenile rheumatoid arthritis?

Still's disease is one type of juvenile rheumatoid arthritis (JRA) and is also known as systemic-onset JRA. By "systemic" it is meant that along with joint inflammation it typically begins with symptoms and signs of systemic (body wide) illness, such as high fevers, gland swelling, and internal organ involvement. Still's disease is named after the English physician Sir George F. Still (1861–1941).

What are symptoms and signs of Still's disease?

Patients with Still's disease usually present with systemic (body wide) symptoms. Extreme fatigue can accompany waves of high fevers that rise to 104 degrees F (41 degrees C) or even higher and rapidly return to normal levels or below. A faint salmon-colored skin rash characteristically comes and goes and usually does not itch (picture of the Still's rash). There is commonly swelling of the lymph glands, enlargement of the spleen and liver, and sore throat. Some patients develop inflammation of the lungs (pleuritis) or around the heart (pericarditis) with occasional fluid accumulation around the lungs (pleural effusion) or heart (pericardial effusion). Although the arthritis may initially be overlooked because of the impressive nature of the systemic symptoms, everyone with Still's disease eventually develops joint pain and swelling. This usually involves many joints (polyarticular arthritis). Any joint can be affected, although there are preferential patterns of joint involvement in Still's disease.

How is Still's disease diagnosed?

Still's disease is diagnosed purely on the basis of the typical clinical features of the illness. Persistent arthritis (arthritis lasting at least 6 weeks) is required to make a firm diagnosis of Still's disease. Other diseases (especially infections, cancers, and other types of arthritis) are excluded.

Many patients with Still's disease develop markedly elevated white blood cell counts, as if they have a serious infection but none is found. Low red blood counts (anemia) and elevated blood tests for inflammation (such as sedimentation rates) are common. However, the classic blood tests for rheumatoid arthritis (rheumatoid factor) and systemic lupus erythematosus (antinuclear antibodies, ANA) are usually negative.

What is the frequency of Still's disease and its features?

Still's disease accounts for 10–20% of all cases of JRA. It affects about 25,000–50,000 children in the United States. It is rare in adults, a majority of whom are between 20 and 35 years of age at onset of symptoms. Of all patients with Still's disease, 100% have high intermittent fever; 100% have joint inflammation and pain, muscle pain with fevers, and develop persistent chronic arthritis. Ninety-five percent (95%) have the faint salmon-colored skin rash.

Eighty-five percent (85%) have swelling of the lymph glands or enlargement of the spleen and liver; and 85% have a marked increase in the white blood cell count. Sixty percent (60%) have inflammation of the lungs (pleuritis) or around the heart (pericarditis). Forty percent

(40%) have severe anemia. And twenty percent (20%) have abdominal pain.

What research is being done on Still's disease?

Diverse types of research are ongoing related to this illness. At one of the latest meetings of the American College of Rheumatology, for example, a paper was presented which demonstrated the effectiveness of intravenous immunoglobulin therapy in adult-onset Still's disease. This was a pilot study. More studies are needed to confirm these results.

What is the outlook with Still's disease?

The fever and other systemic features tend to run their course within several months. The arthritis can be a long-term problem. It usually stays on after the systemic features have gone. The arthritis can then become chronic and persist into adulthood. There are four types of patterns that Still's Disease may take in any patient and this text will attempt to describe them here as best as it can.

How is Still's disease treated?

Still's disease can cause serious damage to the joints, particularly the wrists. It can also impair the function of the heart and lungs. Treatment of Still's disease is directed toward the individual areas of inflammation. Many symptoms are often controlled with anti-inflammatory drugs, such as aspirin or other non-steroid drugs. Cortisone medications (steroids), such as prednisone, are used to treat more severe features of illness. For patients with persistent illness, medications that affect the inflammatory aspects of the immune system are used. Medications now being used are analogous to the classic "second-line" therapies used for patients with rheumatoid arthritis. These include gold, hydroxychloroquine (Plaquenil), penicillamine, azathioprine (Imuran), methotrexate (Rheumatrex), and cyclophosphamide. There is a new class of drugs called biologics that are very promising in treating Still's. Enbrel, Remicade, Kineret, and several others are available and are being used as a first line therapy in treating Still's, meaning you don't have to take methotrexate and fail before you can move on to one of the biologics. Most of the research however shows that when methotrexate is given along with Enbrel or Remicade that the outcome is much better than with either one alone.

Patient and Family Education

Patients and their families should be provided with the necessary information to enable them to have a complete understanding of the disease and its effects on their life. Still's Disease may manifest itself mostly as joint symptoms, especially early in the course of the disease. It is essential that patients with Still's and their families understand that the disease is systemic and may involve many areas of the body.

Patients and their families should understand that the disease is often cyclic in nature, and that they should expect "good" and "bad" days. Further, they should understand that their actions on any given day can cause a "flare" or exacerbation of the disease (that is, a "bad" day). While a patient may never be able to completely stop a bad day, frequently a patient can manage her or his life to reduce the number of bad days.

Central to controlling bad days is planning activities and rest periods. Patients and their families must understand the need for planning virtually every activity of their lives. This is necessary because a patient with this disease can cause a flare by over-working or by increasing physical or emotional stress. Rest is important for the patient with Still's and cannot be overemphasized.

Planning by the patient with Still's should be done on a yearly, monthly, weekly, and daily basis. For example, if the patient is considering a vacation, the dates should be marked on a calendar well in advance so there is ample time to pack and otherwise prepare for the trip. Patients who prepare immediately before the trip may be too fatigued and sore to enjoy the trip, and may initiate a flare. Similarly, weeks should be planned so that there are rest days interspersed with work days. And even the hours of the day should be planned so that after a period of physical activity, a period of rest follows.

Planning should also incorporate changes in body position. Patients should be encouraged to change their position frequently during the course of the day. Ideally, position changes should occur at least every two hours. The patient with Still's who sits most of the day should periodically get up and walk around. The patient who stands most of the day should find some way to periodically sit and rest. It should be acknowledged by all involved that at some point changes in life style may need to be made.

There is some evidence that emotional highs and lows play a part in exacerbation of Still's. Clearly, we cannot plan for every stressful or emotional situation, but there are some instances in which we can.

For example, if the patient with Still's gets emotionally involved with sporting events, then he or she should probably avoid watching the event. If driving at night or in bad weather is stressful for the patient, plan to avoid driving at these times. As noted previously, the disease is cyclic in nature and there are good days as well as bad ones.

One problem with good days, especially in the newly diagnosed patient, is that there may be a tendency for the patient to believe he or she has been "cured" or that the physician may have incorrectly diagnosed the problem. This is why educating the patient and family is important. They must understand the cyclic nature of the disease. Patients who do not understand the disease process may quit taking medication or quit other therapy on good days because they mistakenly believe they are free of the disease. Patients who quit managing the disease are more likely to flare, which can result in further joint destruction or other systemic problems.

Finally, patient education should include a discussion about quackery. There are any number of "rip-off" artists preying on ill-informed patients. There are plenty of devices or gizmos on the market that are advertised as cures for the disease. Further, tabloids sell their issues by printing in large, bold letters purported cures that are "hidden" from the public by the medical establishment. Others claim certain diets and/or vitamin supplements are the best methods to become disease free.

Patients and families are particularly susceptible to these claims if remission of the disease occurs immediately following the use of one of the purported cures. It is the responsibility of health care providers to educate patients about quackery, and this topic should be part of any formal educational program. If patients, families, or practitioners need further information on therapeutic interventions or devices, please have them call the Arthritis Foundation.

Section 8.3

Juvenile Rheumatoid Arthritis and Vision Loss

"Juvenile Rheumatoid Arthritis Cause of Serious Vision Loss," © 2007 Missouri Arthritis Rehabilitation Research and Training Center (MARRTC). Reprinted with permission. For additional information, visit http://marrtc.missouri.edu.

Juvenile rheumatoid arthritis (JRA) causes chronic inflammation of children's joints but what many physicians and parents don't know is that it also causes chronic eye inflammation and is a leading cause of blindness in the United States.

Different parts of the eye can get inflamed and thus harm a child's eyesight. One such part is the uvea, which is the second of three layers of the eye and provides blood to the retina. Inflammation of the uvea (uveitis) is often linked to autoimmune diseases such as JRA.

A recent study by researchers at the National Eye Institute in Bethesda, Maryland, University of Illinois in Chicago, and Oregon Health Sciences University in Portland, Oregon, found a significant rate and range of vision-threatening complications among children with uveitis. They studied the records of close to 500 children with the eye inflammation. On average the children were 9 years old and 20 percent of them had the condition as a result of JRA.

"Usually within a couple of years after arthritis development the eye problems would appear," said Dr. Janine Smith, deputy clinical director at the National Eye Institute and lead author of the study.

"The really important thing about children is they don't complain about eye problems, it's asymptomatic," Smith said. "Children just go with the flow and don't say anything, even with decreased vision."

Because of that, routine eye exams are important, Smith said, and added that 6 percent of the children in the study were discovered to have eye problems with a school exam.

One clue that something may be wrong with the child's eyes is if there are white spots in the pupil, she said. Another way for a parent to check for signs of trouble is to ask the child to cover one eye and read the clock with the other. But the best way to keep eye problems at bay is through regular check-ups, Smith said.

"Remember that those kids are at risk for eye problems and have a minimum of annual eye exams," she said. "The only way you can diagnose it is with an eye exam."

The ultimate payoff of such close attention may be saving the child's vision. Smith and her colleagues found that complications from uveitis were very common and quite often hurt a child's eyesight.

At the time of the first visit to a doctor about eye problems, close to a third of children had already developed cataracts, 15 percent had swelling of the retina, and 5 percent had glaucoma. All these conditions are vision threatening. By 10 years after their first visit, 83 percent of children had developed cataracts and 25 percent had glaucoma.

The main reason for this high rate of complications is that children often go to the eye doctor too late when uveitis has already been going on for some time and the damage is already done and irreversible, Smith said.

"The critical thing is complications may have already damaged eyes despite excellent treatment and control of inflammation."

So how can a child with JRA prevent permanent vision loss? "The number one thing is early treatment," Smith said.

The role of the parents in this ongoing process is crucial. "It's really important to develop good communication with the child in a non-threatening way," Smith said.

Another important aspect of ongoing care is compliance to medication. "They [children] need to understand the disease and why medication is prescribed for uveitis," Smith said. "If your kid needs to use drops every two hours, that's very difficult but it's the parent who's in the best position to ensure that the child is getting it and it has to be worked into the daily life so it's not a big deal."

Communication between parents and children will also help children become good advocates for themselves later in life and prepare them to deal with the disease long term, she said. It will also make the child feel like a partner in the treatment, not a patient.

It is important that parents keep a journal to track the disease and the prescribed treatments and also make sure the child's different physicians talk to one another. Smith said. The study was presented at the 2006 annual meeting of the American College of Rheumatology and is yet to be published.

Section 8.4

Parenting a Child with a Chronic Illness

Parenting a chronically ill child is a challenge. Having a child with a chronic illness is stressful for any family. Parents of a chronically ill child are often faced with difficulties and decisions that other parents will never have to face. A major task for parents of a chronically ill child face is the responsibility of helping their child cope with his or her illness. Here are some suggestions.

Educate yourself about your child's illness. It is very important that parents understand their child's illness. The more parents know about their child's condition, the more they will know about how much can be expected from their child (for example, what activities, sports, and chores their child is physically able to handle). Being knowledgeable about the disorder allows parents to know which behaviors and symptoms are normal, and which are not. Having knowledge about their child's illness will also enable parents to thoroughly answer any questions their child may have about his or her illness. Parents should ask their child's health care providers for information (books, pamphlets, videos) about their child's illness. Parents can also check their local library for information. Parents should not be afraid to ask their child's physician and the other medical staff questions about the illness and treatment plan. Many parents are afraid to say they don't understand something the physician is telling them. Parents should not let this happen to them. Parents should ask questions until they understand. It is also common for parents to have questions they then forget to ask the physician. Some parents find it helpful to keep a small notebook in which they can write down questions (and answers provided by the medical staff when the questions are asked) regarding the illness and treatment plan.

Explain the illness to your child. Many parents of a chronically ill child have a difficult time deciding how much to tell their child about the illness. On one hand, they don't want to cause their child unnecessary anxiety, and on the other hand, they don't want to be misleading. It is usually best for parents to be open and honest with their child about the illness. Children are very perceptive, and they will very likely know when their parents are not being totally honest with them. This may lead to confusion and mistrust. Parents should provide information in simple language their child can understand. Young children sometimes think an illness is punishment for something they have done. Therefore, it is also important to let young children know that the illness is not their fault. Parents should make sure their child knows that they are available to answer any questions the child may have, and they should try to answer questions in an honest and straightforward manner. Parents must be careful, too, not to provide too much information. Parents can do this by gearing their explanations toward their child's level of understanding. The child's health care providers can give parents specific suggestions regarding explaining the particular illness.

Help your child deal with his or her feelings about the illness. Sometimes it's hard to predict how a child will react to the knowledge that he or she has a chronic illness. Parents should make an effort to help their chronically ill child deal with any emotional reactions he or she might have. They can do this by providing support, listening to their child, and discussing their child's feelings. Some children may resist discussing their concerns or feelings in order to protect their parents from becoming upset. It is critical that a chronically ill child feel that he or she can talk to his or her parents about any concerns or feelings without fear of being judged negatively or causing parents to become overly upset. Parents should also keep in mind that a child's thoughts and feelings about the illness may change over time. This is why it is important to keep the lines of communication open at all times.

Prepare your child for medical procedures. Children need to know what to expect in their lives. Facing unknown medical procedures can cause the chronically ill child quite a bit of anxiety. Many parents may think they are protecting their chronically ill child by not telling him or her about upcoming procedures that may be uncomfortable or painful. However, it is usually a good idea for parents or health care staff to take time to prepare children for upcoming procedures. They should explain why the procedure is being done, who will be doing it, what equipment will be used, and whether or not it will be painful or uncomfortable. Obviously, the information provided needs to be geared toward the age level of the child. Providing information often allows children to prepare themselves instead of worrying about the unknown. Most pediatric hospitals have child life specialists who help prepare children for hospitalization, surgery, and various medical procedures. Parents should request information from their health care providers regarding how they can best help prepare their child for specific procedures.

Help your child lead as normal a life as possible. Parents should try as much as possible to treat their chronically ill child like any other child. At the same time, they need to take into consideration their child's illness and any special needs that he or she may have. This can be quite a balancing act for parents. It is very important for parents to encourage participation in various activities that involve other children of the same age.

Don't be afraid to discipline. Many parents are reluctant to set limits with their chronically ill child. However, just like any other child, the chronically ill child needs discipline from his parents. Discipline provides children with structure and security, which is very reassuring to a child. Adequate discipline helps children learn to control their own behavior, too. Parents should make sure that discipline is consistent, both between parents, and from day to day with individual parents. Children need to know what to expect from their parents. Parents should also make sure that other family members and anyone else who cares for their children use consistent discipline, too. Recommended discipline techniques include praising appropriate behavior, using time-out with young children, and restricting privileges for older children.

Give your child responsibilities. Just as the chronically ill child needs discipline, he or she also needs to be given responsibilities. Parents should require that their chronically ill child do his or her share with regard to household chores. Encouraging responsibility is one way to help the chronically ill child lead as normal a life as possible. Parents must use their judgment in assigning chores that their chronically ill child is able to carry out with success. They should be consistent in their requirements, and they should be prepared to provide consequences if chores are not completed. Parents should also remember to acknowledge and offer praise for chores that have been done well.

Maintain family routines as much as possible. Parents should, as much as possible, maintain regular family routines (e.g., wake-up times, mealtimes, bedtimes, regular activities, etc.). Children typically do best when their daily routines are predictable and consistent. Of course, this is not always possible, but an effort should be made to maintain regular routines and schedules for all family members.

Take care of yourself. This may seem like a difficult task for many parents of a chronically ill child. However, it is very important for parents to take care of themselves. They must get the rest and nourishment they need in order to have the energy required to care for their child. Parents who are exhausted and stressed out often have a difficult time making good decisions regarding their child's care and are often unable to provide quality support to their child. Parents must find someone (e.g., a close friend, a clergy member, a counselor, or a support group) to whom they can talk about their concerns, anxieties, and fears. It is critical that parents look after their own physical and mental health for the benefit of their whole family. Children are very perceptive. They know when their parents are upset or worried. If parents of a chronically ill child let their worries and anxieties show, they run the risk of increasing their child's anxieties. Children follow their parents' example on how to react to difficult situations. If parents are not handling the stress well, then the chances are great that their child will also have problems coping.

Prepare your child for the reactions of others. Children with chronic illnesses often don't know how or what to tell others about their illness. Parents can help their children by suggesting various simple and concise explanations of the illness and/or management of the illness. It may help for the parent and child to role-play examples of providing explanations and answering questions others might ask. The issue of how to handle any teasing should be discussed, too. Parents can also demonstrate how to handle teasing (e.g., ignoring, giving a quick humorous response) through role-playing.

Be mindful of what your child can overhear. Parents should try to be careful about what is said within earshot of their child. They should try to avoid letting their child overhear conflicts (between family members or with medical staff) about treatment or other issues that relate to their child's illness (e.g., financial). It is important that children view their family and medical staff as a cohesive team that is competent and supportive.

Let others help. Parents should not try to do everything themselves. They should let family members and friends help. When others ask how they can help, parents should have a list of things that need to be done from which they can choose (e.g., grocery shopping, errands). Parents should have others help in a way that decreases their stress and will allow them some time to relax.

Give your child some choices. Many children with chronic illnesses tend to think they have little control over their lives. Therefore, it is important for parents to help their chronically ill child build a greater sense of control. This can be done by offering the child choices whenever possible (e.g., diet, activities). When appropriate, it can also help to have the child participate in making choices regarding treatment (e.g., what arm to get a shot in, when to do exercises, etc.).

Look for role models. Many children with chronic illnesses feel different and isolated. Being around others with the same illness often helps them in this regard. Many states offer camps for children with specific illnesses that are ideal for helping to nurture friendships between children with the same illness. Parents can ask their child's health care providers for more information about these camps. Parents should also try to contact others in their area with the same illness who are coping well (their child's health care provider may be able to offer advice regarding this subject). Children often benefit from having contact with others who have the same illness and are coping well. Such contact provides exposure to good role models and can provide hope to children who are not coping well. It can also help children to know that someone famous had the same illness they have. Parents should try to do some research and identify people who are very successful despite having the illness.

Handle advice from others appropriately. Often many well-meaning friends and extended family members offer parents advice about how to handle their child's treatment differently (e.g., they disagree with the physician's advice). The best way to handle this is for parents to thank them for their concern and then say that since they (the parents) know all the specifics of their child's medical status, they (the parents) are the ones who will make the medical decisions based on consultation with their child's health care providers.

Help your other children cope. A chronically ill child demands a lot of parental attention. It is no wonder that brothers and sisters often feel jealous, angry, and lonely. Siblings also worry about their ill brother or sister, worry about their parents, and worry that they might get the disorder, too. Therefore, it is important for parents to spend time with their other children to provide a sense of security and to help them cope. Parents should explain the illness to their other children and try to get them to ask questions and to express their concerns. Parents need to maintain open lines of communication with all of their children. It often helps children feel like a more important member of the family to help care for their sibling (when appropriate) in some limited way. Whenever possible, parents should try to schedule and spend individual time with their other children to help them feel important and loved.

Work closely with your child's school. Many chronic illnesses disrupt a child's schooling. It is important for parents to meet with teachers, the counselor, and principal to explain their child's illness and the potential impact on school (e.g., frequent absences, fatigue, activity restrictions). Parents should talk about what the other children in the class should be told about their child's illness. They should try to develop a plan to help their child keep up with schoolwork when he or she can't attend school. Parents should also talk about how special services (e.g., specialized instruction, physical therapy, etc.) can be arranged if necessary.

Hopefully the above suggestions will help your child cope effectively with his or her chronic illness. Parents who are concerned that their child is having significant problems coping should discuss these concerns with their child's health care provider. If necessary, they should request a referral to a mental health professional with experience working with children with the same illness.

Chapter 9

Ankylosing Spondylitis

Genetic Conditions: Ankylosing Spondylitis

What is ankylosing spondylitis?

Ankylosing spondylitis is a form of ongoing joint inflammation (chronic inflammatory arthritis) that primarily affects the spine. This condition is characterized by back pain and stiffness that typically appear in adolescence or early adulthood. Over time, back movement gradually becomes limited as the bones of the spine (vertebrae) fuse together. This progressive bony fusion is called ankylosis.

The earliest symptoms of ankylosing spondylitis result from inflammation of the joints between the pelvic bones (the ilia) and the base of the spine (the sacrum). These joints are called sacroiliac joints, and inflammation of these joints is known as sacroiliitis. The inflammation gradually spreads to the joints between the vertebrae, causing a condition called spondylitis. Ankylosing spondylitis can involve other joints as well, including the shoulders, hips, and, less often, the knees. As the disease progresses, it can affect the joints between the spine and ribs, restricting movement of the chest and making it difficult to

---

This chapter includes text from "Genetic Conditions: Ankylosing Spondylitis," part of the Genetics Home Reference (ghr.nlm.nih.gov), by the National Library of Medicine, February 2009, and "Ankylosing Spondylitis Genes Found," by the National Institute of Arthritis and Musculoskeletal and Skin Diseases (NIAMS, www.niams.nih.gov), part of the National Institutes of Health, March 2008.

breathe deeply. People with advanced disease are also more prone to fractures of the vertebrae.

Ankylosing spondylitis affects the eyes in up to 40 percent of cases, leading to episodes of eye inflammation called acute iritis. Acute iritis causes eye pain and increased sensitivity to light (photophobia). Rarely, ankylosing spondylitis can also cause serious complications involving the heart, lungs, and nervous system.

How common is ankylosing spondylitis?

Ankylosing spondylitis is part of a group of related diseases known as spondyloarthropathies. In the United States, spondyloarthropathies affect 3.5 to 13 per 1,000 people.

What genes are related to ankylosing spondylitis?

Ankylosing spondylitis is likely caused by a combination of genetic and environmental factors, most of which have not been identified. However, researchers have found variations in several genes that influence the risk of developing this disorder.

The HLA-B gene provides instructions for making a protein that plays an important role in the immune system. HLA-B is part of a family of genes called the human leukocyte antigen (HLA) complex. The HLA complex helps the immune system distinguish the body's own proteins from proteins made by foreign invaders (such as viruses and bacteria). The HLA-B gene has many different normal variations, allowing each person's immune system to react to a wide range of foreign proteins. A variation of the HLA-B gene called HLA-B27 increases the risk of developing ankylosing spondylitis.

Although many people with ankylosing spondylitis have the HLA-B27 variation, most people with this version of the HLA-B gene never develop the disorder. It is not known how HLA-B27 increases the risk of developing ankylosing spondylitis.

Variations in several additional genes, including ERAP1, IL1A, and IL23R, have also been associated with ankylosing spondylitis. Although these genes play critical roles in the immune system, it is unclear how variations in these genes affect a person's risk of developing ankylosing spondylitis. Other genes, which have not yet been identified, are also believed to affect the chances of developing ankylosing spondylitis and influence the progression of the disorder. Some of these genes likely play a role in the immune system, while others may have different functions.

Researchers are working to identify these genes and clarify their role in ankylosing spondylitis.

How do people inherit ankylosing spondylitis?

Although ankylosing spondylitis can occur in more than one person in a family, it is not a purely genetic disease. Multiple genetic and environmental factors likely play a part in determining the risk of developing this disorder. As a result, inheriting a genetic variation linked with ankylosing spondylitis does not mean that a person will develop the condition, even in families in which more than one family member has the disorder. For example, about 80 percent of children who inherit HLA-B27 from a parent with ankylosing spondylitis do not develop the disorder.

Ankylosing Spondylitis Genes Found

Work supported by the National Institute of Arthritis and Musculoskeletal Skin Diseases has led to the discovery of two genes responsible for ankylosing spondylitis (AS), an inflammatory and potentially disabling disease of the spine.

The discovery of the two genes—ARTS1 and IL23R—brings the scientific community closer to fully understanding AS, says John D. Reveille, MD, professor and director of the Division of Rheumatology and Clinical Immunogenetics at the University of Texas (UT) Medical School at Houston, who led the study with Matthew A. Brown, MD, professor of immunogenetics at Australia's University of Queensland.

In earlier studies of identical twins, Dr. Brown and his colleagues found that the cause of ankylosing spondylitis is more than 90 percent genetic. With the discovery of the newly identified genes, a large proportion of the genetic risk for AS has now been identified.

The IL23R gene, says Dr. Brown, plays a role in the immune system's response to infection. ARTS1 is involved in processing infectious agents into "bite-size chunks" that can be seen—and fought—by the body's immune system.

The recent discovery is based on work from the largest and most comprehensive genome-wide association scan conducted to date. In this part of the research project, investigators were searching for genetic information related to AS, as well as autoimmune thyroid disease/Graves' disease, breast cancer, and multiple sclerosis.

"This discovery, to me, is the most important since 1973, when HLA-B27 was discovered," says Reveille colleague Frank C. Arnett,

MD, professor of internal medicine and pathology and laboratory medicine at the UT Medical School. HLA-B27 is a powerful predisposing gene that increases the risk of getting AS by more than 100 times.

Dr. Arnett says the location of the genes and the fact they don't coincide with those of autoimmune diseases, such as rheumatoid arthritis, lupus, or juvenile diabetes, helps refute the long-held notion that AS is an autoimmune disease. "It is looking more like AS is not an autoimmune disease, but really an unusual response to infection. These genes working together probably impair the immune system's ability to rid the body of some of these bacteria or their products."

He also believes this discovery could eventually lead to ways to immunize people against AS. "I think these give us the genetic handles to identify the pathways that are involved in AS. Once you know the dysregulated pathway, you can find a drug to either strengthen or inhibit the pathway."

In the meantime, Dr. Reveille says the two genes, along with HLA-B27, could also help physicians identify patients who are at the highest risk for developing AS. "For example, if you have a family member with AS, a simple blood test would be able to tell us if you are also at risk," he says. "We could offer screenings for people with inflammatory back pain. In the past, [testing for the HLA-B27 gene] was all we had. Now we potentially have more tests."

"This is a success story for genetics work," says Dr. Reveille. "I think it will lead the way for other work to be done."

AS is a chronic inflammatory arthritis characterized by joint stiffness, pain, and extra bone growth that can result in partial or complete fusion of the spine. It typically strikes adolescent and young adult males. Currently there is no cure for the disease.

Chapter 10

Behçet Disease

What is Behçet disease?

The disease was first described in 1937 by Dr. Hulusi Behçet, a dermatologist in Turkcy. Behçet disease is now recognized as a chronic condition that causes canker sores or ulcers in the mouth and on the genitals and inflammation in parts of the eye. In some people, the disease also results in arthritis (swollen, painful, stiff joints), skin problems, and inflammation of the digestive tract, brain, and spinal cord.

Who gets Behçet disease?

Behçet disease is common in the Middle East, Asia, and Japan; it is rare in the United States. In Middle Eastern and Asian countries, the disease affects more men than women. In the United States, the opposite is true. Behçet disease tends to develop in people in their twenties or thirties, but people of all ages can develop this disease.

What causes Behçet disease?

The exact cause of Behçet disease is unknown. Most symptoms of the disease are caused by inflammation of the blood vessels. Inflammation

From "Questions and Answers about Behçet Disease," by the National Institute of Arthritis and Musculoskeletal and Skin Diseases (NIAMS, www.niams.nih.gov), part of the National Institutes of Health, April 2009.

is a characteristic reaction of the body to injury or disease and is marked by four signs: swelling, redness, heat, and pain. Doctors think that an autoimmune reaction may cause the blood vessels to become inflamed, but they do not know what triggers this reaction. Under normal conditions, the immune system protects the body from diseases and infections by killing harmful "foreign" substances, such as germs, that enter the body. In an autoimmune reaction, the immune system mistakenly attacks and harms the body's own tissues.

Behçet disease is not contagious; it is not spread from one person to another. Researchers think that two factors are important for a person to get Behçet disease. First, it is believed that abnormalities of the immune system make some people susceptible to the disease. Scientists think that this susceptibility may be inherited; that is, it may be due to one or more specific genes. Second, something in the environment, possibly a bacterium or virus, might trigger or activate the disease in susceptible people.

What are the symptoms of Behçet disease?

Behçet disease affects each person differently. Some people have only mild symptoms, such as canker sores or ulcers in the mouth or on the genitals. Others have more severe signs, such as meningitis, which is an inflammation of the membranes that cover the brain and spinal cord. Meningitis can cause fever, a stiff neck, and headaches. More severe symptoms usually appear months or years after a person notices the first signs of Behçet disease. Symptoms can last for a long time or may come and go in a few weeks. Typically, symptoms appear, disappear, and then reappear. The times when a person is having symptoms are called flares. Different symptoms may occur with each flare; the problems of the disease often do not occur together. To help the doctor diagnose Behçet disease and monitor its course, patients may want to keep a record of which symptoms occur and when. Because many conditions mimic Behçet disease, doctors must observe the lesions (injuries) caused by the disorder to make an accurate diagnosis.

The five most common symptoms of Behçet disease are mouth sores, genital sores, other skin lesions, inflammation of parts of the eye, and arthritis.

- **Mouth sores** (known as oral aphthosis and aphthous stomatitis affect almost all patients with Behçet disease. Individual sores or ulcers are usually identical to canker sores, which are common in many people. They are often the first symptom that a person notices and may occur long before any other symptoms appear. The sores usually have a red border and several may appear at the same time. They may be painful and can make eating difficult. Mouth sores go away in 10 to 14 days but often come back. Small sores usually heal without scarring, but larger sores may scar.

- **Genital sores** affect more than half of all people with Behçet disease and most commonly appear on the scrotum in men and vulva in women. The sores look similar to the mouth sores and may be painful. After several outbreaks, they may cause scarring.

- **Skin problems** are a common symptom of Behçet disease. Skin sores often look red or resemble pus-filled bumps or a bruise. The sores are red and raised, and typically appear on the legs and on the upper torso. In some people, sores or lesions may appear when the skin is scratched or pricked. When doctors suspect that a person has Behçet disease, they may perform a pathergy test, in which they prick the skin with a small needle; 1 to 2 days after the test, people with Behçet disease may develop a red bump where the doctor pricked the skin. However, only half of the Behçet patients in Middle Eastern countries and Japan have this reaction. It is less commonly observed in patients from the United States, but if this reaction occurs, then Behçet disease is likely.

- **Uveitis** involves inflammation of the middle or back part of the eye (the uvea) including the iris, and occurs in more than half of all people with Behçet disease. This symptom is more common among men than women and typically begins within 2 years of the first symptoms. Eye inflammation can cause blurred vision; rarely, it causes pain and redness. Because partial loss of vision or blindness can result if the eye frequently becomes inflamed, patients should report these symptoms to their doctor immediately.

- **Arthritis**, which is inflammation of the joints, occurs in more than half of all patients with Behçet disease. Arthritis causes pain, swelling, and stiffness in the joints, especially in the knees, ankles, wrists, and elbows. Arthritis that results from Behçet disease usually lasts a few weeks and does not cause permanent damage to the joints.

In addition to mouth and genital sores, other skin lesions, eye inflammation, and arthritis, Behçet disease may also cause blood clots and inflammation in the central nervous system and digestive organs.

Blood clots: About 16 percent of patients with Behçet disease have blood clots resulting from inflammation in the veins (thrombophlebitis), usually in the legs. Symptoms include pain and tenderness in the affected area. The area may also be swollen and warm. Because thrombophlebitis can have severe complications, people should report symptoms to their doctor immediately. A few patients may experience artery problems such as aneurysms (balloon-like swelling of the artery wall).

Central nervous system: Behçet disease affects the central nervous system in about 23 percent of all patients with the disease in the United States. The central nervous system includes the brain and spinal cord. Its function is to process information and coordinate thinking, behavior, sensation, and movement. Behçet disease can cause inflammation of the brain and the thin membrane that covers and protects the brain and spinal cord. This condition is called meningoencephalitis. People with meningoencephalitis may have fever, headache, stiff neck, and difficulty coordinating movement, and should report any of these symptoms to their doctor immediately. If this condition is left untreated, a stroke (blockage or rupture of blood vessels in the brain) can result.

Digestive tract: Rarely, Behçet disease causes inflammation and ulceration (sores) throughout the digestive tract that are identical to the aphthous lesions in the mouth and genital area.

This leads to abdominal pain, diarrhea, and/or bleeding. Because these symptoms are very similar to symptoms of other diseases of the digestive tract, such as ulcerative colitis and Crohn disease, careful evaluation is essential to rule out these other diseases.

How is Behçet disease diagnosed?

Diagnosing Behçet disease is very difficult because no specific test confirms it. Less than half of patients initially thought to have Behçet disease actually have it. When a patient reports symptoms, the doctor must examine the patient and rule out other conditions with similar symptoms. Because it may take several months or even years for all the common symptoms to appear, the diagnosis may not be made for a long time. A patient may even visit several different kinds of doctors before the diagnosis is made.

These symptoms are key to a diagnosis of Behçet disease:

- Mouth sores at least three times in 12 months

- Any two of the following symptoms: Recurring genital sores, eye inflammation with loss of vision, characteristic skin lesions, or positive pathergy (skin prick test)

Besides finding these signs, the doctor must rule out other conditions with similar symptoms, such as Crohn disease and reactive arthritis. The doctor also may recommend that the patient see an eye specialist to identify possible complications related to eye inflammation. A dermatologist may perform a biopsy of mouth, genital, or skin lesions to help distinguish Behçet from other disorders.

What kind of doctor treats a patient with Behçet disease?

Because the disease affects different parts of the body, a patient probably will see several different doctors. It may be helpful to both the doctors and the patient for one doctor to manage the complete treatment plan. This doctor can coordinate the treatments and monitor any side effects from the various medications that the patient takes.

A rheumatologist (a doctor specializing in arthritis and other inflammatory disorders) often manages a patient's treatment and treats joint disease. The following specialists also treat other symptoms that affect the different body systems:

- Gynecologist—Treats genital sores in women

- Urologist—Treats genital sores in men and women

- Dermatologist—Treats genital sores in men and women and skin and mucous membrane problems

- Ophthalmologist—Treats eye inflammation

- Gastroenterologist—Treats digestive tract symptoms

- Hematologist—Treats disorders of the blood

- Neurologist—Treats central nervous system symptoms

How is Behçet disease treated?

Although there is no cure for Behçet disease, people usually can control symptoms with proper medication, rest, exercise, and a healthy lifestyle. The goal of treatment is to reduce discomfort and prevent serious complications such as disability from arthritis or blindness. The type of medicine and the length of treatment depend on the person's symptoms and their severity. It is likely that a combination of treatments will be needed to relieve specific symptoms. Patients should tell each of their doctors about all of the medicines they are taking so that the doctors can coordinate treatment.

Topical medicine: Topical medicine is applied directly on the sores to relieve pain and discomfort. For example, doctors prescribe rinses, gels, or ointments. Creams are used to treat skin and genital sores. The medicine usually contains corticosteroids (which reduce inflammation), other anti-inflammatory drugs, or an anesthetic, which relieves pain.

Oral medicine: Doctors also prescribe medicines taken by mouth to reduce inflammation throughout the body, suppress the overactive immune system, and relieve symptoms. Doctors may prescribe one or more of the medicines described below to treat the various symptoms of Behçet disease.

- **Corticosteroids:** Prednisone is a corticosteroid prescribed to reduce pain and inflammation throughout the body for people with severe joint pain, skin sores, eye disease, or central nervous system symptoms. Patients must carefully follow the doctor's instructions about when to take prednisone and how much to take. It also is important not to stop taking the medicine suddenly, because the medicine alters the body's production of the natural corticosteroid hormones. Long-term use of prednisone can have side effects such as osteoporosis (a disease that leads to bone fragility), weight gain, delayed wound healing, persistent heartburn, and elevated blood pressure. However, these side effects are rare when prednisone is taken at low doses for a short time. It is important that patients see their doctor regularly to monitor possible side effects. Corticosteroids are useful in early stages of disease and for acute severe flares. They are of limited use for long-term management of central nervous system and serious eye complications.

- **Immunosuppressive drugs:** These medicines (in addition to corticosteroids) help control an overactive immune system, which occurs in Behçet disease, and reduce inflammation throughout the body and lessen the number of disease flares. Doctors may use immunosuppressive drugs when a person has eye disease or central nervous system involvement. These medicines

140

are very strong and can have serious side effects. Patients must see their doctor regularly for blood tests to detect and monitor side effects. Doctors may use one or more of the following immunosuppressive drugs depending on the person's specific symptoms.

- **Azathioprine:** Most commonly prescribed for people with organ transplants because it suppresses the immune system, azathioprine is now used for people with Behçet disease to treat uveitis and other uncontrolled disease manifestations. This medicine can upset the stomach and may reduce production of new blood cells by the bone marrow.

- **Chlorambucil or cyclophosphamide:** Doctors may use these drugs to treat uveitis and meningoencephalitis. People taking either agent must see their doctor frequently because either can have serious side effects, such as permanent sterility and cancers of the blood. Patients have regular blood tests to monitor blood counts of white cells and platelets.

- **Cyclosporine:** Like azathioprine, doctors prescribe this medicine for people with organ transplants. When used by patients with Behçet disease, cyclosporine reduces uveitis and uncontrolled disease in other organs. To reduce the risk of side effects, such as kidney and liver disease, the doctor can adjust the dose. Patients must tell their doctor if they take any other medicines, because some medicines affect the way the body uses cyclosporine.

- **Colchicine:** Commonly used to treat gout, which is a form of arthritis, colchicine reduces inflammation throughout the body. The medicine sometimes is used to treat arthritis, mucous membrane, and skin symptoms in patients with Behçet disease. A research study in Turkey suggested that the medication works best for males with the disorder. Common side effects of colchicine include nausea, vomiting, and diarrhea. The doctor can decrease the dose to relieve these side effects.

- **Combination treatment:** Cyclosporine is sometimes used with azathioprine when one alone fails. Prednisone along with an immunosuppressive drug is a common combination.

If these medicines do not reduce the symptoms, doctors may use other drugs such as methotrexate. Methotrexate (Rheumatrex, Trexall), which is also used to treat various kinds of cancers as well as rheumatoid arthritis, can relieve Behçet symptoms because it suppresses the immune system and reduces inflammation throughout the body.

Rest and exercise: Although rest is important during flares, doctors usually recommend moderate exercise, such as swimming or walking, when the symptoms have improved or disappeared. Exercise can help people with Behçet disease keep their joints strong and flexible.

What is the prognosis for a person with Behçet disease?

Most people with Behçet disease can lead productive lives and control symptoms with proper medicine, rest, and exercise. Doctors can use many medicines to relieve pain, treat symptoms, and prevent complications. When treatment is effective, flares usually become less frequent. Many patients eventually enter a period of remission (a disappearance of symptoms). In some people, treatment does not relieve symptoms, and gradually more serious symptoms such as eye disease may occur. Serious symptoms may appear months or years after the first signs of Behçet disease.

What are researchers trying to learn about Behçet disease?

Researchers are exploring possible genetic, bacterial, and viral causes of Behçet disease as well as improved drug treatment. For example, genetic studies show strong association of the gene HLA-B51 with the disease, but the exact role of this gene in the development of Behçet is uncertain. Researchers hope to identify genes that increase a person's risk for developing Behçet disease. Studies of these genes and how they work may provide new understanding of the disease and possibly new treatments.

Researchers are also investigating factors in the environment, such as bacteria or viruses, which may trigger Behçet disease. They are particularly interested in whether *Streptococcus*, the bacterium that causes strep throat, is associated with Behçet disease. Many people with Behçet disease have had several strep infections. In addition, researchers suspect that herpesvirus type 1, a virus that causes cold sores, may be associated with Behçet disease.

Finally, researchers are identifying other medicines to better treat Behçet disease. TNF inhibitors are a class of drugs that reduce joint inflammation by blocking the action of a substance called tumor necrosis factor (TNF). Although serious side effects have been reported for TNF inhibitors, they have shown some promise in treating Behçet disease. Examples of TNF inhibitors include etanercept and infliximab. TNF inhibitors belong to a family of drugs called biologics, which target the immune response. Also, interferon alpha, a protein that helps fight infection, has shown promise in treating Behçet disease. Thalidomide, which is believed to be a TNF inhibitor, appears effective in treating severe mouth sores, but its use is experimental and side effects are a concern. Thalidomide is not used to treat women of childbearing age because it causes severe birth defects.

Chapter 11

Bone Spurs, Bursitis, and Tendonitis

Chapter Contents

Section 11.1

Bone Spurs Can Cause Foot Pain

"Foot pain," © 2009 A.D.A.M., Inc. Reprinted with permission.

Definition

Pain or discomfort can be felt anywhere in the foot, including the heel, toes, arch, instep, sole, or ankles.

Causes

Foot pain can be caused by:

- bunions: A protrusion at the base of the big toe, which can become inflamed. Bunions often develop over time from wearing narrow-toed shoes.

- hammer toes: Toes that curl downward into a claw-like position.

- calluses and corns: Thickened skin from friction or pressure. Calluses are on the balls of the feet or heels. Corns appear on your toes.

- plantar warts: From pressure on the soles of your feet.

- fallen arches: Also called flat feet.

Poorly fitting shoes often cause these problems. Aging and being overweight also increase your chances of having foot problems.

Morton neuroma is a type of foot pain that is usually centered between the third and fourth toes. It results from thickening and swelling of tissue around a nerve in the area. Symptoms include tingling and sharp, shooting, or burning pains in the ball of your foot (and sometimes toes), especially when wearing shoes or pressing on the area. Pain gradually gets worse over time. Morton neuroma is more common in women than men.

Other common causes of foot pain include:

- broken bones;

- stress fracture;
- arthritis;
- gout—Common in the big toe, which becomes red, swollen, and very tender;
- plantar fasciitis;
- bone spur;
- sprains;
- bursitis of the heel;
- tendonitis.

Home Care

- Apply ice to reduce pain and swelling. Do this just after an activity that aggravates your pain.
- Elevate your painful foot as much as possible.
- Reduce activity until the problem improves.
- Wear foot pads in areas of friction or pressure. This will prevent rubbing and irritation.
- Take over-the-counter pain medicine, like ibuprofen or acetaminophen. Try this for 2 to 3 weeks (unless you have a history of an ulcer, liver disease, or other condition that does not allow you to take one of these drugs).

For plantar warts, try an over-the-counter wart removal preparation.

For calluses, soak in warm water and then rub them down with a pumice stone. Do not cut or burn corns or calluses.

For foot pain caused by a stress fracture, an extended rest period is often necessary. Crutches may be used for a week or so to take the pressure off, if your foot is particularly painful.

For foot pain due to plantar fasciitis, shoe inserts and stretches may help.

When to Contact a Medical Professional

Call your doctor if:

- You have sudden, severe pain.

- Your pain began following an injury—especially if there is bleeding, bruising, deformity, or you cannot bear weight.

- You have redness or swelling of the joint, an open sore or ulcer on your foot, or a fever.

- You have new foot pain and have been diagnosed with diabetes or peripheral vascular disease (a condition characterized by poor circulation).

- You do not respond to self-care within 1 to 2 weeks.

What to Expect at Your Office Visit

Your doctor will perform a physical examination, paying particular attention to your feet, legs, and back, and your stance, posture, and gait.

To help diagnose the cause of the problem, your doctor will ask medical history questions, such as:

- Are both of your feet affected? If only one, which one?

- Exactly what part of your foot is affected?

- Does the pain move from joint to joint or does it always occur in the same location?

- Did your pain begin suddenly and severely or slowly and mildly, gradually getting worse?

- How long have you had the pain?

- Is it worse at night or when you first wake up in the morning?

- Is it getting better?

- Does anything make your pain feel better or worse?

- Do you have any other symptoms?

X-rays may be useful in making a diagnosis.

For bunions, plantar fasciitis, bone spurs, Morton neuroma, or other conditions, your doctor may inject cortisone. This will be considered if oral medication, changing your shoes, and other measures have not helped. No more than three injections in a year should be attempted in most cases.

A broken foot will be casted. Broken toes will be taped. Orthotics fit by an orthotist or other specialist can help many structurally related problems. Physical therapy is also quite helpful for conditions related to overuse or tight muscles, such as plantar fasciitis or Achilles tendonitis.

Removal of plantar warts, corns, or calluses may be necessary. This may be performed by a medical doctor or a podiatrist.

Surgery may be considered for certain conditions like bunions or hammer toes if the pain interferes with walking or other activities.

Prevention

The following steps can prevent foot problems and foot pain:

- Wear comfortable, properly fitting shoes. They should have good arch support and cushioning.

- Wear shoes with adequate room around the ball of your foot and toe.

- Wear sneakers as often as possible, especially when walking.

- Avoid narrow-toed shoes and high heels.

- Replace running shoes frequently.

- Warm up before exercise, cool down after exercise, and stretch adequately.

- Increase your amount of exercise slowly over time to avoid putting excessive strain on your feet.

- Lose weight if you need to.

- Learn exercises to strengthen your feet and avoid pain. This can help flat feet and other potential foot problems.

- Keep feet dry to avoid friction. This may help prevent corns and calluses.

- Avoid alcohol to prevent attacks of gout.

Section 11.2

Bursitis and Tendonitis

Excerpted from "Questions and Answers About Bursitis and Tendonitis," by the National Institute of Arthritis and Musculoskeletal and Skin Diseases (NIAMS, www.niams.nih.gov), part of the National Institutes of Health, April 2007.

What is bursitis and what is tendonitis?

Bursitis and tendonitis are both common conditions that involve inflammation of the soft tissue around muscles and bones, most often in the shoulder, elbow, wrist, hip, knee, or ankle.

A bursa is a small, fluid-filled sac that acts as a cushion between a bone and other moving parts: muscles, tendons, or skin. Bursae are found throughout the body. Bursitis occurs when a bursa becomes inflamed (redness and increased fluid in the bursa).

A tendon is a flexible band of fibrous tissue that connects muscles to bones. Tendonitis is inflammation of a tendon. Tendons transmit the pull of the muscle to the bone to cause movement. They are found throughout the body, including the hands, wrists, elbows, shoulders, hips, knees, ankles, and feet. Tendons can be small, like those found in the hand, or large, like the Achilles tendon in the heel.

What causes these conditions?

Bursitis is commonly caused by overuse or direct trauma to a joint. Bursitis may occur at the knee or elbow; for example, from kneeling or leaning on the elbows longer than usual on a hard surface. Tendonitis is most often the result of a repetitive injury in the affected area. These conditions occur more often with age. Tendons become less flexible with age, and therefore, more prone to injury.

People such as carpenters, gardeners, musicians, and athletes who perform activities that require repetitive motions or place stress on joints are at higher risk for tendonitis and bursitis.

An infection, arthritis, gout, thyroid disease, and diabetes can also bring about inflammation of a bursa or tendon.

What parts of the body are affected?

Tendonitis causes pain and tenderness just outside a joint. Some common names for tendonitis identify with the sport or movement that typically increases risk for tendon inflammation. They include tennis elbow, golfer's elbow, pitcher's shoulder, swimmer's shoulder, and jumper's knee. Some common examples follow.

Tennis elbow and golfer's elbow: Tennis elbow refers to an injury to the outer elbow tendon. Golfer's elbow is an injury to the inner tendon of the elbow. These conditions can also occur with any activity that involves repetitive wrist turning or hand gripping, such as tool use, hand shaking, or twisting movements. Carpenters, gardeners, painters, musicians, manicurists, and dentists are at higher risk for these forms of tendonitis. Pain occurs near the elbow, sometimes radiating into the upper arm or down to the forearm. Another name for tennis elbow is lateral epicondylitis. Golfer's elbow is also called medial epicondylitis.

Shoulder tendonitis, bursitis, and impingement syndrome: Two types of tendonitis can affect the shoulder. Biceps tendonitis causes pain in the front or side of the shoulder and may travel down to the elbow and forearm. Pain may also occur when the arm is raised overhead. The biceps muscle, in the front of the upper arm, helps stabilize the upper arm bone (humerus) in the shoulder socket. It also helps accelerate and decelerate the arm during overhead movement in activities like tennis or pitching.

Rotator cuff tendonitis causes shoulder pain at the tip of the shoulder and the upper, outer arm. The pain can be aggravated by reaching, pushing, pulling, lifting, raising the arm above shoulder level, or lying on the affected side. The rotator cuff is primarily a group of four muscles that attach the arm to the shoulder girdle/shoulder blade. The rotator cuff attaches the arm to the shoulder joint and allows the arm to rotate and elevate. If the rotator cuff and bursa are irritated, inflamed, and swollen, they may become compressed between the head of the humerus and the acromion, the outer edge of the shoulder blade. Repeated motion involving the arms, or the aging process involving shoulder motion over many years, may also irritate and wear down the tendons, muscles, and surrounding structures. Squeezing of the rotator cuff is called shoulder impingement syndrome.

Inflammation caused by rheumatoid arthritis may cause rotator cuff tendonitis and bursitis. Sports involving overuse of the shoulder and occupations requiring frequent overhead reaching are other potential causes of irritation to the rotator cuff or bursa, and may lead to inflammation and impingement.

Knee tendonitis or jumper's knee: If a person overuses a tendon during activities such as dancing, cycling, or running, it may elongate or undergo microscopic tears and become inflamed. Trying to break a fall may also cause the quadriceps muscles to contract and tear the quadriceps tendon above the knee cap (patella) or the patellar tendon below it. This type of injury is most likely to happen in older people whose tendons tend to be weaker and less flexible. Tendonitis of the patellar tendon is sometimes called jumper's knee because in sports that require jumping, such as basketball, the muscle contraction and force of hitting the ground after a jump strain the tendon. After repeated stress, the tendon may become inflamed or tear.

People with tendonitis of the knee may feel pain during running, hurried walking, or jumping. Knee tendonitis can increase risk for ruptures or large tears to the tendon. A complete rupture of the quadriceps or patellar tendon is not only painful, but also makes it difficult for a person to bend, extend, or lift the leg; or to bear weight on the involved leg.

Achilles tendonitis: Achilles tendon injuries involve an irritation, stretch, or tear to the tendon connecting the calf muscle to the back of the heel. Achilles tendonitis is a common overuse injury, but can also be caused by tight or weak calf muscles or any condition that causes the tendon to become less flexible and more rigid, such as reactive arthritis or normal aging.

Achilles tendon injuries can happen to anyone who regularly participates in an activity that causes the calf muscle to contract, like climbing stairs or using a stair-stepper, but are most common in middle-aged "weekend warriors" who may not exercise regularly or take time to warm up and stretch properly before an activity. Among professional athletes, most Achilles injuries seem to occur in quick-acceleration or jumping sports like football, tennis, and basketball, and almost always end the season's competition for the athlete.

Achilles tendonitis can be a chronic condition. It can also cause what appears to be a sudden injury. Tendonitis is the most common factor contributing to Achilles tendon tears. When a tendon is weakened by age or overuse, trauma can cause it to rupture. These injuries can be so sudden and agonizing that they have been known to bring down charging professional football players in shocking fashion.

How are these conditions diagnosed?

Diagnosis of tendonitis and bursitis begins with a medical history and physical examination. The patient will describe the pain and circumstances in which pain occurs. The location and onset of pain, whether it varies in severity throughout the day, and the factors that relieve or aggravate the pain are all important diagnostic clues. Therapists and physicians will use manual tests called selective tissue tension tests to determine which tendon is involved, and then will palpate (a form of touching the tendon) specific areas of the tendon to pinpoint the area of inflammation. X-rays do not show tendons or bursae, but may be helpful in ruling out problems in the bone or arthritis. In the case of a torn tendon, x-rays may help show which tendon is affected. In a knee injury, for example, an x-ray will show that the patella is lower than normal in a quadriceps tendon tear and higher than normal in a patellar tendon tear. The doctor may also use magnetic resonance imaging (MRI) to confirm a partial or total tear. MRIs detect both bone and soft tissues like muscles, tendons and their coverings (sheaths), and bursae.

An anesthetic-injection test is another way to confirm a diagnosis of tendonitis. A small amount of anesthetic (lidocaine hydrochloride) is injected into the affected area. If the pain is temporarily relieved, the diagnosis is confirmed.

To rule out infection, the doctor may remove and test fluid from the inflamed area.

What kind of health care professional treats these conditions?

A primary care physician or a physical therapist can treat the common causes of tendonitis and bursitis. Complicated cases or those resistant to conservative therapies may require referral to a specialist, such as an orthopaedist or rheumatologist.

How are bursitis and tendonitis treated?

Treatment focuses on healing the injured bursa or tendon. The first step in treating both of these conditions is to reduce pain and inflammation with rest, compression, elevation, and anti-inflammatory medicines such as aspirin, naproxen (Naprosyn, Aleve), or ibuprofen (Advil, Motrin, or Nuprin). Ice may also be used in acute injuries, but most cases of bursitis or tendonitis are considered chronic, and ice is not helpful. When ice is needed, an ice pack can be applied to the affected

153

area for 15–20 minutes every 4–6 hours for 3–5 days. Longer use of ice and a stretching program may be recommended by a health care provider.

Activity involving the affected joint is also restricted to encourage healing and prevent further injury.

In some cases (e.g., in tennis elbow), elbow bands may be used to compress the forearm muscle to provide some pain relief, limiting the pull of the tendon on the bone. Other protective devices, such as foot orthoses for the ankle and foot or splints for the knee or hand, may temporarily reduce stress to the affected tendon or bursa and facilitate quicker healing times, while allowing general activity levels to continue as usual.

The doctor or therapist may use ultrasound (gentle sound-wave vibrations) to warm deep tissues and improve blood flow. Iontophoresis may also be used. This involves using an electrical current to push a corticosteroid medication through the skin directly over the inflamed bursa or tendon. Gentle stretching and strengthening exercises are added gradually. Massage of the soft tissue may be helpful. These may be preceded or followed by use of an ice pack. The type of exercises recommended may vary depending on the location of the affected bursa or tendon.

If there is no improvement, the doctor may inject a corticosteroid medicine into the area surrounding the inflamed bursa or tendon. While corticosteroid injections are a common treatment, they must be used with caution because they may lead to weakening or rupture of the tendon (especially weight-bearing tendons such as the Achilles [ankle], posterior tibial [arch of the foot], and patellar [knee] tendons). If there is still no improvement after 6–12 months, the doctor may perform either arthroscopic or open surgery to repair damage and relieve pressure on the tendons and bursae.

If the bursitis is caused by an infection, the doctor will prescribe antibiotics.

If a tendon is completely torn, surgery may be needed to repair the damage. After surgery on a quadriceps or patellar tendon, for example, the patient will wear a cast for 3–6 weeks and use crutches. For a partial tear, the doctor might apply a cast without performing surgery.

Rehabilitating a partial or complete tear of a tendon requires an exercise program to restore the ability to bend and straighten the knee and to strengthen the leg to prevent repeat injury. A rehabilitation program may last 6 months, although the patient can return to many activities before then.

Can bursitis and tendonitis be prevented?

To help prevent inflammation or reduce the severity of its recurrence, try these tips:

- Warm up or stretch before physical activity.

- Strengthen muscles around the joint.

- Take breaks from repetitive tasks often.

- Cushion the affected joint. Use foam for kneeling or elbow pads. Increase the gripping surface of tools with gloves or padding. Apply grip tape or an oversized grip to golf clubs.

- Use two hands to hold heavy tools; use a two-handed backhand in tennis.

- Don't sit still for long periods.

- Practice good posture and position the body properly when going about daily activities.

- Begin new activities or exercise regimens slowly. Gradually increase physical demands following several well-tolerated exercise sessions.

- If a history of tendonitis is present, consider seeking guidance from your doctor or therapist before engaging in new exercises and activities.

Chapter 12

Carpal Tunnel Syndrome

What is carpal tunnel syndrome (CTS)?

Carpal tunnel syndrome (CTS) is the name for a group of problems that includes swelling, pain, tingling, and loss of strength in your wrist and hand. Your wrist is made of small bones that form a narrow groove or carpal tunnel. Tendons and a nerve called the median nerve must pass through this tunnel from your forearm into your hand. The median nerve controls the feelings and sensations in the palm side of your thumb and fingers. Sometimes swelling and irritation of the tendons can put pressure on the wrist nerve causing the symptoms of CTS. A person's dominant hand is the one that is usually affected. However, nearly half of CTS sufferers have symptoms in both hands.

CTS has become more common in the United States and is quite costly in terms of time lost from work and expensive medical treatment. The U.S. Department of Labor reported that in 2003 the average number of missed days of work due to CTS was 23 days, costing over $2 billion a year. It is thought that about 3.7 percent of the general public in this country suffer from CTS.

What are the symptoms of CTS?

Typically, CTS begins slowly with feelings of burning, tingling, and numbness in the wrist and hand. The areas most affected are the

From "Carpal Tunnel Syndrome," by the Office of Women's Health (www.womenshealth.gov), part of the U.S. Department of Health and Human Services, June 1, 2005.

thumb, index, and middle fingers. At first, symptoms may happen more often at night. Many CTS sufferers do not make the connection between a daytime activity that might be causing the CTS and the delayed symptoms. Also, many people sleep with their wrist bent, which may cause more pain and symptoms at night. As CTS gets worse, the tingling may be felt during the daytime too, along with pain moving from the wrist to your arm or down to your fingers. Pain is usually felt more on the palm side of the hand.

Another symptom of CTS is weakness of the hands that gets worse over time. Some people with CTS find it difficult to grasp an object, make a fist, or hold onto something small. The fingers may even feel like they are swollen even though they are not. Over time, this feeling will usually happen more often.

If left untreated, those with CTS can have a loss of feeling in some fingers and permanent weakness of the thumb. Thumb muscles can actually waste away over time. Eventually, CTS sufferers may have trouble telling the difference between hot and cold temperatures by touch.

What causes CTS and who is more likely to develop it?

Women are three times more likely to have CTS than men. Although there is limited research on why this is the case, scientists have several ideas. It may be that the wrist bones are naturally smaller in most women, creating a tighter space through which the nerves and tendons must pass. Other researchers are looking at genetic links that make it more likely for women to have musculoskeletal injuries such as CTS. Women also deal with strong hormonal changes during pregnancy and menopause that make them more likely to suffer from CTS. Generally, women are at higher risk of CTS between the ages of 45 and 54. Then, the risk increases for both men and women as they age.

There are other factors that can cause CTS, including certain health problems and, in some cases, the cause is unknown.

These are some of the things that might raise your chances of developing CTS:

- **Genetic predisposition:** The carpal tunnel is smaller in some people than others.

- **Repetitive movements:** People who do the same movements with their wrists and hands over and over may be more likely to develop CTS. People with certain types of jobs are more likely to have CTS, including manufacturing and assembly line workers, grocery store checkers, violinists, and carpenters. Some hobbies and sports that use repetitive hand movements can also cause CTS, such as golfing, knitting, and gardening. Whether long-term typing or computer use causes CTS is still being debated. Limited research points to a weak link, but more research is needed.

- **Injury or trauma:** A sprain or a fracture of the wrist can cause swelling and pressure on the nerve, increasing the risk of CTS. Forceful and stressful movements of the hand and wrist can also cause trauma, such as strong vibrations caused by heavy machinery or power tools.

- **Pregnancy:** Hormonal changes during pregnancy and build up of fluid can put pregnant women at greater risk of getting CTS, especially during the last few months. Most doctors treat CTS in pregnant women with wrist splits or rest, rather than surgery, as CTS almost always goes away following childbirth.

- **Menopause:** Hormonal changes during menopause can put women at greater risk of getting CTS. Also, in some postmenopausal women, the wrist structures become enlarged and can press on the wrist nerve.

- **Breast cancer:** Some women who have a mastectomy get lymphedema, the build-up of fluids that go beyond the lymph system's ability to drain it. In mastectomy patients, this causes pain and swelling of the arm. Although rare, some of these women will get CTS due to pressure on the nerve from this swelling.

- **Medical conditions:** People who have diabetes, hypothyroidism, lupus, obesity, and rheumatoid arthritis are more likely to get CTS. In some of these patients, the normal structures in the wrist can become enlarged and lead to CTS.

Also, smokers with CTS usually have worse symptoms and recover more slowly than nonsmokers.

How is CTS treated?

It is important to be treated by a doctor for CTS in order to avoid permanent damage to the wrist nerve and muscles of the hand and thumb. Underlying causes such as diabetes or a thyroid problem should be addressed first. Left untreated, CTS can cause nerve damage that leads to loss of feeling and less hand strength. Over time, the muscles of the thumb can become weak and damaged. You can even lose the ability to feel hot and cold by touch. Permanent injury occurs in about 1 percent of those with CTS.

CTS is much easier to treat early on. Most CTS patients get better after first-step treatments and the following tips for protecting the wrist. Treatments for CTS include the following:

- **Wrist splint:** A splint can be worn to support and brace your wrist in a neutral position so that the nerves and tendons can recover. A splint can be worn 24 hours a day or only at night. Sometimes, wearing a splint at night helps to reduce the pain. Splinting can work the best when done within three months of having any symptoms of CTS.

- **Rest:** For people with mild CTS, stopping or doing less of a repetitive movement may be all that is needed. Your doctor will likely talk to you about steps that you should take to prevent CTS from coming back.

- **Medication:** The short-term use of nonsteroidal anti-inflammatory drugs (NSAIDs) may be helpful to control CTS pain. NSAIDs include aspirin, ibuprofen, and other non-prescription pain relievers. In severe cases, an injection of cortisone may help to reduce swelling. Your doctor may also give you corticosteroids in a pill form. But, these treatments only relieve symptoms temporarily. If CTS is caused by another health problem, your doctor will probably treat that problem first. If you have diabetes, it is important to know that long-term corticosteroid use can make it hard to control insulin levels.

- **Physical therapy:** A physical therapist can help you do special exercises to make your wrist and hand stronger. There are also many different kinds of treatments that can make CTS better and help relieve symptoms. Massage, yoga, ultrasound, chiropractic manipulation, and acupuncture are just a few such options that have been found to be helpful. You should talk with your doctor before trying these alternative treatments.

- **Surgery:** CTS surgery is one of the most common surgeries done in the United States. Generally, surgery is only an option for severe cases of CTS and/or after other treatments have failed for a period of at least six months. Open release surgery is a common approach to CTS surgery and involves making a small incision in the wrist or palm and cutting the ligament to enlarge the carpal tunnel. This surgery is done under a local anesthetic to numb the wrist and hand area and is an outpatient procedure.

Chapter 13

Fibromyalgia

Chapter Contents

Section 13.1

Questions and Answers about Fibromyalgia

From "Frequently Asked Questions about Fibromyalgia," by the
Office of Women's Health (www.womenshealth.gov), part of the U.S.
Department of Health and Human Services, May 1, 2006.

What is fibromyalgia (FM)?

Fibromyalgia is a disorder that causes aches and pain all over the
body. People with FM also are tender throughout the body, which is
most pronounced at certain regions termed "tender points." Tender
points are specific places on the neck, shoulders, back, hips, arms, and
legs. These points hurt when pressure is put on them.

What are the symptoms of fibromyalgia?

People with FM could have the following symptoms:

- Muscle pain
- Fatigue
- Trouble sleeping
- Joint pain and stiffness (sometimes worse in the morning)
- Headaches
- Restless legs
- Tingling or numbness in hands and feet
- Problems with thinking and memory (sometimes called "fibro
fog")
- Leg cramps
- Feeling nervous
- Depression
- Feeling dizzy or lightheaded
- Painful cramping during your period
- Jaw pain

- Upset stomach, cramping, bloating, feeling constipated, or diarrhea
- Trouble swallowing
- Frequent or painful urination

How common is fibromyalgia? Who is mainly affected?

FM affects as many as 1 in 50 Americans. Most people with FM are women (about 80–90%). However, men and children also can have the disorder. Most people are diagnosed during middle age. FM can occur by itself, but people with certain other diseases, such as rheumatoid arthritis and other types of arthritis, may be more likely to have FM. Individuals who have a close relative with FM are more likely to develop FM.

What causes fibromyalgia?

The causes of FM are not known. Researchers think a number of factors might be involved. FM has been linked to the following factors:

- Having a family history of fibromyalgia (i.e., genetics)
- Being exposed to stressful or traumatic events, such as the following:
  - Car accidents
  - Injuries to the body caused by performing the same action over and over again
  - Infections or illnesses
  - Being deployed to war

How is fibromyalgia diagnosed?

People with FM often see many doctors before being diagnosed. One reason for this may be that pain and fatigue, the main symptoms of FM, also are symptoms of many other conditions. Therefore, doctors often must rule out other possible causes of these symptoms before making a diagnosis of FM. FM cannot be detected by a lab test either.

A doctor who knows about FM, however, can make a diagnosis based upon two criteria. One criterion is a history of widespread pain lasting more than 3 months. Pain must be present in both the right and left sides of the body as well as above and below the waist.

Another criteria is the presence of tender points. The body has 18 sites that are possible tender points. For FM diagnosis a person must have 11 or more tender points. To be deemed a tender point, pain must be felt when pressure is applied to the site. People who have FM may feel pain at other sites, too, but those 18 sites on the body are used for diagnosis.

The previous criteria were developed for use to standardize research studies and are not necessary to diagnose individual patients, but if you feel your doctor doesn't know a lot about FM or has doubts about whether it is a "real" illness, see another doctor for a second opinion. Contact a local university medical school or research center for help finding a doctor who has helped others with FM.

How is fibromyalgia treated?

FM can be hard to treat. It's important to find a doctor who has treated others with FM. Many family doctors, general internists, or rheumatologists can treat FM. Rheumatologists are doctors who treat arthritis and other conditions that affect the joints and soft tissues.

Treatment often requires a team approach. The team may include your doctor, a physical therapist, and possibly other health care providers. A pain or rheumatology clinic can be a good place to get treatment.

The U.S. Food and Drug Administration has not yet approved any medicines to treat FM. Doctors treat FM with medicines approved for other purposes. Pain medicines and antidepressants are often used in treatment.

What is the difference between fibromyalgia and chronic fatigue syndrome?

Chronic fatigue syndrome (CFS) and FM are alike in many ways. In fact, it is not uncommon for a person to have both FM and CFS. Some experts believe that FM and CFS are in fact the same disorder, but expressed in slightly different ways. Both CFS and FM have pain and fatigue as symptoms.

The main symptom of CFS is extreme tiredness. CFS often begins after having flu-like symptoms. But people with CFS do not have the tender points that people with FM have. To be diagnosed with CFS, a person must have the following symptoms:

- Extreme fatigue for at least 6 months that cannot be explained by medical tests
- Four or more of the following symptoms:
  - Forgetting things or having a hard time focusing
  - Feeling tired even after sleeping

- Muscle pain or aches
- Pain or aches in joints without swelling or redness
- Feeling discomfort or out of sorts for more than 24 hours after being active
- Headaches of a new type, pattern, or strength
- Tender lymph nodes in the neck or under the arm
- Sore throat

Is there anything I can do to help me feel better?

Besides taking medicine prescribed by your doctor, there are many things you can do to lessen the impact of FM on your life:

- Get enough sleep. Getting enough sleep and the right kind of sleep can help ease the pain and fatigue of FM.
- Get moving. Though pain and fatigue may make exercise and daily activities hard, being active as possible is important. People who have a lot of pain or fatigue should begin with walking or other gentle exercises and slowly build up to more demanding workouts.
- Make changes at work. Most people with FM continue to work, but they may have to make big changes to do so. For example, some people cut down the number of hours, switch to a less demanding job, or adapt a current job.
- Eat right. Try to add more fruits, vegetables, and whole grains to your diet.

What if I can't work because of fibromyalgia?

If you cannot work because of your FM, contact the Social Security Administration for help with disability benefits at 800-772-1213 or www.ssa.gov.

What research is being done on fibromyalgia?

The National Institute of Arthritis and Musculoskeletal and Skin Diseases sponsor research to help understand FM and find better ways to diagnose, treat, and prevent it. Researchers are studying the following topics:

- Why people with FM have are highly sensitive to pain
- The role of stress hormones in the body

- Medicines and behavioral treatments
- Whether there is a gene or genes that make a person more likely to have FM

Section 13.2

Gabapentin Shown Effective for Fibromyalgia Pain

From "Gabapentin Shown Effective for Fibromyalgia Pain," by the National Institute of Arthritis and Musculoskeletal and Skin Diseases (NIAMS, www.niams.nih.gov), part of the National Institutes of Health, June 11, 2007.

New research supported by the National Institutes of Health's National Institute of Arthritis and Musculoskeletal and Skin Diseases (NIAMS) shows that the anticonvulsant medication gabapentin, which is used for certain types of seizures, can be an effective treatment for the pain and other symptoms associated with the common, often hard-to-treat chronic pain disorder, fibromyalgia.

In the NIAMS-sponsored, randomized, double-blind clinical trial of 150 women (90 percent) and men with the condition, Lesley M. Arnold, MD, director of the Women's Health Research Program at the University of Cincinnati College of Medicine, and her colleagues found that those taking gabapentin at dosages of 1,200 to 2,400 mg daily for 12 weeks displayed significantly less pain than those taking placebo. Patients taking gabapentin also reported significantly better sleep and less fatigue. For the majority of participants, the drug was well tolerated. The most common side effects included dizziness and sedation, which were mild to moderate in severity in most cases.

NIAMS Director Stephen I. Katz, MD, PhD, remarked that "While gabapentin does not have Food and Drug Administration approval for fibromyalgia [Note: The FDA approved Lyrica {pregabalin} for treating fibromyalgia on June 21, 2007], I believe this study offers additional insight to physicians considering the drug for their fibromyalgia patients. Fibromyalgia is a debilitating condition for which current treatments are only modestly effective, so a study such as this is potentially good news for people with this common, painful condition."

Fibromyalgia is a chronic disorder characterized by chronic, widespread muscle pain and tenderness, and is frequently accompanied by fatigue, insomnia, depression, and anxiety. It affects three million to six million Americans, mostly women, and can be disabling.

The precise cause of fibromyalgia in not known, but research suggests it is related to a problem with the central nervous system's processing of pain. As with some other chronic pain conditions, people with fibromyalgia often develop a heightened response to stimuli, experiencing pain that would not cause problems in other people. Yet, unlike many other pain syndromes, there is no physical evidence of inflammation or central nervous system damage.

Although gabapentin has little, if any, effect on acute pain, it has shown a robust effect on pain caused by a heightened response to stimuli related to inflammation or nerve injury in animal models of chronic pain syndromes. Researchers have suspected that it might have the same effect in people with fibromyalgia. The new research, published in the April 2007 edition of *Arthritis & Rheumatism*, indicates the suspicions were correct.

Although the researchers cannot say with certainty how gabapentin helps reduce pain, Dr. Arnold says one possible explanation involves the binding of gabapentin to a specific subunit of voltage-gated calcium channels on neurons. "This binding reduces calcium flow into the nerve cell, which reduces the release of some signaling molecules involved in pain processing" she says.

How gabapentin improves sleep and other symptoms is less clear, and there are probably different mechanisms involved in fibromyalgia symptoms. "Gabapentin improved sleep, which is an added benefit to patients with fibromyalgia who often report unrefreshing or disrupted sleep," Dr. Arnold says.

What is important is that people with fibromyalgia now have a potential new treatment option for a condition with few effective treatments. "Studies like this give clinicians evidence-based information to guide their treatment of patients," says Dr. Arnold.

Arnold, LM et al. Gabapentin in the treatment of fibromyalgia; a randomized, double-blind, placebo-controlled multicenter trial. *Arthritis Rheum*. 2007; 56: 1336–1344.

Chapter 14

Gout and Pseudogout

Chapter Contents

Section 14.1

Gout

From "Gout," by the National Institute of Arthritis and
Musculoskeletal and Skin Diseases (NIAMS, www.niams.nih.gov),
part of the National Institutes of Health, December 2006.

What is gout?

Gout is a painful condition that occurs when the bodily waste product uric acid is deposited as needle-like crystals in the joints and/or soft tissues. In the joints, these uric acid crystals cause inflammatory arthritis, which in turn leads to intermittent swelling, redness, heat, pain, and stiffness in the joints.

In many people, gout initially affects the joints of the big toe (a condition called podagra). But many other joints and areas around the joints can be affected in addition to or instead of the big toe. These include the insteps, ankles, heels, knees, wrists, fingers, and elbows. Chalky deposits of uric acid, also known as tophi, can appear as lumps under the skin that surrounds the joints and covers the rim of the ear. Uric acid crystals can also collect in the kidneys and cause kidney stones.

What is uric acid?

Uric acid is a substance that results from the breakdown of purines. A normal part of all human tissue, purines are found in many foods. Normally, uric acid is dissolved in the blood and passed through the kidneys into the urine, where it is eliminated.

If there is an increase in the production of uric acid or if the kidneys do not eliminate enough uric acid from the body, levels of it build up in the blood (a condition called hyperuricemia). Hyperuricemia also may result when a person eats too many high-purine foods, such as liver, dried beans and peas, anchovies, and gravies. Hyperuricemia is not a disease, and by itself it is not dangerous. However, if excess uric acid crystals form as a result of hyperuricemia, gout can develop. The crystals form and accumulate in the joint, causing inflammation.

What are the four stages of gout?

Literally translated, arthritis means "joint inflammation." It refers to more than 100 different diseases that affect the joints. Gout accounts for approximately 5 percent of all cases of arthritis. The disease can progress through four stages:

1. **Asymptomatic (without symptoms) hyperuricemia:** In this stage, a person has elevated levels of uric acid in the blood (hyperuricemia), but no other symptoms. Treatment is usually not required.

2. **Acute gout, or acute gouty arthritis:** In this stage, hyperuricemia has caused the deposit of uric acid crystals in joint spaces. This leads to a sudden onset of intense pain and swelling in the joints, which also may be warm and very tender. An acute attack commonly occurs at night and can be triggered by stressful events, alcohol or drugs, or the presence of another illness. Attacks usually subside within 3 to 10 days, even without treatment, and the next attack may not occur for months or even years. Over time, however, attacks can last longer and occur more frequently.

3. **Interval or intercritical gout:** This is the period between acute attacks. In this stage, a person does not have any symptoms.

4. **Chronic tophaceous gout:** This is the most disabling stage of gout. It usually develops over a long period, such as 10 years. In this stage, the disease may have caused permanent damage to the affected joints and sometimes to the kidneys. With proper treatment, most people with gout do not progress to this advanced stage.

Gout is sometimes confused with other forms of arthritis because the symptoms—acute and episodic attacks of joint warmth, pain, swelling, and stiffness—can be similar. One form of arthritis often confused with gout is called pseudogout. The pain, swelling, and redness of pseudogout can also come on suddenly and may be severe, closely resembling the symptoms of gout. However, the crystals that irritate the joint are calcium phosphate crystals, not uric acid. Therefore, pseudogout is treated somewhat differently and is not reviewed in this text.

What causes gout?

A number of risk factors are associated with hyperuricemia and gout. They include the following risk factors:

- **Genetics:** Twenty percent of people with gout have a family history of the disease.

- **Gender and age:** It is more common in men than in women and more common in adults than in children.

- **Weight:** Being overweight increases the risk of developing hyperuricemia and gout because there is more tissue available for turnover or breakdown, which leads to excess uric acid production.

- **Alcohol consumption:** Drinking too much alcohol can lead to hyperuricemia, because alcohol interferes with the removal of uric acid from the body.

- **Diet:** Eating too many foods that are rich in purines can cause or aggravate gout in some people.

- **Lead exposure:** In some cases, exposure to lead in the environment can cause gout.

- **Other health problems:** Renal insufficiency, or the inability of the kidneys to eliminate waste products, is a common cause of gout in older people. Other medical problems that contribute to high blood levels of uric acid include the following:

  - High blood pressure

  - Hypothyroidism (underactive thyroid gland)

  - Conditions that cause an excessively rapid turnover of cells, such as psoriasis, hemolytic anemia, or some cancers

  - Kelley-Seegmiller syndrome or Lesch-Nyhan syndrome, two rare conditions in which the enzyme that helps control uric acid levels either is not present or is found in insufficient quantities

- **Medications:** A number of medications may put people at risk for developing hyperuricemia and gout. They include the following:

  - Diuretics, such as furosemide (Lasix), hydrochlorothiazide (Esidrix, Hydro-chlor), and metolazone (Diulo, Zaroxolyn), which are taken to eliminate excess fluid from the body in conditions like hypertension, edema, and heart disease, and which decrease the amount of uric acid passed in the urine.

- Salicylate-containing drugs, such as aspirin, may increase the risk of gout.

- Niacin, a vitamin also known as nicotinic acid, may increase the risk of gout.

- Cyclosporine (Sandimmune, Neoral), a medication that suppresses the body's immune system (the system that protects the body from infection and disease). This medication is used in the treatment of some autoimmune diseases, and to prevent the body's rejection of transplanted organs.

- Levodopa (Larodopa) is a medicine used to support communication along nerve pathways in the treatment of Parkinson disease.

Who is likely to develop gout?

Scientists estimate that 6 million adults age 20 and older report having had gout at some time in their lives. It is rare in children and young adults. Men, particularly those between the ages of 40 and 50, are more likely to develop gout than women, who rarely develop the disorder before menopause. People who have had an organ transplant are more susceptible to gout.

How is gout diagnosed?

Gout may be difficult for doctors to diagnose because the symptoms can be vague, and gout often mimics other conditions. Although most people with gout have hyperuricemia at some time during the course of their disease, it may not be present during an acute attack. In addition, having hyperuricemia alone does not mean that a person will get gout. In fact, most people with hyperuricemia do not develop the disease.

To confirm a diagnosis of gout, a doctor may insert a needle into an inflamed joint and draw a sample of synovial fluid, the substance that lubricates a joint. The joint fluid is placed on a slide and examined under a microscope for uric acid crystals. Their absence, however, does not completely rule out the diagnosis.

The doctor also may find it helpful to look for uric acid crystals around joints to diagnose gout. Gout attacks may mimic joint infections, and a doctor who suspects a joint infection (rather than gout) may also culture the joint fluid to see whether bacteria are present.

How is gout treated?

With proper treatment, most people who have gout are able to control their symptoms and live productive lives. Gout can be treated with one or a combination of therapies. The goals of treatment are to ease the pain associated with acute attacks, to prevent future attacks, and to avoid the formation of tophi and kidney stones. Successful treatment can reduce discomfort caused by the symptoms of gout, as well as long-term damage to the affected joints. Treatment will help to prevent disability due to gout.

The most common treatments for an acute attack of gout are nonsteroidal anti-inflammatory drugs (NSAIDs) taken orally (by mouth), or corticosteroids, which are taken orally or injected into the affected joint. NSAIDs reduce the inflammation caused by deposits of uric acid crystals, but have no effect on the amount of uric acid in the body. The NSAIDs most commonly prescribed for gout are indomethacin (Indocin) and naproxen (Anaprox, Naprosyn), which are taken orally every day. Corticosteroids are strong anti-inflammatory hormones. The most commonly prescribed corticosteroid is prednisone. Patients often begin to improve within a few hours of treatment with a corticosteroid, and the attack usually goes away completely within a week or so.

When NSAIDs or corticosteroids do not control symptoms, the doctor may consider using colchicine. This drug is most effective when taken within the first 12 hours of an acute attack. Doctors may ask patients to take oral colchicine as often as every hour until joint symptoms begin to improve or side effects such as nausea, vomiting, abdominal cramps, or diarrhea make it uncomfortable to continue the drug.

For some patients, the doctor may prescribe either NSAIDs or oral colchicine in small daily doses to prevent future attacks. The doctor also may consider prescribing medicine such as allopurinol (Zyloprim) or probenecid (Benemid) to treat hyperuricemia and reduce the frequency of sudden attacks and the development of tophi.

People who have other medical problems, such as high blood pressure or high blood triglycerides (fats), may find that the drugs they take for those conditions can also be useful for gout. Both losartan (Cozaar), a blood pressure medication, and fenofibrate (TriCor), a triglyceride-lowering drug, also help reduce blood levels of uric acid.

The doctor may also recommend losing weight, for those who are overweight; limiting alcohol consumption; and avoiding or limiting high-purine foods, which can increase uric acid levels.

What can people with gout do to stay healthy?

Fortunately, gout can be controlled. People with gout can decrease the severity of attacks and reduce their risk of future attacks by taking their medications as prescribed. Acute gout is best controlled if medications are taken at the first sign of pain or inflammation. Other steps you can take to stay healthy and minimize gout's effect on your life include the following:

- Tell your doctor about all the medicines and vitamins you take. He or she can tell you if any of them increase your risk of hyperuricemia.

- Plan followup visits with your doctor to evaluate your progress.

- Drink plenty of nonalcoholic fluids, especially water. Non-alcoholic fluids help remove uric acid from the body. Alcohol, on the other hand, can raise the levels of uric acid in your blood.

- Exercise regularly and maintain a healthy body weight. Lose weight if you are overweight, but avoid low-carbohydrate diets that are designed for quick weight loss. When carbohydrate intake is insufficient, your body can't completely burn its own fat. As a consequence, substances called ketones form and are released into the bloodstream, resulting in a condition called ketosis. After a short time, ketosis can increase the level of uric acid in your blood.

- Avoid foods that are high in purines.

High-purine foods include the following:

- Anchovies
- Asparagus
- Beef kidneys
- Brains
- Dried beans and peas
- Game meats
- Gravy

- Herring
- Liver
- Mackerel
- Mushrooms
- Sardines
- Scallops
- Sweetbreads

What research is being conducted to help people with gout?

Because uric acid's role in gout is well understood and medications to ease attacks and reduce the risk or severity of future attacks are widely available, gout is one of the most—if not the most—controllable forms of arthritis. But researchers continue to make advances that help people live with gout. Perhaps someday these advances will prevent this extremely painful disease.

Some current areas of gout research include the following:

- **Refining current treatments:** While many medications are available to treat gout, doctors are trying to determine which of the treatments are most effective and at which dosages. Recent studies have compared the effectiveness of different NSAIDs in treating the pain and inflammation of gout and have looked at the optimal dosages of colchicine and allopurinol (a uric-acid-lowering drug) to control and/or prevent painful attacks.

- **Evaluating new therapies:** A number of new therapies have shown promise in recent studies. They include infliximab (Remicade) and other biologic agents that block a chemical called tumor necrosis factor. This chemical is believed to play a role in the inflammation of gout. Another new drug therapy is febuxostat, which works by blocking an enzyme involved in the production of uric acid.

- **Discovering the role of foods:** Gout is the one form of arthritis for which there is proof that specific foods worsen the symptoms. Now research is suggesting that certain foods may also prevent gout. In a study published in the *New England Journal of Medicine*, scientists found that a high intake of low-fat dairy products reduces the risk of gout in men by half. The reason for this protective effect is not yet known. Another study examining the effects of vitamin C on uric acid suggests that it may be beneficial in the prevention and management of gout and other diseases that are associated with uric acid production.

- **Searching for new treatment approaches:** Scientists are also studying the contributions of different types of cells that participate in both the acute and chronic joint manifestations of gout. The specific goals of this research are to better understand how urate crystals activate white blood cells called neutrophils, leading to acute gout attacks; how urate crystals affect the immune system, leading to chronic gout; and how urate crystals interact with bone cells in a way that causes debilitating bone lesions among people with chronic gout. The hope is that a better understanding of the various inflammatory reactions that occur in gout will provide innovative clues for treatment.

- **Examining how genetics and environmental factors can affect hyperuricemia:** Researchers are studying different populations in which gout is prevalent to determine how certain genes and environmental factors may affect blood levels of uric acid, which can leak out and crystallize in the joint, leading to gout.

Section 14.2

Pseudogout

Alternative Names

Calcium pyrophosphate dihydrate deposition disease; CPPD disease

Definition

Pseudogout is a joint disease that can cause attacks of arthritis. Like gout, the condition involves the formation of crystals in the joints. But in pseudogout, the crystals are formed from a salt instead of uric acid.

Causes

Pseudogout is caused by the collection of salt called calcium pyrophosphate dihydrate (CPPD). The buildup of this salt forms crystals in the joints. This leads to attacks of joint swelling and pain in the knees, wrists, ankles, and other joints.

Among older adults, pseudogout is a common cause of sudden (acute) arthritis in one joint.

Pseudogout mainly affects the elderly. However, it can sometimes affect younger patients who have conditions such as:

- acromegaly;
- hemochromatosis;
- ochronosis;
- parathyroid disease;
- thyroid disease;
- Wilson disease.

Because the symptoms are similar, pseudogout can be misdiagnosed as:

- gouty arthritis (gout);
- osteoarthritis;
- rheumatoid arthritis.

Symptoms

- Attacks of joint pain and fluid buildup in the joint, leading to joint swelling
- Chronic (long-term) arthritis
- No symptoms between attacks

Exams and Tests

An examination of joint fluid would show white blood cells and calcium pyrophosphate crystals. Joint x-rays may show joint damage, calcification of cartilage, and calcium deposits in joint spaces.

Careful testing and analysis of crystals found in joints can help the doctor diagnose the condition. Fortunately, because most conditions involving joint pain are treated by the same medicines (such as steroids and nonsteroidal anti-inflammatory drugs), an early mistaken diagnosis does not necessarily result in the wrong treatment.

Treatment

Treatment may involve the removal of fluid to relieve pressure within the joint. A needle is placed into the joint and fluid is removed (aspirated).

Steroid injections may be helpful to treat severely inflamed joints. A course of oral steroids is sometimes used when multiple joints are inflamed.

Nonsteroidal anti-inflammatory medications (NSAIDs) may help ease painful attacks. Colchicine may be useful in some people.

Outlook (Prognosis)

Most people do well with treatment.

Possible Complications

Permanent joint damage can occur without treatment.

When to Contact a Medical Professional

Call for an appointment with your health care provider if you have attacks of joint swelling and joint pain.

Prevention

There is no known way to prevent this disorder. However, treating other problems that may cause pseudogout may make the condition less severe, and may help prevent it from developing in patients who don't already have it.

Chapter 15

Infectious Forms of Arthritis

Chapter Contents

Section 15.1

Arthritis Associated with Lyme Disease

"Fall Is the Season for Lyme Arthritis," by Evren Aken, MD. © 2002 Gillette Children's Specialty Healthcare (www.gillettechildrens.org). Reprinted with permission. Reviewed by David A. Cooke, MD, FACP, June 29, 2009.

Arthritis is a major manifestation of Lyme disease, the most common tick-borne illness in the United States. Lyme arthritis occurs as a result of untreated Lyme infection, which develops when the spirochete called *Borrelia burgdorferi*, the bacteria carried by deer ticks, is transmitted to humans and travels through the bloodstream into various areas of the body, including the joints.

Because early symptoms of Lyme disease aren't always recognized, the disease can go untreated—increasing the chances of developing Lyme arthritis. Sixty percent of untreated children infected with *Borrelia burgdorferi* develop Lyme arthritis.

Lyme arthritis usually presents symptoms during the fall season, several weeks—or even months—after the initial tick bite.

Knowing Early Symptoms Could Prevent Arthritis

The early symptoms of Lyme disease (stage 1 and stage 2) can be mild and easily overlooked. People who are aware of the risk of Lyme disease in their communities, and who don't ignore the sometimes-subtle early symptoms, are most likely to seek medical attention early enough to be assured of a full recovery. Lyme disease is often overlooked—especially in children—because some of the symptoms mimic those of influenza.

Common symptoms seen in early stages of Lyme disease are:

- solid red or bull's-eye rash, called erythema migrans, usually at the bite site (present in 80 to 90 percent of all Lyme disease cases);
- swelling of lymph glands near the bite;
- generalized achiness and headache;
- fever without upper respiratory symptoms (flu-like illness).

Because these symptoms often occur within days of the initial tick bite, testing for Lyme disease may not immediately confirm the infection. Furthermore, ticks that transmit the disease often attach to the scalp, armpits, buttocks, and other inconspicuous areas, so the questioning the patient's whereabouts during the weeks and months prior to developing symptoms, can lead to prompt treatment and prevent the development of Lyme arthritis.

Diagnosing Lyme Arthritis in Children

Symptoms of Lyme arthritis present months—and, in some cases, years—later. Most commonly, the arthritis intermittently attacks one or a few large joints at a time, especially the knee. Nevertheless, numerous joints can be involved, including the temporomandibular joint as originally described by Steer.

Children, especially younger children, may have moderate fevers and increased erythrocyte sedimentation rates. Their first attack of arthritis may last several days to weeks. Although this can mimic septic arthritis, the joint of a child with Lyme arthritis rarely is as painful as that of a child with acute arthritis. Analysis of joint fluid is rarely helpful, because the leukocyte count in synovial fluid can range from fewer than 10,000 to greater than 100,000 cells per milliliter.

Physicians often evaluate joint swelling in active individuals, and suspicion naturally falls first on a patient's activities as a likely cause. Lyme disease is rarely the initial diagnosis, particularly in a patient who recalls none of the disease's usual symptoms. A careful patient history, however, may show that the patient exercised, hiked or camped in a region where Lyme disease is endemic. In such a case, Lyme arthritis may be the initial presentation, and the physician should proceed with appropriate tests to determine proper diagnosis and treatment.

Testing for Lyme Arthritis

Children—especially those with histories of tick bites—who complain of joint pain, a mysterious summer illness, or a rash should undergo specific tests to confirm Lyme disease. Several laboratory tests help diagnose Lyme disease. The most common is the ELISA [enzyme-linked immunosorbent assay] titer test, which measures the amount of antibody to the spirochete. Physicians should be aware that ELISA testing is subject to false-positive results because the spirochete shares certain antigens with other infectious agents. In younger children, false positive ELISA results—particularly of the IgM [immunoglobulin M] type—are common.

Children who have equivocal or positive ELISA results should be tested by Western blot. The Western blot test identifies proteins of the spirochete to which the antibody response is directed. When patients have IgG [immunoglobulin G] reactivity with five or more of 10 particular spirochete proteins, it is highly likely that they have been exposed to the spirochete that carries Lyme disease. However, this test doesn't distinguish between past exposure and present illness. Therefore, results need to be evaluated in the context of clinical symptoms.

During the early stages of Lyme disease, patients often have positive IgM Western blots. Once arthritis develops, the immune response expands to include IgG antibodies. Therefore, a negative IgG Western blot in a patient with arthritis essentially rules out Lyme disease. A positive IgM titer in such a patient is likely a false positive. On the other hand, a positive IgM ELISA titer and a positive IgM Western blot can persist along with a positive IgG for months or years in patients with Lyme disease. It's important to inform patients that they will have positive test results for years (although the titers may drop)—even after they've been treated.

Treatment-Resistant Lyme Arthritis

In cases where arthritis is resistant to treatment, polymerase chair reaction (PCR) testing in the joint may help differentiate non-specific inflammation from ongoing infection.

During antibiotic treatment, children may experience joint discomfort for up to eight weeks. Ibuprofen (30 mg/kg/day) or Naproxen (10–20 mg/kg/day) can be recommended for the first several weeks as adjunct therapy. Despite appropriate treatment, 10 percent of patients may have continued joint swelling more than six months after therapy. That has been termed treatment resistant Lyme arthritis. Such patients deserve evaluation by a rheumatologist to define a further course of action.

Section 15.2

Reactive Arthritis

From "Reactive Arthritis," by the National Institute of Arthritis and Musculoskeletal and Skin Diseases (NIAMS, www.niams.nih.gov), part of the National Institutes of Health, May 2002. Revised by David A. Cooke, MD, FACP, July 29, 2009.

What is reactive arthritis?

Reactive arthritis is a form of arthritis, or joint inflammation, that occurs as a "reaction" to an infection elsewhere in the body. In contrast to septic arthritis, where a microorganism infects a joint in large numbers, reactive arthritis involves few, if any, organisms in the joint. Rather, the presence of harmful organisms elsewhere seems to trigger immune cells to cause inflammation in the joints. Inflammation is a characteristic reaction of tissues to injury or disease and is marked by swelling, redness, heat, and pain.

Reactive arthritis, by definition, occurs during or soon after an infection of one type or another. A number of different types of organisms, mostly but not exclusively bacteria, are known to be triggers for the condition. It is not completely understood how it occurs, but it is thought that the infections may confuse the immune system and lead it to attack healthy tissues. Fortunately, the immune system recovers in most cases and stops its overreaction. The symptoms of reactive arthritis usually last 3 to 12 months, although symptoms can return or develop into a long-term disease in a small percentage of people.

There are a number of discrete types of reactive arthritis. In many patients, reactive arthritis is triggered by a venereal infection in the bladder, the urethra, or, in women, the vagina (the urogenital tract) that is often transmitted through sexual contact. This form of the disorder is sometimes called genitourinary or urogenital reactive arthritis.

Another form of reactive arthritis is caused by an infection in the intestinal tract from eating food or handling substances that are contaminated with bacteria. This form of arthritis is sometimes called enteric or gastrointestinal reactive arthritis.

One distinct form is known as Reiter syndrome, and your doctor may refer to it by yet another term, as a seronegative spondyloarthropathy. The seronegative spondyloarthropathies are a group of disorders that can cause inflammation throughout the body, especially in the spine. (Examples of other disorders in this group include psoriatic arthritis, ankylosing spondylitis, and the kind of arthritis that sometimes accompanies inflammatory bowel disease.) A characteristic feature of Reiter syndrome is that joint symptoms may also be associated with inflammation of the eyes (conjunctivitis) and inflammation of the urinary tract (urethritis). However, these symptoms may occur alone, together, or not at all.

What causes reactive arthritis?

Reactive arthritis typically begins about 1 to 3 weeks after infection.

The bacterium most often associated with Reiter syndrome is *Chlamydia trachomatis*, commonly known as chlamydia. It is usually acquired through sexual contact. Some evidence also shows that respiratory infections with *Chlamydia pneumoniae* may trigger reactive arthritis.

Throat infections caused by group A streptococci (Strep throat) can trigger a reactive arthritis. It is unclear whether this form of arthritis is a limited form of rheumatic fever or a distinct disorder.

Infections in the digestive tract that may trigger reactive arthritis include *Salmonella, Shigella, Yersinia,* and *Campylobacter*. People may become infected with these bacteria after eating or handling improperly prepared food, such as meats that are not stored at the proper temperature.

Doctors do not know exactly why some people exposed to these bacteria develop reactive arthritis and others do not, but they have identified a genetic factor, human leukocyte antigen (HLA) B27, that increases a person's chance of developing reactive arthritis. Approximately 80 percent of people with reactive arthritis test positive for HLA-B27. However, inheriting the HLA-B27 gene does not necessarily mean you will get reactive arthritis. Eight percent of healthy people have the HLA-B27 gene, and only about one-fifth of them will develop reactive arthritis if they contract the triggering infections.

Is reactive arthritis contagious?

Reactive arthritis is not contagious; that is, a person with the disorder cannot pass the arthritis on to someone else. However, the bacteria that can trigger reactive arthritis can be passed from person to person.

Who gets reactive arthritis?

Overall, men between the ages of 20 and 40 are most likely to develop reactive arthritis. However, evidence shows that although men are nine times more likely than women to develop reactive arthritis due to venereally acquired infections, women and men are equally likely to develop reactive arthritis as a result of foodborne infections. Women with reactive arthritis often have milder symptoms than men.

What are the symptoms of reactive arthritis?

Reactive arthritis most typically results in inflammation of the urogenital tract, the joints, and the eyes. Less common symptoms are mouth ulcers and skin rashes. Any of these symptoms may be so mild that patients do not notice them. They usually come and go over a period of several weeks to several months.

Joint symptoms: The arthritis associated with reactive arthritis typically involves pain and swelling in the knees, ankles, and feet. Wrists, fingers, and other joints are affected less often. People with reactive arthritis commonly develop inflammation of the tendons (tendonitis) or at places where tendons attach to the bone (enthesitis). In many people with reactive arthritis, this results in heel pain or irritation of the Achilles tendon at the back of the ankle. Some people with reactive arthritis also develop heel spurs, which are bony growths in the heel that may cause chronic (long-lasting) foot pain. Approximately half of people with reactive arthritis report low-back and buttock pain.

Reactive arthritis also can cause spondylitis (inflammation of the vertebrae in the spinal column) or sacroiliitis (inflammation of the joints in the lower back that connect the spine to the pelvis). People with reactive arthritis who have the HLA-B27 gene are even more likely to develop spondylitis and/or sacroiliitis.

Urogenital tract symptoms: Reactive arthritis often affects the urogenital tract, including the prostate or urethra in men and the urethra, uterus, or vagina in women. Men may notice an increased need to urinate, a burning sensation when urinating, and a fluid discharge from the penis. Some men with reactive arthritis develop prostatitis (inflammation of the prostate gland). Symptoms of prostatitis can include fever and chills, as well as an increased need to urinate and a burning sensation when urinating.

Women with reactive arthritis may develop problems in the urogenital tract, such as cervicitis (inflammation of the cervix) or urethritis (inflammation of the urethra), which can cause a burning sensation during urination. In addition, some women also develop salpingitis (inflammation of the fallopian tubes) or vulvovaginitis (inflammation of the vulva and vagina). These conditions may or may not cause any arthritic symptoms.

Eye involvement: Conjunctivitis, an inflammation of the mucous membrane that covers the eyeball and eyelid, develops in approximately half of people with Reiter syndrome.

Some people may develop uveitis, which is an inflammation of the inner eye. Conjunctivitis and uveitis can cause redness of the eyes, eye pain and irritation, and blurred vision. Eye involvement typically occurs early in the course of Reiter syndrome, and symptoms may come and go.

Other symptoms: Between 20 and 40 percent of men with Reiter syndrome develop small, shallow, painless sores (ulcers) on the end of the penis. A small percentage of men and women develop rashes or small, hard nodules on the soles of the feet and, less often, on the palms of their hands or elsewhere. In addition, some people with Reiter syndrome develop mouth ulcers that come and go. In some cases, these ulcers are painless and go unnoticed.

How is reactive arthritis diagnosed?

Doctors sometimes find it difficult to diagnose reactive arthritis because there is no specific laboratory test to confirm that a person has it. In some cases, the time relationship to a specific infection will be obvious, but in others, it may be more subtle. Blood tests can give clues; there are readily available tests that can indicate whether a person has been recently infection with strep bacteria. If there is strong suspicion, a doctor may order a blood test to detect the genetic factor HLA-B27, but even if the result is positive, the presence of HLA-B27 does not always mean that a person has the disorder.

At the beginning of an examination, the doctor will probably take a complete medical history and note current symptoms as well as any previous medical problems or infections. Before and after seeing the doctor, it is sometimes useful for the patient to keep a record of the symptoms that occur, when they occur, and how long they last. It is especially important to report any flu-like symptoms, such as fever, vomiting, or diarrhea, because they may be evidence of a bacterial infection.

The doctor may use various blood tests besides the HLA-B27 test to help rule out other conditions and confirm a suspected diagnosis of reactive arthritis. For example, the doctor may order rheumatoid factor or antinuclear antibody tests to rule out reactive arthritis. Most people who have reactive arthritis will have negative results on these tests. If a patient's test results are positive, he or she may have some other form of arthritis, such as rheumatoid arthritis or lupus. Doctors also may order a blood test to determine the erythrocyte sedimentation rate (sed rate), which is the rate at which red blood cells settle to the bottom of a test tube of blood. A high sed rate often indicates inflammation somewhere in the body. Typically, people with rheumatic diseases, including reactive arthritis, have an elevated sed rate.

The doctor also is likely to perform tests for infections that might be associated with reactive arthritis. Patients generally are tested for a *Chlamydia* infection because recent studies have shown that early treatment of *Chlamydia*-induced reactive arthritis may reduce the progression of the disease.

The doctor may look for bacterial infections by testing cell samples taken from the patient's throat as well as the urethra in men or cervix in women. Urine and stool samples also may be tested. A sample of synovial fluid (the fluid that lubricates the joints) may be removed from the arthritic joint. Studies of synovial fluid can help the doctor rule out infection in the joint.

Doctors sometimes use x-rays to help diagnose reactive arthritis and to rule out other causes of arthritis. X-rays can detect some of the symptoms of reactive arthritis, including spondylitis, sacroiliitis, swelling of soft tissues, damage to cartilage or bone margins of the joint, and calcium deposits where the tendon attaches to the bone.

What type of doctor treats reactive arthritis?

A person with reactive arthritis probably will need to see several different types of doctors because reactive arthritis affects different parts of the body.

However, it may be helpful to the doctors and the patient for one doctor, usually a rheumatologist (a doctor specializing in arthritis), to manage the complete treatment plan. This doctor can coordinate treatments and monitor the side effects from the various medicines the patient may take. The following specialists treat other features that affect different parts of the body.

- Ophthalmologist: Treats eye disease

- Gynecologist: Treats genital symptoms in women
- Urologist: Treats genital symptoms in men and women
- Dermatologist: Treats skin symptoms
- Orthopedist: Performs surgery on severely damaged joints
- Physiatrist: Supervises exercise regimens

How is reactive arthritis treated?

Although there is no cure for reactive arthritis, some treatments relieve symptoms of the disorder. The doctor is likely to use one or more of the following treatments.

Nonsteroidal anti-inflammatory drugs (NSAIDs): NSAIDs reduce joint inflammation and are commonly used to treat patients with reactive arthritis. Some traditional NSAIDs, such as aspirin and ibuprofen, are available without a prescription, but others that are more effective for reactive arthritis, such as indomethacin and tolmetin, must be prescribed by a doctor.

Corticosteroid injections: For people with severe joint inflammation, injections of corticosteroids directly into the affected joint may reduce inflammation. Doctors usually prescribe these injections only after trying unsuccessfully to control arthritis with NSAIDs.

Topical corticosteroids: These corticosteroids come in a cream or lotion and can be applied directly on the skin lesions, such as ulcers, associated with reactive arthritis. Topical corticosteroids reduce inflammation and promote healing.

Antibiotics: The doctor may prescribe antibiotics to eliminate a bacterial infection that is suspected to have triggered reactive arthritis. The specific antibiotic prescribed depends on the type of bacterial infection present. It is important to follow instructions about how much medicine to take and for how long; otherwise the infection may persist. Typically, an antibiotic is taken for 7 to 10 days or longer. Some doctors may recommend a person with reactive arthritis take antibiotics for a long period of time (up to 3 months). Current research shows that in most cases, this practice is necessary.

Immunosuppressive medicines: A small percentage of patients with reactive arthritis have severe symptoms that cannot be controlled with any of the above treatments. For these people, medicine that suppresses the immune system, such as sulfasalazine or methotrexate, may be effective.

TNF inhibitors: Several relatively new treatments that suppress tumor necrosis factor (TNF), a protein involved in the body's inflammatory response, may be effective for reactive arthritis and other spondyloarthropathies. They include etanercept and infliximab. These treatments were first used to treat rheumatoid arthritis.

Exercise: Exercise, when introduced gradually, may help improve joint function. In particular, strengthening and range-of-motion exercises will maintain or improve joint function. Strengthening exercises build up the muscles around the joint to better support it. Muscle-tightening exercises that do not move any joints can be done even when a person has inflammation and pain. Range-of-motion exercises improve movement and flexibility and reduce stiffness in the affected joint. For patients with spine pain or inflammation, exercises to stretch and extend the back can be particularly helpful in preventing long-term disability. Aquatic exercise also may be helpful. Before beginning an exercise program, patients should talk to a health professional who can recommend appropriate exercises.

What is the prognosis for people who have reactive arthritis?

Most people with reactive arthritis recover fully from the initial flare of symptoms and are able to return to regular activities 2 to 6 months after the first symptoms appear. In such cases, the symptoms of arthritis may last up to 12 months, although these are usually very mild and do not interfere with daily activities. Approximately 20 percent of people with reactive arthritis will have chronic (long-term) arthritis, which usually is mild. Studies show that between 15 and 50 percent of patients will develop symptoms again sometime after the initial flare has disappeared. It is possible that such relapses may be due to reinfection. Back pain and arthritis are the symptoms that most commonly reappear. A small percentage of patients will have chronic, severe arthritis that is difficult to control with treatment and may cause joint deformity.

What are researchers learning about reactive arthritis?

Researchers continue to investigate the causes of reactive arthritis and study treatments for the condition. For example, researchers are trying to better understand the relationship between infection and reactive arthritis. In particular, they are trying to determine why an infection triggers arthritis and why some people who develop infections get reactive arthritis while others do not. Scientists also are studying why people with the genetic factor HLA-B27 are more at risk than others.

Researchers are developing methods to detect the location of the triggering bacteria in the body. Some scientists suspect that after the bacteria enter the body, they are transported to the joints, where they can remain in small amounts indefinitely.

Researchers are testing combination treatments for reactive arthritis. In particular, they are testing the use of antibiotics in combination with TNF inhibitors and with other immunosuppressant medicines, such as methotrexate and sulfasalazine.

Section 15.3

Septic Arthritis

"Septic arthritis," © 2009 A.D.A.M., Inc. Reprinted with permission.

Alternative Names

Bacterial arthritis; Non-gonococcal bacterial arthritis

Definition

Septic arthritis is inflammation of a joint due to a bacterial infection other than gonorrhea (joint infection due to gonorrhea has different symptoms).

Causes

Septic arthritis develops when bacteria spread through the bloodstream to a joint. It may also occur when the joint is directly infected with bacteria by an injury or during surgery. The most common sites for this type of infection are the knee and hip.

Most cases of acute septic arthritis are caused by organisms such as staphylococcus or streptococcus.

Chronic septic arthritis (which is less common) is caused by organisms such as *Mycobacterium tuberculosis* and *Candida albicans*.

The following increase your risk for septic arthritis:

- Artificial joint implants
- Bacterial infection elsewhere in your body
- Chronic illness or disease (such as diabetes, rheumatoid arthritis, and sickle cell disease)
- Intravenous (IV) or injection drug use
- Medications that suppress your immune system
- Recent joint trauma
- Recent joint arthroscopy or other surgery

Septic arthritis may be seen at any age. In children, it occurs most often in those younger than 3 years. The hip is a frequent site of infection in infants.

Septic arthritis is uncommon from age 3 to adolescence. Children with septic arthritis are more likely than adults to be infected with group B streptococcus or Haemophilus influenza, if not immunized.

Symptoms

Symptoms usually come on quickly, with joint swelling, intense joint pain, and low-grade fever.

Symptoms in newborns or infants:

- Cries when infected joint is moved (example: diaper change causes crying if hip joint is infected)
- Irritability
- Fever
- Unable to move the limb with the infected joint (pseudoparalysis)

Symptoms in children and adults:

- Inability to move the limb with the infected joint (pseudoparalysis)
- Intense joint pain
- Joint swelling

- Joint redness
- Low-grade fever

Chills may occur, but are uncommon.

Exams and Tests

- Blood culture
- Joint fluid analysis and culture
- X-ray of affected joint

Treatment

Antibiotics are used to treat the infection.

Rest, immobilization, elevation, and cool compresses may help relieve pain. Performing exercises for the affected joint helps the recovery process.

If joint (synovial) fluid builds up rapidly in the joint as a result of the infection, frequent aspiration of the fluid by inserting a needle into the joint may be needed. Severe cases may need surgery to drain the infected joint fluid.

Outlook (Prognosis)

Recovery is good with prompt antibiotic treatment. If treatment is delayed, permanent joint damage may result.

Possible Complications

- Joint degeneration (arthritis)

When to Contact a Medical Professional

Call for an appointment with your health care provider if you develop symptoms of septic arthritis.

Prevention

Preventive (prophylactic) antibiotics may be helpful for people at high risk.

Chapter 16

Lupus

Defining Lupus

Lupus is one of many disorders of the immune system known as autoimmune diseases. In autoimmune diseases, the immune system turns against parts of the body it is designed to protect. This leads to inflammation and damage to various body tissues. Lupus can affect many parts of the body, including the joints, skin, kidneys, heart, lungs, blood vessels, and brain. Although people with the disease may have many different symptoms, some of the most common ones include extreme fatigue, painful or swollen joints (arthritis), unexplained fever, skin rashes, and kidney problems.

At present, there is no cure for lupus. However, lupus can be effectively treated with drugs, and most people with the disease can lead active, healthy lives. Lupus is characterized by periods of illness, called flares, and periods of wellness, or remission. Understanding how to prevent flares and how to treat them when they do occur helps people with lupus maintain better health. Intense research is underway, and scientists funded by the NIH [National Institutes of Health] are continuing to make great strides in understanding the disease, which may ultimately lead to a cure.

From "Lupus," by the National Institute for Arthritis and Musculoskeletal and Skin Diseases (NIAMS, www.niams.nih.gov), part of the National Institutes of Health, August 2003. Revised by David A. Cooke, MD, FACP, July 5, 2009.

Two of the major questions researchers are studying are who gets lupus and why. We know that many more women than men have lupus. Lupus is three times more common in African American women than in Caucasian women and is also more common in women of Hispanic, Asian, and Native American descent. In addition, lupus can run in families, but the risk that a child or a brother or sister of a patient will also have lupus is still quite low. It is difficult to estimate how many people in the United States have the disease because its symptoms vary widely and its onset is often hard to pinpoint.

There are several kinds of lupus:

- **Systemic lupus erythematosus (SLE)** is the form of the disease that most people are referring to when they say "lupus." The word "systemic" means the disease can affect many parts of the body. The symptoms of SLE may be mild or serious. Although SLE usually first affects people between the ages of 15 and 45 years, it can occur in childhood or later in life as well. This text focuses on SLE.

- **Discoid lupus erythematosus** is a chronic skin disorder in which a red, raised rash appears on the face, scalp, or elsewhere. The raised areas may become thick and scaly and may cause scarring. The rash may last for days or years and may recur. A small percentage of people with discoid lupus have or develop SLE later.

- **Subacute cutaneous lupus erythematosus** refers to skin lesions that appear on parts of the body exposed to sun. The lesions do not cause scarring.

- **Drug-induced lupus** is a form of lupus caused by medications. Many different drugs can cause drug-induced lupus. Symptoms are similar to those of SLE (arthritis, rash, fever, and chest pain) and they typically go away completely when the drug is stopped. The kidneys and brain are rarely involved.

- **Neonatal lupus** is a rare disease that can occur in newborn babies of women with SLE, Sjögren syndrome, or no disease at all. Scientists suspect that neonatal lupus is caused by autoantibodies in the mother's blood called anti-Ro (SSA) and anti-La (SSB). Autoantibodies ("auto" means self) are blood proteins that act against the body's own parts. At birth, the babies have a skin rash, liver problems, and low blood counts. These symptoms gradually go away over several months. In rare instances, babies with neonatal lupus may have a serious heart problem that slows down the natural rhythm of the heart. Neonatal lupus is rare, and most infants of mothers with SLE are entirely healthy. All women who are pregnant and known to have anti-Ro (SSA) or anti-La (SSB) antibodies should be monitored by echocardiograms (a test that monitors the heart and surrounding blood vessels) during the 16th and 30th weeks of pregnancy.

It is important for women with SLE or other related autoimmune disorders to be under a doctor's care during pregnancy. Physicians can now identify mothers at highest risk for complications, allowing for prompt treatment of the infant at or before birth. SLE can also flare during pregnancy, and prompt treatment can keep the mother healthier longer.

Understanding What Causes Lupus

Lupus is a complex disease, and its cause is unknown. It is likely that a combination of genetic, environmental, and possibly hormonal factors work together to cause the disease. Scientists are making progress in understanding lupus. The fact that lupus can run in families indicates that its development has a genetic basis. Recent research suggests that genetics plays an important role; however, no specific "lupus gene" has been identified yet. Studies suggest that several different genes may be involved in determining a person's likelihood of developing the disease, which tissues and organs are affected, and the severity of disease. However, scientists believe that genes alone do not determine who gets lupus and that other factors also play a role. Some of the factors scientists are studying include sunlight, stress, certain drugs, and infectious agents such as viruses.

In lupus, the body's immune system does not work as it should. A healthy immune system produces proteins called antibodies and specific cells called lymphocytes that help fight and destroy viruses, bacteria, and other foreign substances that invade the body. In lupus, the immune system produces antibodies against the body's healthy cells and tissues. These antibodies, called autoantibodies, contribute to the inflammation of various parts of the body and can cause damage to organs and tissues. The most common type of autoantibody that develops in people with lupus is called an antinuclear antibody (ANA) because it reacts with parts of the cell's nucleus (command center). Doctors and scientists do not yet understand all of the factors that cause inflammation and tissue damage in lupus, and researchers are actively exploring them.

Symptoms of Lupus

Each person with lupus has slightly different symptoms that can range from mild to severe and may come and go over time. However, some of the most common symptoms of lupus include painful or swollen joints (arthritis), unexplained fever, and extreme fatigue. A characteristic red skin rash—the so-called butterfly or malar rash—may appear across the nose and cheeks. Rashes may also occur on the face and ears, upper arms, shoulders, chest, and hands. Because many people with lupus are sensitive to sunlight (called photosensitivity), skin rashes often first develop or worsen after sun exposure.

Common symptoms of lupus include the following:

- Painful or swollen joints and muscle pain

- Unexplained fever

- Red rashes, most commonly on the face

- Chest pain upon deep breathing

- Unusual loss of hair

- Pale or purple fingers or toes from cold or stress (Raynaud phenomenon)

- Sensitivity to the sun

- Swelling (edema) in legs or around eyes

- Mouth ulcers

- Swollen glands

- Extreme fatigue

Symptoms can range from mild to severe and may come and go over time.

Other symptoms of lupus include chest pain, hair loss, anemia (a decrease in red blood cells), mouth ulcers, and pale or purple fingers and toes from cold and stress. Some people also experience headaches, dizziness, depression, confusion, or seizures. New symptoms may continue to appear years after the initial diagnosis, and different symptoms can occur at different times. In some people with lupus, only one system of the body, such as the skin or joints, is affected. Other people experience symptoms in many parts of their body. Just how seriously a body system is affected varies from person to person. The following systems in the body also can be affected by lupus.

- **Kidneys:** Inflammation of the kidneys (nephritis) can impair their ability to get rid of waste products and other toxins from the body effectively. There is usually no pain associated with kidney involvement, although some patients may notice swelling in their ankles. Most often, the only indication of kidney disease is an abnormal urine or blood test. Because the kidneys are so important to overall health, lupus affecting the kidneys generally requires intensive drug treatment to prevent permanent damage.

- **Lungs:** Some people with lupus develop pleuritis, an inflammation of the lining of the chest cavity that causes chest pain, particularly with breathing. Patients with lupus also may get pneumonia.

- **Central nervous system:** In some patients, lupus affects the brain or central nervous system. This can cause headaches, dizziness, memory disturbances, vision problems, seizures, stroke, or changes in behavior.

- **Blood vessels:** Blood vessels may become inflamed (vasculitis), affecting the way blood circulates through the body. The inflammation may be mild and may not require treatment or may be severe and require immediate attention.

- **Blood:** People with lupus may develop anemia, leukopenia (a decreased number of white blood cells), or thrombocytopenia (a decrease in the number of platelets in the blood, which assist in clotting). Some people with lupus may have an increased risk for blood clots.

- **Heart:** In some people with lupus, inflammation can occur in the heart itself (myocarditis and endocarditis) or the membrane that surrounds it (pericarditis), causing chest pains or other symptoms. Lupus can also increase the risk of atherosclerosis (hardening of the arteries).

Diagnosing Lupus

Diagnosing lupus can be difficult. It may take months or even years for doctors to piece together the symptoms to diagnose this complex disease accurately. Making a correct diagnosis of lupus requires knowledge and awareness on the part of the doctor and good communication on the part of the patient. Giving the doctor a complete, accurate medical history (for example, what health problems you have had and for how long) is critical to the process of diagnosis. This information, along with a physical examination and the results of laboratory tests, helps the doctor consider other diseases that may mimic lupus, or determine if the patient truly has the disease. Reaching a diagnosis may take time as new symptoms appear.

No single test can determine whether a person has lupus, but several laboratory tests may help the doctor to make a diagnosis. The most useful tests identify certain autoantibodies often present in the blood of people with lupus. For example, the antinuclear antibody (ANA) test is commonly used to look for autoantibodies that react against components of the nucleus, or "command center," of the body's cells. Most people with lupus test positive for ANA; however, there are a number of other causes of a positive ANA besides lupus, including infections, other autoimmune diseases, and occasionally as a finding in healthy people. The ANA test simply provides another clue for the doctor to consider in making a diagnosis. In addition, there are blood tests for individual types of autoantibodies that are more specific to people with lupus, although not all people with lupus test positive for these and not all people with these antibodies have lupus. These antibodies include anti-DNA [deoxyribonucleic acid], anti-Sm, anti-RNP, anti-Ro (SSA), and anti-La (SSB). The doctor may use these antibody tests to help make a diagnosis of lupus.

Some tests are used less frequently but may be helpful if the cause of a person's symptoms remains unclear. The doctor may order a biopsy of the skin or kidneys if those body systems are affected. Some doctors may order a test for anticardiolipin (or antiphospholipid) antibody. The presence of this antibody may indicate increased risk for blood clotting and increased risk for miscarriage in pregnant women with lupus. Again, all these tests merely serve as tools to give the doctor clues and information in making a diagnosis. The doctor will look at the entire picture—medical history, symptoms, and test results—to determine if a person has lupus.

Other laboratory tests are used to monitor the progress of the disease once it has been diagnosed. A complete blood count, urinalysis, blood chemistries, and the erythrocyte sedimentation rate (ESR) test can provide valuable information. Another common test measures the blood level of a group of substances called complement. People with lupus often have increased ESRs and low complement levels, especially during flares of the disease. X-rays and other imaging tests can help doctors see the organs affected by SLE.

Treating Lupus

Diagnosing and treating lupus are often a team effort between the patient and several types of health care professionals. A person with lupus can go to his or her family doctor or internist, or can visit a rheumatologist. A rheumatologist is a doctor who specializes in rheumatic diseases (arthritis and other inflammatory disorders, often involving the immune system). Clinical immunologists (doctors specializing in immune system disorders) may also treat people with lupus. As treatment progresses, other professionals often help. These may include nurses, psychologists, social workers, nephrologists (doctors who treat kidney disease), hematologists (doctors specializing in blood disorders), dermatologists (doctors who treat skin disease), and neurologists (doctors specializing in disorders of the nervous system).

The range and effectiveness of treatments for lupus have increased dramatically, giving doctors more choices in how to manage the disease. It is important for the patient to work closely with the doctor and take an active role in managing the disease. Once lupus has been diagnosed, the doctor will develop a treatment plan based on the patient's age, sex, health, symptoms, and lifestyle. Treatment plans are tailored to the individual's needs and may change over time. In developing a treatment plan, the doctor has several goals: to prevent flares, to treat them when they do occur, and to minimize organ damage and complications. The doctor and patient should reevaluate the plan regularly to ensure it is as effective as possible.

NSAIDs: For people with joint or chest pain or fever, drugs that decrease inflammation, called nonsteroidal anti-inflammatory drugs (NSAIDs), are often used. While some NSAIDs, such as ibuprofen and naproxen, are available over the counter, a doctor's prescription is necessary for others. NSAIDs may be used alone or in combination with other types of drugs to control pain, swelling, and fever. Even though some NSAIDs may be purchased without a prescription, it is important that they be taken under a doctor's direction. Common side effects of NSAIDs can include stomach upset, heartburn, diarrhea, and fluid retention. Some people with lupus also develop liver, kidney, or even neurological complications, making it especially important to stay in close contact with the doctor while taking these medications.

Antimalarials: Antimalarials are another type of drug commonly used to treat lupus. These drugs were originally used to treat malaria, but doctors have found that they also are useful for lupus. A common antimalarial used to treat lupus is hydroxychloroquine (Plaquenil). It may be used alone or in combination with other drugs and generally is used to treat fatigue, joint pain, skin rashes, and inflammation of the lungs. Clinical studies have found that continuous treatment with antimalarials may prevent flares from recurring. Side effects of antimalarials can include stomach upset and, extremely rarely, damage to the retina of the eye.

Corticosteroids: The mainstay of lupus treatment involves the use of corticosteroid hormones, such as prednisone (Deltasone), hydrocortisone, methylprednisolone (Medrol), and dexamethasone (Decadron, Hexadrol). Corticosteroids are related to cortisol, which is a natural anti-inflammatory hormone. They work by rapidly suppressing inflammation. Corticosteroids can be given by mouth, in creams applied to the skin, or by injection. Because they are potent drugs, the doctor will seek the lowest dose with the greatest benefit. Short-term side effects of corticosteroids include swelling, increased appetite, and weight gain. These side effects generally stop when the drug is stopped. It is dangerous to stop taking corticosteroids suddenly, so it is very important that the doctor and patient work together in changing the corticosteroid dose. Sometimes doctors give very large amounts of corticosteroid by vein over a brief period of time (days) ("bolus" or "pulse" therapy). With this treatment, the typical side effects are less likely and slow withdrawal is unnecessary.

Long-term side effects of corticosteroids can include stretch marks on the skin, weakened or damaged bones (osteoporosis and osteonecrosis), high blood pressure, damage to the arteries, high blood sugar (diabetes), infections, and cataracts. Typically, the higher the dose and the longer they are taken, the greater the risk and severity of side effects. Researchers are working to develop ways to limit or offset the use of corticosteroids. For example, corticosteroids may be used in combination with other, less potent drugs, or the doctor may try to slowly decrease the dose once the disease is under control. People with lupus who are using corticosteroids should talk to their doctors about taking supplemental calcium and vitamin D or other drugs to reduce the risk of osteoporosis (weakened, fragile bones).

Immunosuppressives: For some patients whose kidneys or central nervous systems are affected by lupus, a type of drug called an immunosuppressive may be used. Immunosuppressives, such as cyclophosphamide (Cytoxan) and mycophenolate mofetil (CellCept), restrain the overactive immune system by blocking the production of immune cells. These drugs may be given by mouth or by infusion (dripping the drug into the vein through a small tube). Side effects may include nausea, vomiting, hair loss, bladder problems, decreased fertility, and increased risk of cancer and infection. The risk for side effects increases with the length of treatment. As with other treatments for lupus, there is a risk of relapse after the immunosuppressives have been stopped.

Other therapies: In some patients, methotrexate (Folex, Mexate, Rheumatrex), a disease-modifying antirheumatic drug, may be used to help control the disease. Working closely with the doctor helps ensure that treatments for lupus are as successful as possible. Because some treatments may cause harmful side effects, it is important to report any new symptoms to the doctor promptly. It is also important not to stop or change treatments without talking to the doctor first.

Alternative and complementary therapies: Because of the nature and cost of the medications used to treat lupus and the potential for serious side effects, many patients seek other ways of treating the disease. Some alternative approaches people have tried include special diets, nutritional supplements, fish oils, ointments and creams, chiropractic treatment, and homeopathy. Although these methods may not be harmful in and of themselves, and may be associated with symptomatic or psychosocial benefit, no research to date shows that they affect the disease process or prevent organ damage. Some alternative or complementary approaches may help the patient cope or reduce some of the stress associated with living with a chronic illness. If the doctor feels the approach has value and will not be harmful, it can be incorporated into the patient's treatment plan. However, it is important not to neglect regular health care or treatment of serious symptoms. An open dialogue between the patient and physician about the relative values of complementary and alternative therapies allows the patient to make an informed choice about treatment options.

Lupus and Quality of Life

Despite the symptoms of lupus and the potential side effects of treatment, people with lupus can maintain a high quality of life overall. One key to managing lupus is to understand the disease and its impact. Learning to recognize the warning signs of a flare can help the patient take steps to ward it off or reduce its intensity. Many people with lupus experience increased fatigue, pain, a rash, fever, abdominal discomfort, headache, or dizziness just before a flare. Developing strategies to prevent flares can also be helpful, such as learning to recognize your warning signals and maintaining good communication with your doctor.

It is also important for people with lupus to receive regular health care, instead of seeking help only when symptoms worsen. Results from a medical exam and laboratory work on a regular basis allow the doctor to note any changes and to identify and treat flares early. The treatment plan, which is tailored to the individual's specific needs and circumstances, can be adjusted accordingly. If new symptoms are identified early, treatments may be more effective. Other concerns also can be addressed at regular checkups. The doctor can provide guidance about such issues as the use of sunscreens, stress reduction, and the importance of structured exercise and rest, as well as birth control and family planning. Because people with lupus can be more susceptible to infections, the doctor may recommend yearly influenza vaccinations or pneumococcal vaccinations for some patients.

Women with lupus should receive regular preventive health care, such as gynecological and breast examinations. Men with lupus should consider whether to have the prostate-specific antigen (PSA) test. Both men and women need to have their blood pressure and cholesterol checked on a regular basis. Due to a markedly elevated risk of cardiovascular disease, many experts recommend that all patients with lupus should take a type of cholesterol-lowering medication, known as a statin. If a person is taking corticosteroids or antimalarial medications, an eye exam should be done at least yearly to screen for and treat eye problems.

Staying healthy requires extra effort and care for people with lupus, so it becomes especially important to develop strategies for maintaining wellness. Wellness involves close attention to the body, mind, and spirit. One of the primary goals of wellness for people with lupus is coping with the stress of having a chronic disorder. Effective stress management varies from person to person. Some approaches that may help include exercise, relaxation techniques such as meditation, and setting priorities for spending time and energy.

Developing and maintaining a good support system is also important. A support system may include family, friends, medical professionals, community organizations, and support groups. Participating in a support group can provide emotional help, boost self-esteem and morale, and help develop or improve coping skills.

Warning Signs of a Flare

- Increased fatigue
- Pain
- Rash
- Fever
- Abdominal discomfort
- Headache
- Dizziness

Preventing a Flare

- Learn to recognize your warning signals.
- Maintain good communication with your doctor.
- Learning more about lupus may also help. Studies have shown that patients who are well-informed and participate actively in their own care experience less pain, make fewer visits to the doctor, build self-confidence, and remain more active.

Tips for Working with Your Doctor

- Seek a health care provider who is familiar with SLE and who will listen to and address your concerns.
- Provide complete, accurate medical information.
- Make a list of your questions and concerns in advance.
- Be honest and share your point of view with the health care provider.
- Ask for clarification or further explanation if you need it.
- Talk to other members of the health care team, such as nurses, therapists, or pharmacists.
- Do not hesitate to discuss sensitive subjects (for example, birth control, intimacy) with your doctor.
- Discuss any treatment changes with your doctor before making them.

Pregnancy for Women with Lupus

Although a lupus pregnancy is considered high risk, most women with lupus carry their babies safely to the end of their pregnancy. Women with lupus have a higher rate of miscarriage and premature births compared with the general population. In addition, women who have antiphospholipid antibodies are at a greater risk of miscarriage in the second trimester because of their increased risk of blood clotting in the placenta. Lupus patients with a history of kidney disease have a higher risk of preeclampsia (hypertension with a buildup of excess watery fluid in cells or tissues of the body). Pregnancy counseling and planning before pregnancy are important. Ideally, a woman should have no signs or symptoms of lupus and be taking no medications for at least 6 months before she becomes pregnant.

Some women may experience a mild to moderate flare during or after their pregnancy; others do not. Pregnant women with lupus, especially those taking corticosteroids, also are more likely to develop high blood pressure, diabetes, hyperglycemia (high blood sugar), and kidney complications, so regular care and good nutrition during pregnancy are essential. It is also advisable to have access to a neonatal (newborn) intensive care unit at the time of delivery in case the baby requires special medical attention.

Current Research

Lupus is the focus of intense research as scientists try to determine what causes the disease and how it can best be treated. Some of the questions they are working to answer include: Why are women more likely than men to have the disease? Why are there more cases of lupus in some racial and ethnic groups? What goes wrong in the immune system, and why? How can we correct the way the immune system functions once something goes wrong? What treatment approaches will work best to lessen lupus symptoms? How do we cure lupus?

To help answer these questions, scientists are developing new and better ways to study the disease. They are doing laboratory studies that compare various aspects of the immune systems of people with lupus with those of other people both with and without lupus. They also use mice with disorders resembling lupus to better understand the abnormalities of the immune system that occur in lupus and to identify possible new therapies.

The National Institute of Arthritis and Musculoskeletal and Skin Diseases (NIAMS), a component of the Department of Health and

Human Services' National Institutes of Health (NIH), has a major focus on lupus research in its on-campus program in Bethesda, Maryland. By evaluating patients with lupus and their relatives, researchers on campus are learning more about how lupus develops and changes over time. The NIAMS also funds many lupus researchers across the United States. Some of these researchers are studying the genetic factors that increase a person's risk for developing lupus. To help scientists gain new knowledge, the NIAMS also has established Specialized Centers of Research devoted specifically to lupus research. In addition, the NIAMS is funding lupus registries that gather medical information as well as blood and tissue samples from patients and their relatives. This gives researchers across the country access to information and materials they can use to help identify genes that determine susceptibility to the disease.

Identifying genes that play a role in the development of lupus is an active area of research. For example, researchers suspect that a genetic defect in a cellular process called apoptosis, or "programmed cell death," exists in people with lupus. Apoptosis is similar to the process that causes leaves to turn color in autumn and fall from trees; it allows the body to eliminate cells that have fulfilled their function and typically need to be replaced. If there is a problem in the apoptosis process, harmful cells may stay around and do damage to the body's own tissues. For example, in a mutant mouse strain that develops a lupus-like illness, one of the genes that control apoptosis is defective. When it is replaced by a normal gene, the mice no longer develop signs of the disease. Scientists are studying what role genes involved in apoptosis may play in human disease development.

Studying genes for complement, a series of proteins in the blood that play an important part in the immune system, is another active area of lupus research. Complement acts as a backup for antibodies, helping them destroy foreign substances that invade the body. If there is a decrease in complement, the body is less able to fight or destroy foreign substances. If these substances are not removed from the body, the immune system may become overactive and begin to make autoantibodies.

Recent large studies of families with lupus have identified a number of genetic regions that appear to be associated with risk of SLE. Although the specific genes and their function remain unknown, intensive work in mapping the entire human genome offers promise that these genes will be identified in the near future. This should provide knowledge of the complex factors that contribute to lupus susceptibility.

NIAMS-funded researchers are uncovering the impact of genetic, socioeconomic, and cultural factors on the course and outcome of lupus in Hispanics, African Americans, and Caucasians. Preliminary data show that African American and Hispanic lupus patients typically have more kidney damage compared with Caucasians. In addition, NIAMS-funded researchers found that African American lupus patients have more skin damage compared with Hispanics and Caucasians, and that the death rate from lupus is higher in African Americans and Hispanics compared with Caucasians.

It is thought that autoimmune diseases, such as lupus, occur when a genetically susceptible individual encounters an unknown environmental agent or trigger. In this circumstance, an abnormal immune response can be initiated that leads to the signs and symptoms of lupus. Research has focused on both the genetic susceptibility and the environmental trigger. Although the environmental trigger remains unknown, microbial agents such as Epstein-Barr virus and others have been considered.

Researchers also are studying other factors that may affect a person's susceptibility to lupus. For example, because lupus is more common in women than in men, some researchers are investigating the role of hormones and other male-female differences in the development and course of the disease. Two recent studies funded by the NIH that focused on the safety and effectiveness of oral contraceptives (birth control pills) and hormone replacement therapy in women with lupus concluded they did not increase the risk of flares. Doctors have worried about the wisdom of prescribing oral contraceptives or estrogen replacement therapy for women with lupus because of a widely held view that estrogens can make the disease worse. Scientists do not know the effects of oral contraceptives on women with antiphospholipid antibody syndrome. Interestingly, other data suggests that women who take oral contraceptives may be more likely to develop lupus in the first place, so scientists' understanding of these relationships remain incomplete.

Patients with lupus are at risk of developing atherosclerotic vascular disease (hardening of the blood vessels that can cause heart attack, angina, or stroke). The increased risk is due partly to having lupus and partly to steroid therapy. Preventing atherosclerotic vascular disease in lupus patients is a new area of study. NIAMS-funded researchers are studying the most effective ways to manage cardiovascular risk factors and prevent cardiovascular disease in adult lupus patients.

In childhood lupus, researchers are evaluating the safety and effectiveness of drugs called statins that lower LDL (or bad) cholesterol levels as a method of preventing fat buildup in the blood vessels.

One out of five lupus patients experiences symptoms such as headaches, dizziness, memory disturbances, stroke, or changes in behavior that result from changes in the brain or other parts of the central nervous system. Such lupus patients have what is called "neuropsychiatric" lupus. NIAMS-funded scientists are applying new tools such as brain imaging techniques to discover cellular activity and specific genes that may cause neuropsychiatric lupus. By uncovering the mechanisms responsible for central nervous system damage in lupus patients, researchers hope to move closer to improved diagnosis and treatment for patients with neuropsychiatric lupus.

Researchers are focusing on finding better treatments for lupus. A primary goal of this research is to develop treatments that can effectively minimize the use of corticosteroids. Scientists are trying to identify combination therapies that may be more effective than single treatment approaches. Another goal is to improve the treatment and management of lupus in the kidneys and central nervous system. For example, a 20-year study supported by the NIAMS and the NIH found that combining cyclophosphamide with prednisone helped delay or prevent kidney failure, a serious complication of lupus.

On the basis of new information about the disease process, scientists are using novel "biologic agents" to selectively block parts of the immune system. Development and testing of these new drugs, which are based on compounds that occur naturally in the body, comprise an exciting and promising new area of lupus research. The hope is that these treatments not only will be effective, but also will have fewer side effects. Preliminary research suggests that white blood cells known as B cells may play a key role in the development of lupus. Biologics that interfere with B cell function or block the interactions of immune cells are active areas of research. These targeted treatments hold promise because they have the advantage of reduced side effects and adverse reactions compared with conventional therapies. Clinical trials have tested the safety and effectiveness of rituximab (also called anti-CD20 or Rituxan®) and abatacept (Orencia®) in treating people with lupus. Rituximab is a genetically engineered antibody that blocks the production of B cells, and abatacept blocks production of several inflammatory hormones. Results have been disappointing to date, but other studies are still in progress. Other treatment options currently being explored include reconstructing the immune system by bone marrow transplantation. In the future, gene therapy also may play an important role in lupus treatment.

Chapter 17

Myositis

Dermatomyositis

What is dermatomyositis?

Dermatomyositis is one of a group of muscle diseases known as the inflammatory myopathies, which are characterized by chronic muscle inflammation accompanied by muscle weakness. Dermatomyositis' cardinal symptom is a skin rash that precedes or accompanies progressive muscle weakness. The rash looks patchy, with bluish-purple or red discolorations, and characteristically develops on the eyelids and on muscles used to extend or straighten joints, including knuckles, elbows, heels, and toes. Red rashes may also occur on the face, neck, shoulders, upper chest, back, and other locations, and there may be swelling in the affected areas. The rash sometimes occurs without obvious muscle involvement. Adults with dermatomyositis may experience weight loss or a low-grade fever, have inflamed lungs, and be sensitive to light. Children and adults with dermatomyositis may develop calcium deposits, which appear as hard bumps under the skin or in the muscle (called calcinosis). Calcinosis most often occurs 1–3 years after the disease begins. These deposits are seen more often in children with

This chapter contains text from "Dermatomyositis Information Page," "Inclusion Body Myositis Information Page," and "Polymyositis Information Page," by the National Institute of Neurological Disorders and Stroke (NINDS, www.ninds.nih.gov), part of the National Institutes of Health, January 29, 2009.

211

dermatomyositis than in adults. In some cases of dermatomyositis, distal muscles (muscles located away from the trunk of the body, such as those in the forearms and around the ankles and wrists) may be affected as the disease progresses. Dermatomyositis may be associated with collagen-vascular or autoimmune diseases, such as lupus.

Is there any treatment?

There is no cure for dermatomyositis, but the symptoms can be treated. Options include medication, physical therapy, exercise, heat therapy (including microwave and ultrasound), orthotics and assistive devices, and rest. The standard treatment for dermatomyositis is a corticosteroid drug, given either in pill form or intravenously. Immunosuppressant drugs, such as azathioprine and methotrexate, may reduce inflammation in people who do not respond well to prednisone. Periodic treatment using intravenous immunoglobulin can also improve recovery. Other immunosuppressive agents used to treat the inflammation associated with dermatomyositis include cyclosporine A, cyclophosphamide, and tacrolimus. Physical therapy is usually recommended to prevent muscle atrophy and to regain muscle strength and range of motion. Many individuals with dermatomyositis may need a topical ointment, such as topical corticosteroids, for their skin disorder. They should wear a high-protection sunscreen and protective clothing. Surgery may be required to remove calcium deposits that cause nerve pain and recurrent infections.

What is the prognosis?

Most cases of dermatomyositis respond to therapy. The disease is usually more severe and resistant to therapy in individuals with cardiac or pulmonary problems.

What research is being done?

The National Institute of Neurological Disorders and Stroke (NINDS) and other institutes of the National Institutes of Health (NIH) conduct research relating to dermatomyositis in laboratories at the NIH and support additional research through grants to major medical institutions across the country. Currently funded research is exploring patterns of gene expression among the inflammatory myopathies, the role of viral infection as a precursor to the disorders, and the safety and efficacy of various treatment regimens.

Inclusion Body Myositis

What is inclusion body myositis?

Inclusion body myositis (IBM) is one of a group of muscle diseases known as the inflammatory myopathies, which are characterized by chronic muscle inflammation accompanied by muscle weakness. The onset of muscle weakness in IBM is generally gradual (over months or years) and affects both proximal (close to the trunk of the body) and distal (further away from the trunk) muscles. Muscle weakness may affect only one side of the body. Falling and tripping are usually the first noticeable symptoms of IBM. For some individuals, the disorder begins with weakness in the wrists and fingers that causes difficulty with pinching, buttoning, and gripping objects. There may be weakness of the wrist and finger muscles and atrophy (thinning or loss of muscle bulk) of the forearm muscles and quadriceps muscles in the legs. Difficulty swallowing occurs in approximately half of IBM cases. Symptoms of the disease usually begin after the age of 50, although the disease can occur earlier. IBM occurs more frequently in men than in women.

Is there any treatment?

There is no cure for IBM, nor is there a standard course of treatment. The disease is generally unresponsive to corticosteroids and immunosuppressive drugs. Some evidence suggests that intravenous immunoglobulin may have a slight, but short-lasting, beneficial effect in a small number of cases.

Physical therapy may be helpful in maintaining mobility. Other therapy is symptomatic and supportive.

What is the prognosis?

IBM is generally resistant to all therapies and its rate of progression appears to be unaffected by currently available treatments.

Polymyositis

What is polymyositis?

Polymyositis is one of a group of muscle diseases known as the inflammatory myopathies, which are characterized by chronic muscle inflammation accompanied by muscle weakness. Polymyositis affects skeletal muscles (those involved with making movement) on both sides of the body. It is rarely seen in persons under age 18; most cases are in adults between the ages of 31 and 60. Slow, but progressive muscle weakness starts in the proximal muscles (muscles closest to the trunk of the body), which eventually leads to difficulties climbing stairs, rising from a sitting position, lifting objects, or reaching overhead. People with polymyositis may also experience arthritis, shortness of breath, difficulty swallowing and speaking, and heart arrhythmias. In some cases of polymyositis, distal muscles (muscles further away from the trunk of the body, such as those in the forearms and around the ankles and wrists) may be affected as the disease progresses. Polymyositis may be associated with collagen-vascular or autoimmune diseases, such as lupus. Polymyositis may also be associated with infectious disorders, such as HIV (human immunodeficiency virus) or AIDS (acquired immunodeficiency syndrome).

Is there any treatment?

There is no cure for polymyositis, but the symptoms can be treated. Options include medication, physical therapy, exercise, heat therapy (including microwave and ultrasound), orthotics and assistive devices, and rest. The standard treatment for polymyositis is a corticosteroid drug, given either in pill form or intravenously. Immunosuppressant drugs, such as azathioprine and methotrexate, may reduce inflammation in people who do not respond well to prednisone. Periodic treatment using intravenous immunoglobulin can also improve recovery. Other immunosuppressive agents used to treat the inflammation associated with polymyositis include cyclosporine A, cyclophosphamide, and tacrolimus. Physical therapy is usually recommended to prevent muscle atrophy and to regain muscle strength and range of motion.

What is the prognosis?

The prognosis for polymyositis varies. Most people respond fairly well to therapy, but some have a more severe disease that does not respond adequately to therapies and are left with significant disability. In rare cases individuals with severe and progressive muscle weakness will develop respiratory failure or pneumonia. Difficulty swallowing may cause weight loss and malnutrition.

Chapter 18

Osteoporosis

Chapter Contents

Section 18.1

Understanding Osteoporosis

From "Handout on Health: Osteoporosis," by the National Institute on Arthritis and Musculoskeletal and Skin Diseases (NIAMS, www.niams .nih.gov), part of the National Institutes of Health, April 2007.

Defining Osteoporosis

Osteoporosis is a disease marked by reduced bone strength leading to an increased risk of fractures, or broken bones. Bone strength has two main features: bone mass (amount of bone) and bone quality. Osteoporosis is the major underlying cause of fractures in postmenopausal women and the elderly. Fractures occur most often in bones of the hip, spine, and wrist, but any bone can be affected. Some fractures can be permanently disabling, especially when they occur in the hip.

Osteoporosis is often called a "silent disease" because it usually progresses without any symptoms until a fracture occurs or one or more vertebrae (bones in the spine) collapse. Collapsed vertebrae may first be felt or seen when a person develops severe back pain, loss of height, or spine malformations such as a stooped or hunched posture. Bones affected by osteoporosis may become so fragile that fractures occur spontaneously or as the result of minor bumps, falls, or normal stresses and strains such as bending, lifting, or even coughing.

Many people think that osteoporosis is a natural and unavoidable part of aging. However, medical experts now believe that osteoporosis is largely preventable. Furthermore, people who already have osteoporosis can take steps to prevent or slow further progress of the disease and reduce their risk of future fractures. Although osteoporosis was once viewed primarily as a disease of old age, it is now recognized as a disease that can stem from less than optimal bone growth during childhood and adolescence, as well as from bone loss later in life.

The Occurrence and Impact of Osteoporosis

In the United States today, an estimated 10 million people over age 50 have osteoporosis and nearly 34 million have low bone mass that puts them at increased risk for developing the disease. Four out of five people who have osteoporosis are women, but about 2 million men in the United States also have the disease and 14 million more have low bone mass that puts them at risk for it. One in two women and as many as one in four men over age 50 will have an osteoporosis-related fracture in their lifetime.

Osteoporosis can strike at any age, although the risk for developing the disease increases as you get older. In the future, more people will be at risk for developing osteoporosis because people are living longer and the number of elderly people in the population is increasing.

Osteoporosis affects women and men of all races and ethnic groups. It is most common in non-Hispanic white women and Asian women. African American women have a lower risk of developing osteoporosis, but they are still at significant risk. For Hispanic and Native American women the data aren't clear. Among men, osteoporosis is more common in non-Hispanic whites and Asians than in men of other ethnic or racial groups.

The cost of osteoporosis to society is high. In 2002 dollars, between $12.2 billion and $17.9 billion was spent in the United States on hospitals and nursing homes for people with osteoporosis-related and associated fractures, and the costs are rising. The indirect costs of the disease, such as those resulting from reduced productivity and lost wages, are unknown. In addition to the financial costs, osteoporosis takes a toll in terms of reduced quality of life for many people who suffer fractures. It can also affect the lives of family members and friends who serve as caregivers.

Of all fractures, hip fractures have the most serious impact. Most hip fractures require hospitalization and surgery; some hip fracture patients require nursing home placement. Fifty percent of people who fracture a hip will be unable to walk without assistance. About one in five hip fracture patients over age 50 die in the year following their fracture as a result of associated medical complications. Vertebral fractures also can have serious consequences, including chronic back pain and disability. They have also been linked to increased mortality in older people.

Bone Basics

Bone is a living tissue that supports our muscles, protects vital internal organs, and stores most of the body's calcium. It consists mainly of a framework of tough, elastic fibers of a protein called collagen and crystals of calcium phosphate mineral that harden and strengthen the framework. The combination of collagen and calcium phosphate makes bones strong yet flexible to hold up under stress.

Bone also contains living cells, including some that nourish the tissue and others that control the process known as bone remodeling. Throughout life, our bones are constantly being renewed by means of this remodeling process, in which old bone is removed (bone resorption) and replaced by new bone (bone formation). Bone remodeling is carried out through the coordinated actions of bone-removing cells called osteoclasts and bone-forming cells called osteoblasts.

During childhood and the teenage years, new bone is added to the skeleton faster than old bone is removed, or resorbed. As a result, bones grow in both size and strength. After you stop growing taller, bone formation continues at a faster pace than resorption until around the early twenties, when women and men reach their peak bone mass, or maximum amount of bone. Peak bone mass is influenced by various genetic and external, or environmental, factors, including whether you are male or female (your sex), hormones, nutrition, and physical activity. Genetic factors may determine as much as 50 to 90 percent of bone mass; environmental factors account for the remaining 10 to 50 percent. This means you have some control over your peak bone mass.

After your early twenties, your bone mass may remain stable or decrease very gradually for a period of years, depending on a variety of lifestyle factors such as diet and physical activity. Starting in midlife, both men and women experience an age-related decline in bone mass. Women lose bone rapidly in the first 4 to 8 years after menopause (the completion of a full year without a menstrual period), which usually occurs between ages 45 and 55. By age 65, men and women tend to be losing bone tissue at the same rate, and this more gradual bone loss continues throughout life.

Causes of Osteoporosis

A major cause of osteoporosis is less than optimal bone growth during childhood and adolescence, resulting in failure to reach optimal peak bone mass. Thus, peak bone mass attained early in life is one of the most important factors affecting your risk of osteoporosis in later years. People who start out with greater reserves of bone (higher peak bone mass) are less likely to develop osteoporosis when bone loss occurs as a result of aging, menopause, or other factors. Other causes of osteoporosis are bone loss due to a greater than expected rate of bone resorption, a decreased rate of bone formation, or both.

Deterioration of bone quality, which reflects the internal structure, or architecture, of bone as well as other factors, is also thought to contribute to decreased bone strength and increased fracture risk. Scientists do not yet clearly understand all the factors that affect bone quality and the relationship between these factors and the risk of osteoporosis and fractures. However, this is an active area of research.

A major contributor to bone loss in women during later life is the reduction in estrogen production that occurs with menopause. Estrogen is a sex hormone that plays a critical role in building and maintaining bone. Decreased estrogen, whether due to natural menopause, surgical removal of the ovaries, or chemotherapy or radiation treatments for cancer, can lead to bone loss and eventually osteoporosis. After menopause, the rate of bone loss speeds up as the amount of estrogen produced by a woman's ovaries drops dramatically. Bone loss is most rapid in the first few years after menopause but continues into the postmenopausal years.

In men, sex hormone levels also decline after middle age, but the decline is more gradual. These declines probably also contribute to bone loss in men after around age 50.

Osteoporosis can also result from bone loss that may accompany a wide range of disease conditions, eating disorders, and certain medications and medical treatments. For instance, osteoporosis may be caused by long-term use of some antiseizure medications (anticonvulsants) and glucocorticoid medications such as prednisone and cortisone. Glucocorticoids are anti-inflammatory drugs used to treat many diseases, including rheumatoid arthritis, lupus, asthma, and Crohn disease. Other causes of osteoporosis include alcoholism, anorexia nervosa, abnormally low levels of sex hormones, hyperthyroidism, kidney disease, and certain gastrointestinal disorders. Sometimes osteoporosis results from a combination of causes.

Risk Factors for Osteoporosis

Factors that are linked to the development of osteoporosis or contribute to an individual's likelihood of developing the disease are called risk factors. Many people with osteoporosis have several risk factors for the disease, but others who develop osteoporosis have no identified risk factors. There are some risk factors that you cannot change, and others that you can or may be able to change.

Risk factors you cannot change include the following:

- **Sex:** Your chances of developing osteoporosis are greater if you are a woman. Women have lower peak bone mass and smaller bones than men. They also lose bone more rapidly than men in middle age because of the dramatic reduction in estrogen levels that occurs with menopause.

- **Age:** The older you are, the greater your risk of osteoporosis. Bone loss builds up over time, and your bones become weaker as you age.

- **Body size:** Slender, thin-boned women are at greater risk, as are, surprisingly, taller women.

- **Race:** Caucasian (white) and Asian women are at highest risk. African American and Hispanic women have a lower but significant risk. Among men, Caucasians are at higher risk than others. These differences in risk can be explained in part—although not entirely—by differences in peak bone mass among these groups.

- **Family history:** Susceptibility to osteoporosis and fractures appears to be, in part, hereditary. People whose parents have a history of fractures also tend to have reduced bone mass and an increased risk for fractures.

Risk factors you can or may be able to change include the following:

- **Sex hormone deficiencies:** The most common manifestation of estrogen deficiency in premenopausal women is amenorrhea, the abnormal absence of menstrual periods. Missed or irregular periods can be caused by various factors, including hormonal disorders as well as extreme levels of physical activity combined with restricted calorie intake—for example, in female marathon runners, ballet dancers, and women who spend a great deal of time and energy working out at the gym. Low estrogen levels in women after menopause and low testosterone levels in men also increase the risk of osteoporosis. Lower than normal estrogen levels in men may also play a role. Low testosterone and estrogen levels are often a cause of osteoporosis in men being treated with certain medications for prostate cancer.

- **Diet:** From childhood into old age, a diet low in calcium and vitamin D can increase your risk of osteoporosis and fractures. Excessive dieting or inadequate caloric intake can also be bad for bone health. People who are very thin and do not have much body fat to cushion falls have an increased risk of fracture.

- **Certain medical conditions:** In addition to sex hormone problems and eating disorders, other medical conditions—including a variety of genetic, endocrine, gastrointestinal, blood, and rheumatic disorders—are associated with an increased risk for osteoporosis. Anorexia nervosa, for example, is an eating disorder that leads to abnormally low body weight, malnutrition, amenorrhea, and other effects on the body that adversely affect bone health. Late onset of puberty and early menopause reduce lifetime estrogen exposure in women and also increase the risk of osteoporosis.

- **Medications:** Long-term use of certain medications, including glucocorticoids and some anticonvulsants, leads to bone loss and increased risk of osteoporosis. Other drugs that may lead to bone loss include anticlotting drugs, such as heparin; drugs that suppress the immune system, such as cyclosporine; and drugs used to treat prostate cancer.

- **An inactive lifestyle or extended bed rest:** Low levels of physical activity and prolonged periods of inactivity can contribute to an increased rate of bone loss. They also leave you in poor physical condition, which can increase your risk of falling and breaking a bone.

- **Excessive use of alcohol:** Chronic heavy drinking is a significant risk factor for osteoporosis.

- **Smoking:** Most studies indicate that smoking is a risk factor for osteoporosis and fracture, although the exact reasons for the harmful effects of tobacco use on bone health are still unclear.

Risk Factors for Osteoporosis-Related Fractures

Although low bone mass (or low bone density) plays an important role in determining a person's risk of osteoporosis, it is only one of many risk factors for fractures. Fracture risk results from a combination of bone-dependent and bone-independent factors. Various aspects of "bone geometry," such as tallness, hip structure, and thighbone (femur) length, can also affect your chances of breaking a bone if you fall. Increasing age, excessive weight loss, a history of fractures since age 45, having an existing spine fracture, and having a mother who fractured her hip all increase the risk of hip fracture independent of a person's bone density, and individuals with more risk factors have a higher chance of suffering a hip fracture.

Factors that increase the likelihood of falling and the severity of falls also contribute to fracture risk. These include decreased muscle strength, poor balance, impaired eyesight, and impaired mental abilities. The angle at which you fall also affects your risk of fracture. Use of certain medications, such as tranquilizers and muscle relaxants, and hazardous elements in your living environment, such as slippery throw rugs and icy sidewalks, can also increase your risk of falls.

Diagnosing Osteoporosis

Diagnosing osteoporosis involves several steps, starting with a physical exam and a careful medical history, blood and urine tests, and possibly a bone mineral density assessment. When recording information about your medical history, your doctor will ask questions to find out whether you have risk factors for osteoporosis and fractures. The doctor may ask about any fractures you have had, your lifestyle (including diet, exercise habits, and whether you smoke), current or past health problems and medications that could contribute to low bone mass and increased fracture risk, your family history of osteoporosis and other diseases, and, for women, your menstrual history. The doctor will also do a physical exam that should include checking for loss of height and changes in posture and may include checking your balance and gait (the way you walk).

If you have back pain or have experienced a loss in height or a change in posture, the doctor may request an x-ray of your spine to look for spinal fractures or malformations due to osteoporosis. However, x-rays cannot necessarily detect osteoporosis. The results of laboratory tests of blood and urine samples can help your doctor identify conditions that may be contributing to bone loss, such as hormonal problems or vitamin D deficiency. If the results of your physical exam, medical history, x-rays, or laboratory tests indicate that you may have osteoporosis or that you have significant risk factors for the disease, your doctor may recommend a bone density test.

Mineral is what gives hardness to bones, and the density of mineral in the bones is an important determinant of bone strength. Bone mineral density (BMD) testing can be used to definitively diagnose osteoporosis, detect low bone mass before osteoporosis develops, and help predict your risk of future fractures. In general, the lower your bone density, the higher your risk for fracture. The results of a bone density test will help guide decisions about starting therapy to prevent or treat osteoporosis. BMD testing may also be used to monitor the effectiveness of ongoing therapy.

The most widely recognized test for measuring bone mineral density is a quick, painless, noninvasive technology known as dual-energy x-ray absorptiometry (DXA). This technique, which uses low levels of x-rays, involves passing a scanner over your body while you are lying on a cushioned table. DXA can be used to determine BMD of the entire skeleton and at various sites that are prone to fracture, such as the hip, spine, or wrist. Bone density measurement by DXA at the hip and spine is generally considered the most reliable way to diagnose osteoporosis and predict fracture risk.

The doctor will compare your BMD test results to the average bone density of young, healthy people and to the average bone density of other people of your age, sex, and race. For both women and men, the diagnosis of osteoporosis using DXA measurements of BMD is currently based on a number called a T-score. Your T-score represents the extent to which your bone density differs from the average bone density of young, healthy people. If you are diagnosed with osteoporosis or very low bone density, or if your bone density is below a certain level and you have other risk factors for fractures, the doctor will talk with you about options for treatment or prevention of osteoporosis.

The U.S. Preventive Services Task Force, an independent panel of experts in primary care and prevention, recommends that all women age 65 and older be screened for osteoporosis. The task force also recommends that routine screening begin at age 60 for women at increased risk for fractures due to osteoporosis (for instance, those who have additional risk factors). If you have not been checked for osteoporosis and you are a woman over age 65, or if you suspect that you have significant risk factors for the disease, you may want to talk to your doctor about being evaluated. For example, if you are over 50 and have broken a bone, you may have osteoporosis or be at increased risk for the disease. You should also ask your doctor about osteoporosis if you notice that you have lost height or your posture has become stooped or hunched, or if you experience sudden back pain. You may also want to be evaluated for osteoporosis and fracture risk if you have a chronic disease or eating disorder known to increase the risk of osteoporosis, are taking one or more medications known to cause bone loss, or have multiple risk factors for osteoporosis and osteoporosis-related fractures.

Treating Osteoporosis

The primary goal in treating people with osteoporosis is preventing fractures. A comprehensive treatment program includes a focus on proper nutrition, exercise, and prevention of falls that may result in fractures. Your doctor may also prescribe one of several medications that have been shown to slow or stop bone loss or build new bone, increase bone density, and reduce fracture risk. If you take medication to prevent or treat osteoporosis, it is still essential that you obtain the recommended amounts of calcium and vitamin D. Exercising and maintaining other aspects of a healthy lifestyle are also important.

For people with osteoporosis resulting from another condition, the best approach is to identify and treat the underlying cause. If you are taking a medication that causes bone loss, your doctor may be able to reduce the dose of that medication or switch you to another medication that is effective but not harmful to your bones. If you have a disease that requires long-term glucocorticoid therapy, such as rheumatoid arthritis or lupus, you can also take certain medications approved for the prevention or treatment of osteoporosis associated with aging or menopause. Staying as active as possible, eating a healthy diet that includes adequate calcium and vitamins, and avoiding smoking and excess alcohol use are also important for people with osteoporosis resulting from other conditions. Children and adolescents with such conditions as juvenile rheumatic diseases and asthma can also be diagnosed with this kind of osteoporosis.

Medical specialists who treat osteoporosis include family physicians, internists, endocrinologists, geriatricians, gynecologists, orthopedic surgeons, rheumatologists, and physiatrists (doctors specializing in physical medicine and rehabilitation). Physical and occupational therapists and nurses may also participate in the care of people with osteoporosis.

Nutrition

A healthy, balanced diet that includes plenty of fruits and vegetables; enough calories; and adequate calcium, vitamin D, and vitamin K is essential for minimizing bone loss and maintaining overall health. Calcium and vitamin D are especially important for bone health. Calcium is the most important nutrient for preventing osteoporosis and for reaching peak bone mass. For healthy postmenopausal women who are not consuming enough calcium (1,200 mg per day) in their diet, calcium and vitamin D supplements help to preserve bone mass and prevent hip fracture. Calcium is also needed for the heart, muscles, and nerves to work properly and for blood to clot normally. We take in calcium from our diet and lose it from the body mainly through urine, feces, and sweat. The body depends on dietary calcium to build healthy new bone and avoid excessive loss of calcium from bone to meet other needs. The Institute of Medicine of the National Academy of Sciences recommends specific amounts of dietary calcium and vitamin D for various stages of life. Adults need 1,000 milligrams of calcium per day, and the recommendation increases to 1,200 milligrams after age 50.

Many people in the United States consume much less than the recommended amount of calcium in their diets. Good sources of calcium include low-fat dairy products; dark green leafy vegetables, including broccoli, bok choy, collards, and turnip greens; sardines and salmon with bones; soy beans, tofu, and other soy products; and calcium-fortified foods such as orange juice, cereals, and breads. If you have trouble getting enough calcium in your diet, you may need to take a calcium supplement such as calcium carbonate, calcium phosphate, or calcium citrate. Your daily calcium intake should not exceed 2,500 milligrams because too much calcium can cause problems such as kidney stones. Calcium coming from food sources provides better protection from kidney stones. Anyone who has had a kidney stone should increase their dietary calcium and decrease the amount from supplements as well as increase fluid intake.

Vitamin D is required for proper absorption of calcium from the intestine. It is made in the skin after exposure to sunlight. Fifteen minutes in the sun every day without sunscreen and with some of your skin exposed is enough to meet the body's needs for vitamin D. Only a few foods naturally contain significant amounts of vitamin D, including fatty fish and fish oils. Foods fortified with vitamin D, such as milk and cereals, are a major dietary source of vitamin D. Although many people obtain enough vitamin D naturally, studies show that vitamin D production decreases in older adults, in people who are housebound, and during the winter—especially in northern latitudes. If you are at risk for vitamin D deficiency, you can take multivitamins or calcium supplements that contain vitamin D to meet the recommended daily intake of 400 International Units (IU) for men and women age 51 to 70 and 600 IU for people over 70. Doses of more than 2,000 IU per day are not advised unless under the supervision of a doctor. Larger doses can be given initially to people who are deficient as a way to replenish stores of vitamin D.

Lifestyle

In addition to a healthy diet, a healthy lifestyle is important for optimizing bone health. You should avoid smoking and, if you drink alcohol, do so in moderation (no more than one drink per day is a good general guideline). It is also important to recognize that some prescription medications can cause bone loss or increase your risk of falling and breaking a bone. Talk to your doctor if you have concerns about any medications you are taking.

Exercise

Exercise is an important part of an osteoporosis treatment program. Physical activity is needed to build and maintain bone throughout adulthood, and complete bed rest leads to serious bone loss. The evidence suggests that the most beneficial physical activities for bone health include strength training or resistance training. Exercise can help maintain or even modestly increase bone density in adulthood and, together with adequate calcium and vitamin D intake, can help minimize age-related bone loss in older people. Exercise of various sorts has other important benefits for people with osteoporosis. It can reduce your risk of falling by increasing muscle mass and strength and improving coordination and balance. In older people, exercise also improves function and delays loss of independence.

Although exercise is beneficial for people with osteoporosis, it should not put any sudden or excessive strain on your bones. If you have osteoporosis, you should avoid high-impact exercise. To help ensure against fractures, a physical therapist or rehabilitation medicine specialist can recommend specific exercises to strengthen and support your back, teach you safe ways of moving and carrying out daily activities, and recommend an exercise program that is tailored to your circumstances. Other trained exercise specialists, such as exercise physiologists, may also be able to help you develop a safe and effective exercise program.

Fall Prevention

Fall prevention is a critical concern for men and women with osteoporosis. Falls increase your likelihood of fracturing a bone in the hip, wrist, spine, or other part of the skeleton. Fractures can affect your quality of life and lead to loss of independence and even premature death. A host of factors can contribute to your risk of falling.

Falls can be caused by impaired vision or balance, loss of muscle mass, and chronic or short-term illnesses that impair your mental or physical functioning. They can also be caused by the effects of certain medications, including sedatives or tranquilizers, sleeping pills, antidepressants, anticonvulsants, muscle relaxants, some heart medicines, blood pressure pills, and diuretics. Use of four or more prescription medications has also been shown to increase the risk for falling. Drinking alcoholic beverages is another risk factor. If you have osteoporosis, it is important to be aware of any physical changes you may be experiencing that affect your balance or gait and to discuss these changes with your doctor or other health care provider. It is also important to have regular checkups and tell your doctor if you have had problems with falling.

The force or impact of a fall (how hard you land) plays a major role in determining whether you will break a bone. Catching yourself so that you land on your hands or grabbing onto an object as you fall can prevent a hip fracture. You may break your wrist or arm instead, but the consequences are not as serious as if you break your hip. Studies have shown that wearing a specially designed garment that contains hip padding may reduce hip fractures resulting from falls in frail, elderly people living in nursing homes or residential care facilities, but use of the garments by residents is often low.

Falls can also be caused by factors in your environment that create unsafe conditions.

Outdoors and away from home, try these tips to reduce falls:

- Use a cane or walker for added stability.

- Wear shoes that give good support and have thin nonslip soles. Avoid wearing slippers and athletic shoes with deep treads.

- Walk on grass when sidewalks are slippery; in winter, sprinkle salt or kitty litter on slippery sidewalks.

- Be careful on highly polished floors that are slick and dangerous, especially when wet, and walk on plastic or carpet runners when possible.

- Stop at curbs and check their height before stepping up or down.

Indoors, try these tips to reduce falls:

- Keep rooms free of clutter, especially on floors.

- Keep floor surfaces smooth but not slippery.

- Wear shoes that give good support and have thin nonslip soles. Avoid wearing slippers and athletic shoes with deep treads.

- Be sure carpets and area rugs have skid-proof backing or are tacked to the floor. Use double-stick tape to keep rugs from slipping.

- Be sure stairwells are well lit and that stairs have handrails.

- Install grab bars on bathroom walls near tub, shower, and toilet.

- Use a rubber bath mat or slip-proof seat in the shower or tub.

- Improve the lighting in your home. Use a night light or flashlight if you get up at night.

- Use stepladders that are stable and have a handrail.

- Install ceiling fixtures or lamps that can be turned on by a switch near the room's entrance.

- If you live alone (or spend large amounts of time alone), consider purchasing a cordless phone; you won't have to rush to answer the phone when it rings and you can call for help if you do fall.

- Consider having a personal emergency-response system; you can use it to call for help if you fall.

Medications

The U.S. Food and Drug Administration (FDA) has approved several medications for prevention or treatment of osteoporosis, based on their ability to reduce fractures. Alendronate (Fosamax), raloxifene (Evista), risedronate (Actonel), and ibandronate (Boniva) are approved for the prevention and treatment of postmenopausal osteoporosis. Teriparatide (Forteo) is approved for treatment of the disease in postmenopausal women and men who are at high risk for fracture. Calcitonin (Miacalcin, Fortical) is also approved for treatment. Estrogen (hormone therapy) is approved for the prevention of postmenopausal osteoporosis, but has associated health risks that may outweigh its benefits. In addition, alendronate and risedronate are approved for treating osteoporosis in men and for use by men and women with glucocorticoid-induced osteoporosis.

Alendronate, risedronate, and ibandronate belong to a group of drugs known as bisphosphonates, which reduce the activity of cells that cause bone loss. In postmenopausal women with osteoporosis, the bisphosphonate drugs reduce bone loss, increase bone density in both the spine and hip, and reduce the risk of fracture. Side effects may include digestive system problems.

Raloxifene is also approved for the treatment and prevention of osteoporosis. It is one of a relatively new group of drugs known as selective estrogen receptor modulators (SERMs). These drugs are not estrogens, but they have estrogen-like effects on some tissues and estrogen-blocking effects on other tissues. Raloxifene mimics the effects of estrogen on bones, but does not have estrogen's potentially harmful effects on breast tissue or the uterus. Raloxifene has been shown to prevent bone loss, have beneficial effects on bone mass, and reduce the risk of spine fractures. It is taken as a tablet once a day. Side effects may include hot flashes, sweating, clot formation in some blood vessels, muscle soreness, weight gain, or a rash.

Teriparatide is an injectable form of human parathyroid hormone (PTH) that is approved for postmenopausal women and men with osteoporosis who are at high risk for having a fracture. It is the first approved agent for the treatment of osteoporosis that stimulates new bone formation. Teriparatide is taken by once-daily injection into the thigh or abdomen. This treatment stimulates new bone formation in both the spine and hip and reduces the risk of fractures in postmenopausal women and men. Side effects include nausea, dizziness, and leg cramps. Use of teriparatide for more than 2 years is not recommended because the effects of long-term treatment are not yet known. Following PTH treatment with a bisphosphonate drug will preserve the bone mass gains.

Calcitonin is approved for the treatment of osteoporosis in women who are at least 5 years beyond menopause. Calcitonin is a hormone involved in calcium regulation and bone metabolism. It is taken as a single daily nasal spray or as an injection under the skin. In women who are at least 5 years beyond menopause, calcitonin slows bone loss and increases spinal bone density. Some patients report that calcitonin also relieves pain from bone fractures. The effects of calcitonin on fracture risk are still unclear. Injected calcitonin does not affect other organs or systems in the body besides bone, but it may cause an allergic reaction. Side effects may include flushing of the face and hands, increased frequency of urination, nausea, and skin rash. The only side effects reported with nasal calcitonin are a runny nose and other signs of nasal irritation.

Estrogen and combined estrogen and progestin (hormone therapy) are approved for the prevention of postmenopausal osteoporosis as well as the treatment of moderate to severe hot flashes and vaginal dryness that may accompany menopause. Estrogen without an added progestin is recommended only for women who have had a hysterectomy (surgery to remove the uterus), because estrogen increases the risk of developing cancer of the uterine lining and progestin reduces that risk. Studies have shown that hormone therapy can increase bone density and prevent bone loss, and that estrogen plus progestin prevents osteoporosis-related fractures in the hip and other sites in postmenopausal women. Results of the NIH-sponsored Women's Health Initiative, a large, long-term study of disease prevention strategies in postmenopausal women, show that both estrogen alone as well as estrogen plus progestin prevent osteoporosis and fractures when used at the commonly administered doses. The drugs used in these trials were conjugated equine estrogens (CEE, 0.625 mg /day) and medroxyprogesterone acetate (MPA, 2.5 mg/day). At these doses, there was no protection from cardiovascular disease and an increase in strokes and blood clots. In the trial of combination therapy, there was also an increase in breast cancer. On the basis of these findings, medical experts concluded that, in most women, the harmful effects of long-term use of hormone therapy are likely to outweigh the disease prevention benefits. The Food and Drug Administration has recommended that women use hormone therapy at the lowest dose and for the shortest time. The risks and benefits of low-dose hormone therapy and estrogen patches are still unclear. Women who use, or are considering, hormone therapy (either estrogen plus progestin or estrogen alone) solely for the prevention of osteoporosis should carefully consider and discuss with their doctor other approved treatments. They should also talk to the doctor about whether the benefits of hormone therapy outweigh the potential harms in view of their personal preferences and individual risk factors for various diseases and consider whether lower doses of hormone therapy may be appropriate.

Alternative Therapies

Many people are interested in the use of natural estrogens, particularly phytoestrogens, as an alternative to hormone therapy for the prevention of osteoporosis. Phytoestrogens are compounds from plants that have weak estrogen-like effects. One form of phytoestrogen is found in flaxseed (linseed), rye, berries, fruits, vegetables, and whole grains. Another form is present in red clover and beans, especially soybeans and soy products. Some animal studies with phytoestrogens have had promising results, but no effects on bone density or fracture reduction in humans have yet been shown. A study of ipriflavone, a synthetic phytoestrogen derivative used as an osteoporosis therapy outside of the United States, showed that this compound did not reduce bone loss in postmenopausal women. In addition, ipriflavone use was linked to low white blood cell counts. NIH is sponsoring clinical trials designed to provide information on whether dietary phytoestrogens might be a safe and effective alternative to estrogen therapy for preventing bone loss in postmenopausal women.

Preventing Osteoporosis

Preventing osteoporosis is a lifelong endeavor. To reach optimal peak bone mass and minimize loss of bone as you get older, there are several factors you should consider. Addressing all of these factors is the best way to optimize bone health throughout life.

Calcium

An inadequate supply of calcium over a lifetime is thought to play a significant role in the development of osteoporosis. Many published studies show that low calcium intakes are associated with low bone mass, rapid bone loss, and high fracture rates. National surveys suggest that the average calcium intake of individuals is far below the levels recommended for optimal bone health. Individuals who consume adequate amounts of calcium and vitamin D throughout life are more likely to achieve optimal skeletal mass early in life and are less likely to lose bone later in life.

Calcium needs change during your lifetime. The body's demand for calcium is greater during childhood and adolescence, when the skeleton is growing rapidly, and in women during pregnancy and breast-feeding. Postmenopausal women and older men also need to consume more calcium. Increased calcium requirements in older people may be related to vitamin D deficiencies that reduce intestinal absorption of calcium. Also, as you age, your body becomes less efficient at absorbing calcium and other nutrients. Older adults are also more likely to have chronic medical problems and to use medications that may impair calcium absorption. Calcium and vitamin D supplements may help slow bone loss and prevent hip fracture. Results from the Women's Health Initiative Calcium with Vitamin D trial showed that for postmenopausal women, particularly those over age 60, a daily dose of 1,000 mg of calcium carbonate combined with 400 IUs of vitamin D3 led to improvements in hip bone density and a reduction in hip fracture.

Adolescence is the most critical period for building bone mass that helps protect against osteoporosis later in life. Yet studies show that among children age 9 to 19 in the United States, few meet the recommended levels. Therefore, it is especially important for parents, other caregivers, and pediatricians to talk to children and young teens about developing bone-healthy habits, including eating calcium-rich foods and getting enough exercise.

Vitamin D

Vitamin D plays an important role in calcium absorption and bone health. It is made in the skin after exposure to sunlight and can also be obtained through the diet, as described in the section of this booklet on treating osteoporosis. Although many people are able to obtain enough vitamin D naturally, vitamin D production decreases in the elderly, in people who are housebound or do not get enough sun, and in some people with chronic neurological or gastrointestinal diseases. These individuals and others at risk for vitamin D deficiency may require vitamin D supplementation. The recommended daily intake of vitamin D is 200 International Units (IU) for infants, children, and adults up to age 50; 400 IU for men and women age 51 to 70; and 600 IU for people over 70. Consuming more than 2,000 IU of vitamin D per day (or 1,000 IU for infants) can cause serious health problems.

Overall Nutrition

A healthy, balanced diet that includes lots of fruits and vegetables and enough calories is also important for lifelong bone health.

Exercise

Like muscle, bone is living tissue that responds to exercise by becoming stronger. There is good evidence that physical activity early in life contributes to higher peak bone mass. (However, remember that excessive exercise can be bad for bone health.) The best exercise for building and maintaining bone mass is weight-bearing exercise: exercise that you do on your feet and that forces you to work against gravity. Weight-bearing exercises include jogging, aerobics, hiking, walking, stair climbing, gardening, weight training, tennis, and dancing. High-impact exercises may provide the most benefit. Bicycling and swimming are not weight-bearing exercises, but they have other health benefits. Exercise machines that provide some degree of weight-bearing exercise include treadmills, stair-climbing machines, ski machines, and exercise bicycles.

Strength training to build and maintain muscle mass and exercises that help with coordination and balance are also important. Later in life, the benefits of exercise for building and maintaining bone mass are not nearly as great, but staying active and doing weight-bearing exercise is still important. A properly designed exercise program that builds muscles and improves balance and coordination provides other benefits for older people, including helping to prevent falls and maintaining overall health and independence. Experts recommend 30 minutes or more of moderate physical activity on most (preferably all) days of the week, including a mix of weight-bearing exercises, strength training (two or three times a week), and balance training.

Smoking

Smoking is bad for your bones and for your heart and lungs. Women who smoke have lower levels of estrogen compared to nonsmokers and frequently go through menopause earlier.

Alcohol

People who drink heavily are more prone to bone loss and fractures because of poor nutrition and harmful effects on calcium balance and hormonal factors. Drinking too much also increases the risk of falling, which is likely to increase fracture risk.

Medications That Cause Bone Loss

The long-term use of glucocorticoids can lead to a loss of bone density and fractures. Other forms of drug therapy that can cause bone loss include long-term treatment with certain antiseizure drugs, such as phenytoin (Dilantin) and barbiturates; some drugs used to treat endometriosis; excessive use of aluminum-containing antacids; certain cancer treatments; and excessive thyroid hormone. It is important to discuss the use of these drugs with your doctor, and not to stop or alter your medication dose on your own.

Prevention Medications

Various medications are available for the prevention, as well as treatment, of osteoporosis.

Osteoporosis and Quality of Life

Aside from its effects on your bones, osteoporosis can change your life in many other ways. Osteoporosis affects each person differently and to different degrees. For example, people with a single fracture and those who have had multiple fractures do not face the same challenges. The particular site of a fracture (hip, spine, etc.) may also influence a person's life in different ways. The effects of osteoporosis on quality of life can include the following:

- Anxiety and depression
- Reduced self-image
- Limitations in the ability to work and enjoy leisure activities
- Acute or chronic pain
- Difficulties in performing the activities of daily life
- Loss of independence
- Changes in relationships with family and friends

Because osteoporosis has such wide-ranging effects, experts say that doctors and other health care providers should treat the whole person, not only the disease. Various measures are available to address the impact of osteoporosis on an individual's quality of life, including the emotional, physical, and functional effects of the disease as well as its social aspects. Some of these issues and how to address them are outlined below.

Emotional Impacts of Osteoporosis

- If you are nervous about the risk of breaking a bone when you go out to crowded places such as malls, movie theaters, or museums, try going at less crowded times. Take breaks and sit down when you feel tired.

- If you have been feeling symptoms of depression—such as loss of appetite, hopelessness, feeling useless and helpless, or having thoughts of suicide—for more than 2 weeks, consult a doctor, social worker, or therapist.

- Medications and counseling are available to fight depression. If you are feeling self-conscious about changes in your appearance, such as the curvature (kyphosis) that occurs in the upper spine after multiple vertebral fractures, look for styles of clothing that minimize figure changes.

Functional and Physical Aspects of Osteoporosis

- If you have trouble working, doing chores around the house, or other routine activities such as grocery shopping, try breaking them into short segments.

- Get up from sitting every half hour or so to ease muscle strain and reposition your skeleton. Also be aware of your posture, and avoid bending and twisting at the same time.

- Look for ways to modify sports and leisure activities that you enjoy to protect your bones, or cultivate new forms of physical activity that put less stress on your skeleton.

- If you experience pain after a fracture, try such pain-relief strategies as hot and cold compresses, biofeedback, and other relaxation strategies. Avoid long periods of inactivity or bed rest, which will worsen osteoporosis.

- Consult your health care professional about the use of analgesics such as acetaminophen (Tylenol or other brands).

- For chronic (long-term) back pain or tiredness caused by fractures in the spine, consult a physical therapist or rehabilitation specialist for exercises to strengthen the back muscles, which may minimize or relieve pain. You will need to continue these exercises faithfully to maintain their benefits.

Social Aspects of Osteoporosis

- Support groups, friends, and family members can help you manage the social challenges and limitations resulting from osteoporosis.

- Don't be afraid to ask others for help in dealing with the effects of osteoporosis on your life. For example, you may need to ask a family member, friend, or neighbor to help you bring groceries into your house or apartment. Find ways to give to others who help you so that you do not feel forced to choose between feeling that you are taking too much help and not taking any help at all.

- Remember that it is normal to want and need help from others as well as to help other people. You can work to keep relationships balanced so that no one does most of the taking over a long period of time, and keep in mind that we all help others throughout life. Friends and family are probably happy to help you, just as you feel good when you help others.

- Concern about experiencing or causing fractures can affect intimate relations between a husband and wife when one or both of you have osteoporosis. Although these topics can be difficult to discuss, couples can look for ways to achieve intimacy without increasing fracture risk. Most physical therapists have been trained to address this issue and can offer advice.

- If tension builds up between you and your spouse as you try to cope with limitations that result from living with osteoporosis, talk with your spouse about these feelings and discuss ways that you might handle the situation. Simply acknowledging and sharing your mutual concerns can often be helpful.

Section 18.2

Osteoporosis and Arthritis: Two Common But Different Conditions

From "Osteoporosis and Arthritis: Two Common but Different Conditions," by the National Institute of Arthritis and Musculoskeletal and Skin Diseases (NIAMS, www.niams.nih.gov), part of the National Institutes of Health, January 2009.

Many people confuse osteoporosis and some types of arthritis. This text discusses the similarities and differences between these conditions.

Osteoporosis

Osteoporosis is a condition in which the bones become less dense and more likely to fracture. Osteoporosis is a major health threat for an estimated 44 million Americans, 68 percent of whom are women. In osteoporosis, there is a loss of bone tissue that leaves bones less dense and more likely to fracture. It can result in a loss of height, severe back pain, and change in one's posture. Osteoporosis can impair a person's ability to walk and can cause prolonged or permanent disability.

Osteoporosis is known as a silent disease because it can progress undetected for many years without symptoms until a fracture occurs. Osteoporosis is diagnosed by a bone mineral density test, which is a safe and painless way to detect low bone density.

Although there is no cure for the disease, the Food and Drug Administration has approved several medications to prevent and treat osteoporosis. In addition, a diet rich in calcium and vitamin D, regular weight-bearing exercise, and a healthy lifestyle can prevent or lessen the effects of the disease.

Arthritis

Arthritis is a general term for conditions that affect the joints and surrounding tissues. Joints are places in the body where bones come together, such as the knees, wrists, fingers, toes, and hips. The two most common types of arthritis are osteoarthritis and rheumatoid arthritis.

- **Osteoarthritis (OA)** is a painful, degenerative joint disease that often involves the hips, knees, neck, lower back, or small joints of the hands. OA usually develops in joints that are injured by repeated overuse from performing a particular task or playing a favorite sport or from carrying around excess body weight. Eventually this injury or repeated impact thins or wears away the cartilage that cushions the ends of the bones in the joint. As a result, the bones rub together, causing a grating sensation. Joint flexibility is reduced, bony spurs develop, and the joint swells. Usually, the first symptom of OA is pain that worsens following exercise or immobility. Treatment usually includes analgesics, topical creams, or nonsteroidal anti-inflammatory drugs (known as NSAIDs); appropriate exercises or physical therapy; joint splinting; or joint replacement surgery for seriously damaged larger joints, such as the knee or hip.

- **Rheumatoid arthritis (RA)** is an autoimmune inflammatory disease that usually involves various joints in the fingers, thumbs, wrists, elbows, shoulders, knees, feet, and ankles. An autoimmune disease is one in which the body releases enzymes that attack its own healthy tissues. In RA, these enzymes destroy the linings of joints. This causes pain, swelling, stiffness, malformation, and reduced movement and function. People with RA also may have systemic symptoms, such as fatigue, fever, weight loss, eye inflammation, anemia, subcutaneous nodules (bumps under the skin), or pleurisy (a lung inflammation).

Although osteoporosis and osteoarthritis are two very different medical conditions with little in common, the similarity of their names

Table 18.1. Similarities and Differences among Osteoporosis, Osteoarthritis, and Rheumatoid Arthritis (*continued on next page*)

	Osteoporosis	Osteoarthritis	Rheumatoid Arthritis
Risk Factors			
Age-related	X	X	
Menopause	X		
Family history	X	X	X
Use of certain medications (e.g., glucocorticoids, seizure medications)	X		
Calcium deficiency or inadequate vitamin D	X		
Inactivity	X		
Overuse of joints		X	
Smoking	X		
Excessive alcohol	X		
Anorexia nervosa	X		
Excessive weight		X	
Physical Effects			
Affects entire skeleton	X		
Affects joints		X	X
Is an autoimmune disease			X
Bony spurs		X	X
Enlarged or malformed joints		X	X
Height loss	X		
Treatment Options			
Raloxifene	X		
Bisphosphonates (e.g., alendronate, risedronate, ibandronate, and zoledronic acid)	X		
Calcitonin	X		
Teriparatide	X		
Estrogen	X		
Calcium and vitamin D	X		
Weight management		X	

Table 18.1. Similarities and Differences among Osteoporosis, Osteoarthritis, and Rheumatoid Arthritis (*continued*)

	Osteoporosis	Osteoarthritis	Rheumatoid Arthritis
Treatment Options (continued)			
Glucocorticoids			X
NSAIDs	X	X	X
Methotrexate			X
Disease-modifying anti-rheumatic drugs, biologic response modifiers, tumor necrosis factor inhibitors			X
Pain Management			
Pain medication (e.g., NSAIDs, narcotics, muscle relaxants)	X	X	X
Rehabilitation	X	X	X
Support groups	X	X	X
Exercises: postural	X	X	X
Exercises: isometric, isotonic, isokinetic	X	X	X
Joint splinting		X	X
Physical therapy	X	X	X
Passive exercises		X	X
Hip fracture surgical repair (may include hip replacement depending on type of fracture)	X		
Joint replacement surgery (usually for pain, malformation, or impaired mobility)		X	X
Heat and cold	X	X	X
Massage therapy	X	X	X
Acupuncture	X	X	X
Psychological approaches (e.g., relaxation, visualization, biofeedback)	X	X	X
Tai chi	X	X	X
Low stress yoga	X	X	X

causes great confusion. These conditions develop differently, have different symptoms, are diagnosed differently, and are treated differently. Studies show that people with OA are less likely than average to develop osteoporosis. On the other hand, people with RA may be more likely to develop osteoporosis. This is especially true because some medications used to treat RA can contribute to osteoporosis.

Osteoporosis and arthritis do share many coping strategies. With either or both of these conditions, many people benefit from exercise programs that may include physical therapy and rehabilitation. In general, exercises that emphasize stretching, strengthening, posture, and range of motion are appropriate. Examples include low-impact aerobics, swimming, tai chi, and low-stress yoga. However, people with osteoporosis must take care to avoid activities that include bending forward from the waist, twisting the spine, or lifting heavy weights. People with arthritis must compensate for limited movement in affected joints. Always check with your doctor to determine whether a certain exercise or exercise program is safe for your specific medical situation.

Most people with arthritis will use pain management strategies at some time. This is not always true for people with osteoporosis. Usually, people with osteoporosis need pain relief when they are recovering from a fracture. In cases of severe osteoporosis with multiple spine fractures, pain control also may become part of daily life. Regardless of the cause, pain management strategies are similar for people with osteoporosis, OA, and RA.

Table 18.1 provides an overview of some of the similarities and differences among osteoporosis, OA, and RA. Some individuals with these conditions may have a different experience or may require a different medical approach to manage their disorder.

Section 18.3

What People with RA Need to Know about Osteoporosis

Excerpted from "What People with Rheumatoid Arthritis Need to Know About Osteoporosis," by the National Institute of Arthritis and Musculoskeletal and Skin Diseases (NIAMS, www.niams.nih.gov), part of the National Institutes of Health, January 2009.

What is rheumatoid arthritis?

Rheumatoid arthritis is an autoimmune disease, a disorder in which the body attacks its own healthy cells and tissues. When someone has rheumatoid arthritis, the membranes around his or her joints become inflamed and release enzymes that cause the surrounding cartilage and bone to wear away. In severe cases, other tissues and body organs also can be affected.

Individuals with rheumatoid arthritis often experience pain, swelling, and stiffness in their joints, especially those in the hands and feet. Motion can be limited in the affected joints, curtailing one's ability to accomplish even the most basic everyday tasks. About one-quarter of those with rheumatoid arthritis develop nodules (bumps) that grow under the skin, usually close to the joints. Fatigue, anemia (low red blood cell count), neck pain, and dry eyes and dry mouth also can occur in individuals with the disease.

Scientists estimate that about 1.3 million people in the United States have rheumatoid arthritis. The disease occurs in all racial and ethnic groups, but affects two to three times as many women as men. Rheumatoid arthritis is more commonly found in older individuals, although the disease typically begins in middle age. Children and young adults can also be affected.

What is juvenile arthritis?

Juvenile arthritis occurs in children 16 years of age or younger. Children with severe juvenile arthritis may be candidates for glucocorticoid medication, the use of which has been linked to bone loss in children as well as adults. Physical activity can be challenging in children with juvenile arthritis because it may cause pain. Incorporating physical activities recommended by the child's doctor and a diet rich in calcium and vitamin D is especially important, so that these children can build adequate bone mass and reduce the risk of future fracture.

What is the link between rheumatoid arthritis and osteoporosis?

Studies have found an increased risk of bone loss and fracture in individuals with rheumatoid arthritis. People with rheumatoid arthritis are at increased risk for osteoporosis for many reasons. To begin with, the glucocorticoid medications often prescribed for the treatment of rheumatoid arthritis can trigger significant bone loss. In addition, pain and loss of joint function caused by the disease can result in inactivity, further increasing osteoporosis risk. Studies also show that bone loss in rheumatoid arthritis may occur as a direct result of the disease. The bone loss is most pronounced in areas immediately surrounding the affected joints. Of concern is the fact that women, a group already at increased risk for osteoporosis, are two to three times more likely than men to have rheumatoid arthritis as well.

What are some osteoporosis management strategies?

Strategies for preventing and treating osteoporosis in people with rheumatoid arthritis are not significantly different from the strategies for those who do not have the disease.

Nutrition: A well-balanced diet rich in calcium and vitamin D is important for healthy bones. Good sources of calcium include low-fat dairy products; dark green, leafy vegetables; and calcium-fortified foods and beverages. Supplements can help ensure that you get adequate amounts of calcium each day, especially in people with a proven milk allergy. The Institute of Medicine recommends a daily calcium intake of 1,000 mg (milligrams) for men and women, increasing to 1,200 mg for those ages 50 and older.

Vitamin D plays an important role in calcium absorption and bone health. It is synthesized in the skin through exposure to sunlight. Food sources of vitamin D include egg yolks, saltwater fish, and liver. Many people obtain enough vitamin D by getting about 15 minutes of sunlight each day. Others, especially those who are older or housebound, may need vitamin D supplements to achieve the recommended intake of 400 to 600 IU (International Units) each day.

Exercise: Like muscle, bone is living tissue that responds to exercise by becoming stronger. The best activity for your bones is weight-bearing exercise that forces you to work against gravity. Some examples include walking, climbing stairs, weight training, and dancing.

Exercising can be challenging for people with rheumatoid arthritis, and it needs to be balanced with rest when the disease is active. However, regular exercise, such as walking, can help prevent bone loss and, by enhancing balance and flexibility, can reduce the likelihood of falling and breaking a bone. Exercise is also important for preserving joint mobility.

Healthy lifestyle: Smoking is bad for bones as well as the heart and lungs. Women who smoke tend to go through menopause earlier, resulting in earlier reduction in levels of the bone-preserving hormone estrogen and triggering earlier bone loss. In addition, smokers may absorb less calcium from their diets. Alcohol also can have a negative effect on bone health. Those who drink heavily are more prone to bone loss and fracture, because of both poor nutrition and increased risk of falling.

Bone density test: A bone mineral density (BMD) test measures bone density in various parts of the body. This safe and painless test can detect osteoporosis before a fracture occurs and can predict one's chances of fracturing in the future. The BMD test can help determine whether medication should be considered. People with rheumatoid arthritis, particularly those who have been receiving glucocorticoid therapy for 2 months or more, should talk to their doctor about whether a BMD test is appropriate.

Medication: Like rheumatoid arthritis, osteoporosis has no cure. However, medications are available to prevent and treat osteoporosis. The Food and Drug Administration has approved several medications (alendronate, risedronate, ibandronate, zoledronic acid, raloxifene, calcitonin, teriparatide, and estrogen/hormone therapy) for the prevention and/or treatment of osteoporosis in postmenopausal women. Alendronate and risedronate also are approved for use in men. For people with rheumatoid arthritis who have or are at risk for glucocorticoid-induced osteoporosis, alendronate (for treatment) and risedronate (for prevention and treatment) are approved.

Chapter 19

Paget Disease of Bone

What is Paget disease of bone?

Paget disease is a chronic disorder that can result in enlarged and misshapen bones. The excessive breakdown and formation of bone tissue causes affected bone to weaken—resulting in bone pain, misshapen bones, fractures, and arthritis in the joints near the affected bones. Paget disease typically is localized, affecting just one or a few bones, as opposed to osteoporosis, for example, which affects all the bones in the body.

Scientists do not know for sure what causes Paget disease. In some cases, the disease runs in families, and so far two genes have been identified that predispose affected people to develop Paget disease. In most cases, however, scientists suspect that environmental factors play a role. For example, scientists are studying the possibility that a slow-acting virus may cause Paget disease.

Who is affected?

An estimated 1 million people in the United States have Paget disease, or about 1.3 people per 100 men and women age 45 to 74. The disease is more common in older people and those of northern European heritage. Men are about twice as likely as women to have the disease.

From "Information for Patients About Paget's Disease of Bone," by the National Institute of Arthritis and Musculoskeletal and Skin Diseases (NIAMS, www.niams.nih.gov), part of the National Institutes of Health, January 2009.

Research suggests that a close relative of someone with Paget disease is seven times more likely to develop the disease than someone without an affected relative.

What are the symptoms?

Many patients do not know they have Paget disease because they have no symptoms. Sometimes the symptoms may be confused with those of arthritis or other disorders. In other cases, the diagnosis is made only after the patient has developed complications.

Symptoms can include the following:

- Pain, which can occur in any bone affected by the disease or result from arthritis, a complication that develops in some patients

- Headaches and hearing loss, which may occur when Paget disease affects the skull

- Pressure on nerves, which may occur when Paget disease affects the skull or spine

- Increased head size, bowing of a limb, or curvature of the spine, which may occur in advanced cases

- Hip pain, which may occur when Paget disease affects the pelvis or thighbone

- Damage to cartilage of joints, which may lead to arthritis

Any bone or bones can be affected, but Paget disease occurs most frequently in the spine, pelvis, legs, or skull. Generally, symptoms progress slowly, and the disease does not spread to normal bones.

How is it diagnosed?

Paget disease is almost always diagnosed using x-rays but may be discovered initially by either of the following tests:

- **Alkaline phosphatase blood test:** An elevated level of alkaline phosphatase in the blood can be suggestive of Paget disease.

- **Bone scans:** Bone scans are useful in determining the extent and activity of the condition.

If a blood test or bone scan suggests Paget disease, the affected bone(s) should be x-rayed to confirm the diagnosis.

Early diagnosis and treatment are important to minimize complications. Siblings and children of people with Paget disease may wish to have an alkaline phosphatase blood test every 2 or 3 years starting around the age of 40. If the alkaline phosphatase level is higher than normal, a bone scan may be used to identify which bone or bones are affected and an x-ray of these bones is used to verify the diagnosis of Paget disease.

What is the prognosis?

The outlook for people diagnosed with Paget disease is generally good, particularly if treatment is given before major changes have occurred in the affected bones. Treatment can reduce symptoms but is not a cure. Osteogenic sarcoma, a form of bone cancer, is an extremely rare complication that occurs in less than 1 percent of all patients with Paget disease.

What other medical conditions may it lead to?

Paget disease may lead to other medical conditions, including:

- **Arthritis:** Long bones in the leg may bow, distorting alignment and increasing pressure on nearby joints. In addition, pagetic bone may enlarge, causing joint surfaces to undergo excessive wear and tear. In these cases, pain may be caused by a combination of Paget disease and osteoarthritis.

- **Hearing loss:** Loss of hearing in one or both ears may occur when Paget disease affects the skull and the bone that surrounds the inner ear. Treating Paget disease may slow or stop hearing loss. Hearing aids also may help.

- **Heart disease:** In severe Paget disease, the heart works harder to pump blood to affected bones. This usually does not result in heart failure except in some people who also have hardening of the arteries.

- **Kidney stones:** Kidney stones are more common in patients with Paget disease.

- **Nervous system problems:** Pagetic bone can cause pressure on the brain, spinal cord, or nerves and reduced blood flow to the brain and spinal cord.

- **Sarcoma:** Rarely, Paget disease is associated with the development of a malignant tumor of the bone. When there is a sudden onset or worsening of pain, sarcoma should be considered.

- **Loose teeth:** When Paget disease affects the facial bones, the teeth may loosen. This may make chewing more difficult.

- **Vision loss:** Rarely, when the skull is involved, the nerves to the eye may be affected, causing some loss of vision.

Paget disease is not associated with osteoporosis. Although Paget disease and osteoporosis can occur in the same patient, they are completely different disorders. Despite their marked differences, several medications for Paget disease also are used to treat osteoporosis.

Who treats it?

The following types of medical specialists are generally knowledgeable about treating Paget disease:

- **Endocrinologists:** Doctors who specialize in hormonal and metabolic disorders

- **Rheumatologists:** Doctors who specialize in joint and muscle disorders

- **Others:** Orthopaedic surgeons, neurologists, and otolaryngologists (doctors who specialize in ear, nose, and throat disorders) may be called on to evaluate specialized symptoms.

How is it treated?

Drug therapy: The Food and Drug Administration has approved several medications to treat Paget disease. The medications work by controlling the excessive breakdown and formation of bone that occurs in the disease. The goal of treatment is to relieve bone pain and prevent progression of the disease. People with Paget disease should talk to their doctors about which medication is right for them. It is also important to get adequate calcium and vitamin D through diet and supplements as prescribed by your doctor, except for patients who have had kidney stones.

- **Bisphosphonates:** Bisphosphonates are a class of drugs used to treat a variety of bone diseases. Of the six bisphosphonates currently available to treat Paget disease, the most commonly prescribed are the four most potent: Actonel, Fosamax, Aredia, and Reclast. Didronel and Skelid may be appropriate therapies for selected patients, but are less commonly used. People with severe kidney disease should not use any of these drugs.

- **Calcitonin:** Calcitonin is a naturally occurring hormone made by the thyroid gland. The medication may be appropriate for certain patients but is less effective than bisphosphonates and seldom used. The nasal spray form of this medication is not approved for the treatment of Paget disease.

Surgery: Medical therapy before surgery helps decrease bleeding and other complications. Patients who are having surgery should discuss pretreatment with their doctor. Surgery may be advised for three major complications of Paget disease:

- **Fractures:** Surgery may allow fractures to heal in better position.

- **Severe degenerative arthritis:** Hip or knee replacement may be considered if disability is severe and medication and physical therapy are no longer helpful.

- **Bone deformity:** Cutting and realigning pagetic bone (a procedure called an osteotomy) may reduce the pain in weight-bearing joints, especially the knees.

Complications resulting from enlargement of the skull or spine may injure the nervous system. However, most neurological symptoms, even those that are moderately severe, can be treated with medication and do not require neurosurgery.

Diet and exercise: There is no special diet to prevent or help treat Paget disease. However, according to the National Academy of Sciences, everyone age 50 and older should get 1,200 mg of calcium and at least 400 IU (International Units) of vitamin D every day to maintain a healthy skeleton. People age 70 and older need to increase their vitamin D intake to 600 IU. People with a history of kidney stones should discuss calcium and vitamin D intake with their doctor.

Exercise is important because it helps preserve skeletal health, prevent weight gain, and maintain joint mobility. Patients should discuss any new exercise program with their doctor before beginning, to avoid any undue stress on affected bones.

Chapter 20

Polymyalgia Rheumatica and Giant Cell Arteritis

What is polymyalgia rheumatica?

Polymyalgia rheumatica is a rheumatic disorder associated with moderate-to-severe musculoskeletal pain and stiffness in the neck, shoulder, and hip area. Stiffness is most noticeable in the morning or after a period of inactivity, and typically lasts longer than 30 minutes. This disorder may develop rapidly; in some people it comes on literally overnight. But for most people, polymyalgia rheumatica develops more gradually.

The cause of polymyalgia rheumatica is not known. But it is associated with immune system problems, genetic factors, and an event, such as an infection, that triggers symptoms. The fact that polymyalgia rheumatica is rare in people under the age of 50 and becomes more common as age increases suggests that it may be linked to the aging process.

Polymyalgia rheumatica usually resolves within 1 to 2 years. The symptoms of polymyalgia rheumatica are quickly controlled by treatment with corticosteroids, but symptoms return if treatment is stopped too early. Corticosteroid treatment does not appear to influence the length of the disease.

From "Polymyalgia Rheumatica and Giant Cell Arteritis," by the National Institute of Arthritis and Musculoskeletal and Skin Diseases (NIAMS, www.niams.nih.gov), part of the National Institutes of Health, December 2006.

What is giant cell arteritis?

Giant cell arteritis, also known as temporal arteritis and cranial arteritis, is a disorder that results in inflammation of arteries of the scalp (most apparent in the temporal arteries, which are located on the temples on each side of the head), neck, and arms. This inflammation causes the arteries to narrow, impeding adequate blood flow. For a good prognosis, it is critical to receive early treatment, before irreversible tissue damage occurs.

How are polymyalgia rheumatica and giant cell arteritis related?

It is unclear how or why polymyalgia rheumatica and giant cell arteritis frequently occur together. But some people with polymyalgia rheumatica also develop giant cell arteritis either simultaneously, or after the musculoskeletal symptoms have disappeared. Other people with giant cell arteritis also have polymyalgia rheumatica at some time while the arteries are inflamed.

When undiagnosed or untreated, giant cell arteritis can cause potentially serious problems, including permanent vision loss and stroke. So regardless of why giant cell arteritis might occur along with polymyalgia rheumatica, it is important that doctors look for symptoms of the arteritis in anyone diagnosed with polymyalgia rheumatica.

Patients, too, must learn and watch for symptoms of giant cell arteritis, because early detection and proper treatment are key to preventing complications. Any symptoms should be reported to your doctor immediately.

What are the symptoms of polymyalgia rheumatica?

In addition to the musculoskeletal stiffness mentioned earlier, people with polymyalgia rheumatica also may have flu-like symptoms, including fever, weakness, and weight loss.

What are the symptoms of giant cell arteritis?

Early symptoms of giant cell arteritis may resemble flu symptoms such as fatigue, loss of appetite, and fever. Symptoms specifically related to the inflamed arteries of the head include headaches, pain and tenderness over the temples, double vision or visual loss, dizziness or problems with coordination, and balance. Pain may also affect the jaw and tongue, especially when eating, and opening the mouth wide may become difficult. In rare cases, giant cell arteritis causes ulceration of the scalp.

Who is at risk for these conditions?

Caucasian women over the age of 50 have the highest risk of developing polymyalgia rheumatica and giant cell arteritis. While women are more likely than men to develop the conditions, research suggests that men with giant cell arteritis are more likely to suffer potentially blinding eye involvement. Both conditions almost exclusively affect people over the age of 50. The incidence of both peaks between 70 and 80 years of age.

Polymyalgia rheumatica and giant cell arteritis are both quite common, according to the National Arthritis Data Work Group. In the United States, it is estimated that 700 per 100,000 people in the general population over 50 years of age develop polymyalgia rheumatica. An estimated 200 per 100,000 people over 50 years of age develop giant cell arteritis.

How are polymyalgia rheumatica and giant cell arteritis diagnosed?

A diagnosis of polymyalgia rheumatica is based primarily on the patient's medical history and symptoms, and on a physical examination. No single test is available to definitively diagnose polymyalgia rheumatica. However, doctors often use lab tests to confirm a diagnosis or rule out other diagnoses or possible reasons for the patient's symptoms.

The most typical laboratory finding in people with polymyalgia rheumatica is an elevated erythrocyte sedimentation rate, commonly referred to as the sed rate. This test measures inflammation by determining how quickly red blood cells fall to the bottom of a test tube of unclotted blood. Rapidly descending cells (an elevated sed rate) indicate inflammation in the body. While the sed rate measurement is a helpful diagnostic tool, it alone does not confirm polymyalgia rheumatica. An abnormal result indicates only that tissue is inflamed, but this is also a symptom of many forms of arthritis and other rheumatic diseases.

Before making a diagnosis of polymyalgia rheumatica, the doctor may order additional tests. For example, the C-reactive protein test is another common means of measuring inflammation. There is also a common test for rheumatoid factor, an antibody (a protein made by the immune system) that is sometimes found in the blood of people with rheumatoid arthritis. While polymyalgia rheumatica and rheumatoid arthritis share many symptoms, those with polymyalgia rheumatica rarely test positive for rheumatoid factor. Therefore, a positive rheumatoid factor might suggest a diagnosis of rheumatoid arthritis instead of polymyalgia rheumatica.

As with polymyalgia rheumatica, a diagnosis of giant cell arteritis is based largely on symptoms and a physical examination. The exam may reveal that the temporal artery is inflamed and tender to the touch, and that it has a reduced pulse.

Any doctor who suspects giant cell arteritis should order a temporal artery biopsy. In this procedure, a small section of the artery is removed through an incision in the skin over the temple area and examined under a microscope. A biopsy that is positive for giant cell arteritis will show abnormal cells in the artery walls. Some patients showing symptoms of giant cell arteritis will have negative biopsy results. In such cases, the doctor may suggest a second biopsy.

How are they treated?

The treatment of choice for both polymyalgia rheumatica and giant cell arteritis is corticosteroid medication, usually prednisone.

Polymyalgia rheumatica responds to a low daily dose of prednisone that is increased as needed until symptoms disappear. At this point, the doctor may gradually reduce the dosage to determine the lowest amount needed to alleviate symptoms. Most patients can discontinue medication after 6 months to 2 years. If symptoms recur, prednisone treatment is required again.

Nonsteroidal anti-inflammatory drugs (NSAIDs), such as aspirin and ibuprofen (Advil, Motrin), also may be used to treat polymyalgia rheumatica. The medication must be taken daily, and long-term use may cause stomach irritation. For most patients, NSAIDs alone are not enough to relieve symptoms.

Even without treatment, polymyalgia rheumatica usually disappears in one to several years. With treatment, however, symptoms disappear quickly, usually in 24 to 48 hours. If prednisone doesn't bring improvement, the doctor is likely to consider other possible diagnoses.

Giant cell arteritis is treated with high doses of prednisone. If not treated promptly, the condition carries a small but definite risk of blindness, so prednisone should be started as soon as possible, perhaps even before confirming the diagnosis with a temporal artery biopsy.

As with polymyalgia rheumatica, the symptoms of giant cell arteritis quickly disappear with treatment; however, high doses of prednisone are typically maintained for one month.

Once symptoms disappear and the sed rate is normal, there is much less risk of blindness. At that point, the doctor can begin to gradually reduce the prednisone dose.

In both polymyalgia rheumatica and giant cell arteritis, an increase in symptoms may develop when the prednisone dose is reduced to lower levels. The physician may need to hold the lower dose for a longer period of time or even modestly increase it again, temporarily, to control the symptoms. Once the symptoms are in remission and the prednisone has been discontinued for several months, recurrence is less common.

Whether taken on a long-term basis for polymyalgia rheumatica or for a shorter period for giant cell arteritis, prednisone carries a risk of side effects. While long-term use and/or higher doses carry the greatest risk, people taking the drug at any dose or for any length of time should be aware of the potential side effects, which include the following:

- Fluid retention and weight gain
- Rounding of the face
- Delayed wound healing
- Bruising easily
- Diabetes
- Myopathy (muscle wasting)
- Glaucoma
- Increased blood pressure
- Decreased calcium absorption in the bones, which can lead to osteoporosis
- Irritation of the stomach
- Increase in infections

People taking corticosteroids may have some side effects or none at all. Anyone who experiences side effects should report them to his or her doctor. When the medication is stopped, the side effects disappear. Because prednisone and other corticosteroid drugs reduce the body's natural production of corticosteroid hormones, which are necessary for the body to function properly, it is important not to stop taking the medication unless instructed by a doctor to do so. The patient and doctor must work together to gradually reduce the medication.

What is the outlook?

Most people with polymyalgia rheumatica and giant cell arteritis lead productive, active lives. The duration of drug treatment differs by patient. Once treatment is discontinued, polymyalgia may recur; but once again, symptoms respond rapidly to prednisone. When properly treated, giant cell arteritis rarely recurs.

Chapter 21

Psoriasis and Psoriatic Arthritis

Chapter Contents

Section 21.1

Psoriasis

From "Questions and Answers About Psoriasis," by the National Institute of Arthritis and Musculoskeletal and Skin Diseases (NIAMS, www.niams .nih.gov), part of the National Institutes of Health, May 2003. Reviewed and revised by David A. Cooke, MD, FACP, July 26, 2009.

What is psoriasis?

Psoriasis is a chronic (long-lasting) skin disease of scaling and inflammation that affects 2 to 2.6 percent of the United States population, or between 5.8 and 7.5 million people. Although the disease occurs in all age groups, it primarily affects adults. It appears about equally in males and females. Psoriasis occurs when skin cells quickly rise from their origin below the surface of the skin and pile up on the surface before they have a chance to mature. Usually this movement (also called turnover) takes about a month, but in psoriasis it may occur in only a few days. In its typical form, psoriasis results in patches of thick, red (inflamed) skin covered with silvery scales. These patches, which are sometimes referred to as plaques, usually itch or feel sore. They most often occur on the elbows, knees, other parts of the legs, scalp, lower back, face, palms, and soles of the feet, but they can occur on skin anywhere on the body.

The disease may also affect the fingernails, the toenails, and the soft tissues of the genitals and inside the mouth. While it is not unusual for the skin around affected joints to crack, approximately 1 million people with psoriasis experience joint inflammation that produces symptoms of arthritis. This condition is called psoriatic arthritis.

How does psoriasis affect quality of life?

Individuals with psoriasis may experience significant physical discomfort and some disability. Itching and pain can interfere with basic functions, such as self-care, walking, and sleep. Plaques on hands and feet can prevent individuals from working at certain occupations, playing some sports, and caring for family members or a home. The frequency of medical care is costly and can interfere with an employment or school schedule. People with moderate to severe psoriasis may feel self-conscious about their appearance and have a poor self-image that stems from fear of public rejection and psychosexual concerns. Psychological distress can lead to significant depression and social isolation.

What causes psoriasis?

Psoriasis is a skin disorder driven by the immune system, especially involving a type of white blood cell called a T cell. Normally, T cells help protect the body against infection and disease. In the case of psoriasis, T cells are put into action by mistake and become so active that they trigger other immune responses, which lead to inflammation and to rapid turnover of skin cells. In about one third of the cases, there is a family history of psoriasis. Researchers have studied a large number of families affected by psoriasis and identified genes linked to the disease. (Genes govern every bodily function and determine the inherited traits passed from parent to child.) People with psoriasis may notice that there are times when their skin worsens, then improves. Conditions that may cause flare-ups include infections, stress, and changes in climate that dry the skin. Also, certain medicines, including lithium and beta blockers, which are prescribed for high blood pressure, may trigger an outbreak or worsen the disease.

How is psoriasis diagnosed?

Occasionally, doctors may find it difficult to diagnose psoriasis, because it often looks like other skin diseases. It may be necessary to confirm a diagnosis by examining a small skin sample under a microscope. There are several forms of psoriasis. Some of these include the following:

- **Plaque psoriasis:** Skin lesions are red at the base and covered by silvery scales.

- **Guttate psoriasis:** Small, drop-shaped lesions appear on the trunk, limbs, and scalp. Guttate psoriasis is most often triggered by upper respiratory infections (for example, a sore throat caused by streptococcal bacteria).

- **Pustular psoriasis:** Blisters of noninfectious pus appear on the skin. Attacks of pustular psoriasis may be triggered by medications, infections, stress, or exposure to certain chemicals.

- **Inverse psoriasis:** Smooth, red patches occur in the folds of the skin near the genitals, under the breasts, or in the armpits. The symptoms may be worsened by friction and sweating.

- **Erythrodermic psoriasis:** Widespread reddening and scaling of the skin may be a reaction to severe sunburn or to taking corticosteroids (cortisone) or other medications. It can also be caused by a prolonged period of increased activity of psoriasis that is poorly controlled.

- **Psoriatic arthritis:** Joint inflammation that produces symptoms of arthritis in patients who have or will develop psoriasis.

How is psoriasis treated?

Doctors generally treat psoriasis in steps based on the severity of the disease, size of the areas involved, type of psoriasis, and the patient's response to initial treatments. This is sometimes called the "1-2-3" approach. In step 1, medicines are applied to the skin (topical treatment). Step 2 uses light treatments (phototherapy). Step 3 involves taking medicines by mouth or injections that treat the whole immune system (called systemic therapy).

Over time, affected skin can become resistant to treatment, especially when topical corticosteroids are used. Also, a treatment that works very well in one person may have little effect in another. Thus, doctors often use a trial-and-error approach to find a treatment that works, and they may switch treatments periodically (for example, every 12 to 24 months) if a treatment does not work or if adverse reactions occur.

Topical treatment: Treatments applied directly to the skin may improve its condition. Doctors find that some patients respond well to ointment or cream forms of corticosteroids, vitamin D_3, retinoids, coal tar, or anthralin. Bath solutions and moisturizers may be soothing, but they are seldom strong enough to improve the condition of the skin. Therefore, they usually are combined with stronger remedies.

- Corticosteroids: These drugs reduce inflammation and the turnover of skin cells, and they suppress the immune system. Available in different strengths, topical corticosteroids (cortisone) are usually applied to the skin twice a day. Short-term treatment is often effective in improving, but not completely eliminating, psoriasis. Long-term use or overuse of highly potent (strong) corticosteroids can cause thinning of the skin, internal side effects, and resistance to the treatment's benefits. If less than 10 percent of the skin is involved, some doctors will prescribe a high-potency corticosteroid ointment. High-potency corticosteroids may also be prescribed for plaques that don't improve with other treatment, particularly those on the hands or feet. In situations where the objective of treatment is comfort, medium-potency corticosteroids may be prescribed for the broader skin areas of the torso or limbs. Low-potency preparations are used on delicate skin areas.

- Calcipotriene: This drug is a synthetic form of vitamin D_3 that can be applied to the skin. Applying calcipotriene ointment (for example, Dovonex) twice a day controls the speed of turnover of skin cells. Because calcipotriene can irritate the skin, however, it is not recommended for use on the face or genitals. It is sometimes combined with topical corticosteroids to reduce irritation. Use of more than 100 grams of calcipotriene per week may raise the amount of calcium in the body to unhealthy levels.

- Retinoid: Topical retinoids are synthetic forms of vitamin A. The retinoid tazarotene (Tazorac) is available as a gel or cream that is applied to the skin. If used alone, this preparation does not act as quickly as topical corticosteroids, but it does not cause thinning of the skin or other side effects associated with steroids. However, it can irritate the skin, particularly in skin folds and the normal skin surrounding a patch of psoriasis. It is less irritating and sometimes more effective when combined with a corticosteroid. Because of the risk of birth defects, women of childbearing age must take measures to prevent pregnancy when using tazarotene.

- Coal tar: Preparations containing coal tar (gels and ointments) may be applied directly to the skin, added (as a liquid) to the bath, or used on the scalp as a shampoo. Coal tar products are available in different strengths, and many are sold over the counter (not requiring a prescription). Coal tar is less effective than corticosteroids and many other treatments and, therefore, is sometimes combined with ultraviolet B (UVB) phototherapy for a better result. The most potent form of coal tar may irritate the skin, is messy, has a strong odor, and may stain the skin or clothing. Thus, it is not popular with many patients.

- Anthralin: Anthralin reduces the increase in skin cells and inflammation. Doctors sometimes prescribe a 15- to 30-minute application of anthralin ointment, cream, or paste once each day to treat chronic psoriasis lesions. Afterward, anthralin must be washed off the skin to prevent irritation. This treatment often fails to adequately improve the skin, and it stains skin, bathtub, sink, and clothing brown or purple. In addition, the risk of skin irritation makes anthralin unsuitable for acute or actively inflamed eruptions.

- Salicylic acid: This peeling agent, which is available in many forms such as ointments, creams, gels, and shampoos, can be applied to reduce scaling of the skin or scalp. Often, it is more effective when combined with topical corticosteroids, anthralin, or coal tar.

- Clobetasol propionate: This is a foam topical medication (Olux), which has been approved for the treatment of scalp and body psoriasis. The foam penetrates the skin very well, is easy to use, and is not as messy as many other topical medications.

- Bath solutions: People with psoriasis may find that adding oil when bathing, then applying a moisturizer, soothes their skin. Also, individuals can remove scales and reduce itching by soaking for 15 minutes in water containing a coal tar solution, oiled oatmeal, Epsom salts, or Dead Sea salts.

- Moisturizers: When applied regularly over a long period, moisturizers have a soothing effect. Preparations that are thick and greasy usually work best because they seal water in the skin, reducing scaling and itching.

Light therapy: Natural ultraviolet light from the sun and controlled delivery of artificial ultraviolet light are used in treating psoriasis.

- Sunlight: Much of sunlight is composed of bands of different wavelengths of ultraviolet (UV) light. When absorbed into the skin, UV light suppresses the process leading to disease, causing activated T cells in the skin to die. This process reduces inflammation and slows the turnover of skin cells that causes scaling. Daily, short, nonburning exposure to sunlight clears or improves psoriasis in many people. Therefore, exposing affected skin to sunlight is one initial treatment for the disease.

- Ultraviolet B (UVB) phototherapy: UVB is light with a short wavelength that is absorbed in the skin's epidermis. An artificial source can be used to treat mild and moderate psoriasis. Some physicians will start treating patients with UVB instead of topical agents. A UVB phototherapy, called broadband UVB, can be used for a few small lesions, to treat widespread psoriasis, or for lesions that resist topical treatment. This type of phototherapy is normally given in a doctor's office by using a light panel or light box. Some patients use UVB light boxes at home under a doctor's guidance. A newer type of UVB, called narrowband UVB, emits the part of the ultraviolet light spectrum band that is most helpful for psoriasis. Narrowband UVB treatment is superior to broadband UVB, but it is less effective than PUVA treatment. It is gaining in popularity because it does help and is more convenient than PUVA. At first, patients may require several treatments of narrowband UVB spaced close together to improve their skin. Once the skin has shown improvement, a maintenance treatment once each week may be all that is necessary. However, narrowband UVB treatment is not without risk. It can cause more severe and longer lasting burns than broadband treatment.

- Psoralen and ultraviolet A phototherapy (PUVA): This treatment combines oral or topical administration of a medicine called psoralen with exposure to ultraviolet A (UVA) light. UVA has a long wavelength that penetrates deeper into the skin than UVB. Psoralen makes the skin more sensitive to this light. PUVA is normally used when more than 10 percent of the skin is affected or when the disease interferes with a person's occupation (for example, when a teacher's face or a salesperson's hands are involved). Compared with broadband UVB treatment, PUVA treatment taken two to three times a week clears psoriasis more consistently and in fewer treatments. However, it is associated with more short-term side effects, including nausea, headache, fatigue, burning, and itching. Care must be taken to avoid sunlight after ingesting psoralen to avoid severe sunburns, and the eyes must be protected for one to two days with UVA-absorbing glasses. Long-term treatment is associated with an increased risk of squamous cell and, possibly, melanoma skin cancers. Simultaneous use of drugs that suppress the immune system, such as cyclosporine, have little beneficial effect and increase the risk of cancer.

- Light therapy combined with other therapies: Studies have shown that combining ultraviolet light treatment and a retinoid, like acitretin, adds to the effectiveness of UV light for psoriasis. For this reason, if patients are not responding to light therapy, retinoids may be added. UVB phototherapy, for example, may be combined with retinoids and other treatments. One combined therapy program, referred to as the Ingram regime, involves a coal tar bath, UVB phototherapy, and application of an anthralin-salicylic acid paste that is left on the skin for 6 to 24 hours. A similar regime, the Goeckerman treatment, combines coal tar ointment with UVB phototherapy. Also, PUVA can be combined with some oral medications (such as retinoids) to increase its effectiveness.

Systemic treatment: For more severe forms of psoriasis, doctors sometimes prescribe medicines that are taken internally by pill or injection. This is called systemic treatment. Recently, attention has been given to a group of drugs called biologics which are made from proteins produced by living cells instead of chemicals. They interfere with specific immune system processes.

- Methotrexate: Like cyclosporine, methotrexate slows cell turn-over by suppressing the immune system. It can be taken by pill or injection. Patients taking methotrexate must be closely monitored because it can cause liver damage and/or decrease the production of oxygen-carrying red blood cells, infection-fighting white blood cells, and clot-enhancing platelets. As a precaution, doctors do not prescribe the drug for people who have had liver disease or anemia (an illness characterized by weakness or tiredness due to a reduction in the number or volume of red blood cells that carry oxygen to the tissues). It is sometimes combined with PUVA or UVB treatments. Methotrexate should not be used by pregnant women, or by women who are planning to get pregnant, because it may cause birth defects.

- Retinoids: A retinoid, such as acitretin (Soriatane), is a compound with vitamin A-like properties that may be prescribed for severe cases of psoriasis that do not respond to other therapies. Because this treatment also may cause birth defects, women must protect themselves from pregnancy beginning 1 month before through 3 years after treatment with acitretin. Most patients experience a recurrence of psoriasis after these products are discontinued.

- Cyclosporine: Taken orally, cyclosporine acts by suppressing the immune system to slow the rapid turnover of skin cells. It may provide quick relief of symptoms, but the improvement stops when treatment is discontinued. The best candidates for this therapy are those with severe psoriasis who have not responded to, or cannot tolerate, other systemic therapies. Its rapid onset of action is helpful in avoiding hospitalization of patients whose psoriasis is rapidly progressing. Cyclosporine may impair kidney function or cause high blood pressure (hypertension). Therefore, patients must be carefully monitored by a doctor. Also, cyclosporine is not recommended for patients who have a weak immune system or those who have had skin cancers as a result of PUVA treatments in the past. It should not be given with phototherapy.

- 6-Thioguanine: This drug is nearly as effective as methotrexate and cyclosporine. It has fewer side effects, but there is a greater likelihood of anemia. This drug must also be avoided by pregnant women and by women who are planning to become pregnant, because it may cause birth defects.

- Hydroxyurea (Hydrea): Compared with methotrexate and cyclosporine, hydroxyurea is somewhat less effective. It is sometimes combined with PUVA or UVB treatments. Possible side effects include anemia and a decrease in white blood cells and platelets. Like methotrexate and retinoids, hydroxyurea must be avoided by pregnant women or those who are planning to become pregnant, because it may cause birth defects.

- Alefacept (Amevive): This is the first biologic drug approved specifically to treat moderate to severe plaque psoriasis. It is administered by a doctor, who injects the drug once a week for 12 weeks. The drug is then stopped for a period of time while changes in the skin are observed and a decision is made regarding the need or further treatment. Because alefacept suppresses the immune system, the skin often improves, but there is also an increased risk of infection or other problems, possibly including cancer. Monitoring by a doctor is required, and a patient's blood must be tested weekly around the time of each injection to make certain that T cells and other immune system cells are not overly depressed.

- Etanercept (Enbrel), Infliximab (Remicade), Adalimumab (Humira), and Golimumab (Simponi): These drugs are approved treatments for psoriatic arthritis where the joints swell and become inflamed. Etanercept (Enbrel) and Infliximab (Remicade) are also approved for treatment of plaque psoriasis, although they are generally reserved for severe cases. Like alefacept, they are biologic response modifiers, which after injection blocks interactions between certain cells in the immune system. They all limit the action of a specific protein called tumor necrosis factor

265

(TNF) that is overproduced in the lubricating fluid of the joints and surrounding tissues, causing inflammation. Because this same protein is overproduced in the skin of people with psoriatic arthritis, patients receiving these drugs also may notice an improvement in their skin. Individuals should not receive treatment with these medications if they have an active infection, a history of recurring infections, or an underlying condition, such as diabetes, that increases their risk of infection. Screening for tuberculosis infection prior to starting therapy is also important, as these drugs can cause a latent infection to activate. The risk for serious fungal infections and certain types of cancers are also increased by these medications. Those who have psoriasis and certain neurological conditions, such as multiple sclerosis, cannot be treated with these drugs. Added caution is needed for psoriasis patients who have rheumatoid arthritis or are receiving other biological modifier drugs; these patients should follow the advice of a rheumatologist regarding this treatment.

- Antibiotics: These medications are not indicated in routine treatment of psoriasis. However, antibiotics may be employed when an infection, such as that caused by the bacteria *Streptococcus*, triggers an outbreak of psoriasis, as in certain cases of guttate psoriasis.

Combination therapy: There are many approaches for treating psoriasis. Combining various topical, light, and systemic treatments often permits lower doses of each and can result in increased effectiveness. Therefore, doctors are paying more attention to combination therapy.

Psychological support: Some individuals with moderate to severe psoriasis may benefit from counseling or participation in a support group to reduce self-consciousness about their appearance or relieve psychological distress resulting from fear of social rejection.

Section 21.2

Psoriatic Arthritis

Up to 30 percent of people with psoriasis also develop psoriatic arthritis, which causes pain, stiffness and swelling in and around the joints.

Psoriatic arthritis can develop at any time, but it most commonly appears between the ages of 30 and 50 and affects men at a higher rate than women. Genes, the immune system, and environmental factors are all believed to play a role in the onset of the disease.

Early recognition, diagnosis, and treatment of psoriatic arthritis are critical to relieve pain and inflammation and help prevent progressive joint damage.

Types of Psoriatic Arthritis

There are five types of psoriatic arthritis: symmetric, asymmetric, distal interphalangeal predominant (DIP), spondylitis, and arthritis mutilans.

Symmetric arthritis is much like rheumatoid arthritis but generally milder with less deformity. It usually affects multiple symmetric pairs of joints (occurs in the same joints on both sides of the body) and can be disabling.

Asymmetric arthritis can involve a few or many joints and does not occur in the same joints on both sides of the body. It can affect any joint, such as the knee, hip, ankle, or wrist. The hands and feet may have enlarged "sausage" digits. The joints may also be warm, tender, and red. Individuals may experience periodic joint pain which is usually responsive to medical therapy. This form is generally mild, although some people might develop disabling disease.

Distal interphalangeal predominant (DIP) although the "classic" type, occurs in only about 5 percent of people with psoriatic arthritis. Primarily, it involves the distal joints of the fingers and toes (the joint closest to the nail). Sometimes it is confused with osteoarthritis, but nail changes are usually prominent.

Spondylitis is inflammation of the spinal column. In about 5 percent of individuals with psoriatic arthritis, spondylitis is the predominant symptom. Inflammation with stiffness of the neck, lower back, sacroiliac, or spinal vertebrae are common symptoms in a larger number of patients, making motion painful and difficult. Peripheral disease can be present in the hands, arms, hips, legs, and feet.

Arthritis mutilans is a severe, deforming, and destructive arthritis that affects fewer than 5 percent of people with psoriatic arthritis. It principally affects the small joints of the hands and feet, though there is frequently associated neck or lower back pain.

Diagnosing Psoriatic Arthritis

Psoriatic arthritis can develop slowly with mild symptoms, or it can develop quickly and be severe. Early recognition, diagnosis, and treatment of psoriatic arthritis can help prevent or limit extensive joint damage that occurs in later stages of the disease.

Generally, one or more of the following symptoms appears:

- Generalized fatigue
- Tenderness, pain, and swelling over tendons
- Swollen fingers and toes
- Stiffness, pain, throbbing, swelling, and tenderness in one or more joints
- A reduced range of motion
- Morning stiffness and tiredness
- Nail changes: For example, the nail separates from the nail bed and/or becomes pitted and mimics fungus infections.
- Redness and pain of the eye, such as conjunctivitis

The disease can develop in a joint after an injury and may mimic a cartilage tear. The diagnosis of psoriatic arthritis may sometimes be made only after repeated episodes. Muscle or joint pain can occur without joint inflammation (swelling). Tendonitis and bursitis may be prominent features.

Swelling of the fingers and toes can suggest a "sausage-like" appearance, known as dactylitis. Psoriatic arthritis usually affects the distal joints (those closest to the nail) in fingers or toes. The lower back, wrists, knees, or ankles also may be affected.

In 85 percent of patients, skin disease precedes joint disease. Therefore, it is important to tell your dermatologist if you have any aches and pains. It is important to note that having a severe case of psoriasis does not necessarily mean a person will have a severe case of psoriatic arthritis. A person could have few skin lesions, but have many joints affected by the arthritis.

Diagnosing Psoriatic Arthritis: Tests to Confirm the Diagnosis

A person with joint aches and pains should talk to a doctor about diagnosis and treatment. Primary-care doctors or dermatologists can treat psoriatic arthritis, but psoriatic arthritis patients should consider seeing a rheumatologist, a doctor who specializes in arthritis.

There is no definitive test for psoriatic arthritis. The diagnosis is made mostly on a clinical basis and by a process of elimination. Medical history, physical examination, blood tests, MRIs [magnetic resonance imaging tests], and x-rays of the joints that have symptoms may be used to diagnose psoriatic arthritis. It is important to communicate your history of psoriasis to your doctor.

The symptoms of psoriatic arthritis are similar to those of three other arthritic diseases: rheumatoid arthritis, gout, and reactive arthritis. Rheumatoid arthritis generally involves joints symmetrically distributed on both sides of the body, and it may produce bumps under the skin that are not present in psoriatic arthritis. However, some forms of psoriatic arthritis look very similar. The simultaneous presence of psoriasis on the skin and nail changes supports a diagnosis of psoriatic arthritis.

A certain antibody, called a rheumatoid factor, is normally present in rheumatoid arthritis. The rheumatoid factor is not usually found in the blood of psoriatic arthritis patients. A blood test for that antibody may help distinguish between the two diseases. A person can have rheumatoid arthritis and psoriatic arthritis, but that is rare. Many of the treatments for psoriatic arthritis and rheumatoid arthritis overlap.

Likewise, it is possible to have gout along with psoriasis and psoriatic arthritis. If you have an excruciatingly painful attack in a joint, particularly in the big toe, you may want to have a test for gout. Fluid drawn from the affected joint is examined to resolve the diagnosis of gout or psoriatic arthritis. Psoriatic arthritis patients are commonly misdiagnosed as having gout, because they often have elevated serum uric acid levels, which also can be caused by taking low-dose aspirin or by increased skin cell turnover. It is important to distinguish between the two forms of arthritis, because they may be treated with different medications.

In the very early stages of the disease, x-rays usually do not reveal signs of arthritis and may not help in making a diagnosis. In the later stages, x-rays may show changes that are characteristic of psoriatic arthritis but not found with other types of arthritis, such as the "pencil in cup" phenomenon where the end of the bone gets whittled down to a sharp point. Changes in the peripheral joints and in the spine support the diagnosis of psoriatic arthritis. However, most of the changes occur in the later stages of the disease.

Chapter 22

Scleroderma

What is scleroderma?

Derived from the Greek words "sklerosis," meaning hardness, and "derma," meaning skin, scleroderma literally means hard skin. Although it is often referred to as if it were a single disease, scleroderma is really a symptom of a group of diseases that involve the abnormal growth of connective tissue, which supports the skin and internal organs. It is sometimes used, therefore, as an umbrella term for these disorders. In some forms of scleroderma, hard, tight skin is the extent of this abnormal process. In other forms, however, the problem goes much deeper, affecting blood vessels and internal organs, such as the heart, lungs, and kidneys.

Scleroderma is called both a rheumatic disease and a connective tissue disease. The term rheumatic disease refers to a group of conditions characterized by inflammation or pain in the muscles, joints, or fibrous tissue. A connective tissue disease is one that affects tissues such as skin, tendons, and cartilage.

What are the different types of scleroderma?

The group of diseases we call scleroderma falls into two main classes: localized scleroderma and systemic sclerosis. (Localized diseases affect

Excerpted from "Handout on Health: Scleroderma," by the National Institute on Arthritis and Musculoskeletal and Skin Diseases (NIAMS, www.niams .nih.gov), part of the National Institutes of Health, July 2006.

271

only certain parts of the body; systemic diseases can affect the whole body.) Both groups include subgroups. Although there are different ways these groups and subgroups may be broken down or referred to (and your doctor may use different terms from what you see here), the following is a common way of classifying these diseases.

Localized scleroderma: Localized types of scleroderma are those limited to the skin and related tissues and, in some cases, the muscle below. Internal organs are not affected by localized scleroderma, and localized scleroderma can never progress to the systemic form of the disease. Often, localized conditions improve or go away on their own over time, but the skin changes and damage that occurs when the disease is active can be permanent. For some people, localized scleroderma is serious and disabling.

There are two generally recognized types of localized scleroderma:

- **Morphea:** Morphea comes from a Greek word that means "form" or "structure." The word refers to local patches of scleroderma. The first signs of the disease are reddish patches of skin that thicken into firm, oval-shaped areas. The center of each patch becomes ivory colored with violet borders. These patches sweat very little and have little hair growth. Patches appear most often on the chest, stomach, and back. Sometimes they appear on the face, arms, and legs. Morphea can be either localized or generalized. Localized morphea limits itself to one or several patches, ranging in size from a half-inch to 12 inches in diameter. The condition sometimes appears on areas treated by radiation therapy. Some people have both morphea and linear scleroderma. The disease is referred to as generalized morphea when the skin patches become very hard and dark and spread over larger areas of the body. Regardless of the type, morphea generally fades out in 3 to 5 years; however, people are often left with darkened skin patches and, in rare cases, muscle weakness.

- **Linear scleroderma:** As suggested by its name, the disease is characterized by a single line or band of thickened or abnormally colored skin. Usually, the line runs down an arm or leg, but in some people it runs down the forehead. People sometimes use the French term *en coup de sabre*, or "sword stroke," to describe this highly visible line.

Systemic scleroderma (also known as systemic sclerosis): This is the term for the form of the disease that not only includes the skin, but also involves the tissues beneath, the blood vessels, and the major organs.

Systemic sclerosis is typically broken down into limited cutaneous scleroderma and diffuse cutaneous scleroderma. Some doctors break systemic sclerosis down into a third subset called systemic sclerosis sine (Latin for "without") scleroderma. This means that patients have other manifestations of scleroderma but they do not have any overt skin thickening.

Limited cutaneous scleroderma: Limited cutaneous scleroderma typically comes on gradually and affects the skin only in certain areas: the fingers, hands, face, lower arms, and legs. Most people with limited disease have Raynaud phenomenon for years before skin thickening starts. Telangiectasia and calcinosis often follow. Gastrointestinal involvement occurs commonly, and some patients have severe lung problems, even though the skin thickening remains limited. People with limited disease often have all or some of the symptoms that some doctors call CREST, which stands for the following:

- **Calcinosis:** The formation of calcium deposits in the connective tissues, which can be detected by x-ray. These deposits are typically found on the fingers, hands, face, and trunk and on the skin above elbows and knees. When the deposits break through the skin, painful ulcers can result.

- **Raynaud phenomenon:** A condition in which the small blood vessels of the hands or feet contract in response to cold or anxiety. As the vessels contract, the hands or feet turn white and cold, then blue. As blood flow returns, they become red. Fingertip tissues may suffer damage, leading to ulcers, scars, or gangrene.

- **Esophageal dysfunction:** Impaired function of the esophagus (the tube connecting the throat and the stomach) that occurs when smooth muscles in the esophagus lose normal movement. In the upper and lower esophagus, the result can be swallowing difficulties. In the lower esophagus, the result can be chronic heartburn or inflammation.

- **Sclerodactyly:** Thick and tight skin on the fingers, resulting from deposits of excess collagen within skin layers. The condition makes it harder to bend or straighten the fingers. The skin may also appear shiny and darkened, with hair loss.

- **Telangiectasia:** A condition caused by the swelling of tiny blood vessels, in which small red spots appear on the hands and face.

Although not painful, these red spots can create cosmetic problems.

Diffuse cutaneous scleroderma: This condition typically comes on suddenly. Skin thickening begins in the hands and spreads quickly and over much of the body, affecting the hands, face, upper arms, upper legs, chest, and stomach in a symmetrical fashion (for example, if one arm or one side of the trunk is affected, the other is also affected). Some people may have more area of their skin affected than others. Internally, this condition can damage key organs such as the intestines, lungs, heart, and kidneys.

People with diffuse disease often are tired, lose appetite and weight, and have joint swelling or pain. Skin changes can cause the skin to swell, appear shiny, and feel tight and itchy.

The damage of diffuse scleroderma typically occurs over a few years. After the first 3 to 5 years, people with diffuse disease often enter a stable phase lasting for varying lengths of time. During this phase, symptoms subside: joint pain eases, fatigue lessens, and appetite returns. Progressive skin thickening and organ damage decrease.

Gradually, however, the skin may begin to soften, which tends to occur in reverse order of the thickening process: the last areas thickened are the first to begin softening. Some patients' skin returns to a somewhat normal state, while other patients are left with thin, fragile skin without hair or sweat glands. Serious new damage to the heart, lungs, or kidneys is unlikely to occur, although patients are left with whatever damage they have in specific organs.

People with diffuse scleroderma face the most serious long-term outlook if they develop severe kidney, lung, digestive, or heart problems. Fortunately, less than one-third of patients with diffuse disease develop these severe problems. Early diagnosis and continual and careful monitoring are important.

What causes scleroderma?

Although scientists don't know exactly what causes scleroderma, they are certain that people cannot catch it from or transmit it to others. Studies of twins suggest it is also not inherited. Scientists suspect that scleroderma comes from several factors that may include:

- **Abnormal immune or inflammatory activity:** Like many other rheumatic disorders, scleroderma is believed to be an autoimmune disease. An autoimmune disease is one in which the immune system, for unknown reasons, turns against one's own body. In scleroderma, the immune system is thought to stimulate cells called fibroblasts so they produce too much collagen. The collagen forms thick connective tissue that builds up within the skin and internal organs and can interfere with their functioning. Blood vessels and joints can also be affected.

- **Genetic makeup:** Although genes seem to put certain people at risk for scleroderma and play a role in its course, the disease is not passed from parent to child like some genetic diseases.

- **Environmental triggers:** Research suggests that exposure to some environmental factors may trigger scleroderma-like disease (which is not actually scleroderma) in people who are genetically predisposed to it. Suspected triggers include viral infections, certain adhesive and coating materials, and organic solvents such as vinyl chloride or trichloroethylene. But no environmental agent has been shown to cause scleroderma. In the past, some people believed that silicone breast implants might have been a factor in developing connective tissue diseases such as scleroderma. But several studies have not shown evidence of a connection.

- **Hormones:** By the middle to late childbearing years (age 30 to 55), women develop scleroderma 7 to 12 times more often than men. Because of female predominance at these and all ages, scientists suspect that hormonal differences between women and men play a part in the disease. However, the role of estrogen or other female hormones has not been proven.

Who gets scleroderma?

Although scleroderma is more common in women, the disease also occurs in men and children. It affects people of all races and ethnic groups. However, there are some patterns by disease type.

Localized forms of scleroderma are more common in people of European descent than in African Americans. Morphea usually appears between the ages of 20 and 40, and linear scleroderma usually occurs in children or teenagers.

Systemic scleroderma, whether limited or diffuse, typically occurs in people from 30 to 50 years old. It affects more women of African American than European descent.

Because scleroderma can be hard to diagnose and it overlaps with or resembles other diseases, scientists can only estimate how many cases there actually are.

Estimates for the number of people in the United States with systemic sclerosis range from 40,000 to 165,000. By contrast, a survey that included all scleroderma-related disorders, including Raynaud phenomenon, suggested a number between 250,000 and 992,500.

For some people, scleroderma (particularly the localized forms) is fairly mild and resolves with time. But for others, living with the disease and its effects day to day has a significant impact on their quality of life.

How is scleroderma diagnosed?

Depending on your particular symptoms, a diagnosis of scleroderma may be made by a general internist, a dermatologist (a doctor who specializes in treating diseases of the skin, hair, and nails), an orthopedist (a doctor who treats bone and joint disorders), a pulmonologist (a lung specialist), or a rheumatologist (a doctor specializing in treatment of musculoskeletal disorders and rheumatic diseases). A diagnosis of scleroderma is based largely on the medical history and findings from the physical exam. To make a diagnosis, your doctor will ask you a lot of questions about what has happened to you over time and about any symptoms you may be experiencing. Are you having a problem with heartburn or swallowing? Are you often tired or achy? Do your hands turn white in response to anxiety or cold temperatures?

Once your doctor has taken a thorough medical history, he or she will perform a physical exam. Finding one or more of the following factors can help the doctor diagnose a certain form of scleroderma:

- Changed skin appearance and texture, including swollen fingers and hands and tight skin around the hands, face, mouth, or elsewhere
- Calcium deposits developing under the skin
- Changes in the tiny blood vessels (capillaries) at the base of the fingernails
- Thickened skin patches

Finally, your doctor may order lab tests to help confirm a suspected diagnosis. At least two proteins, called antibodies, are commonly found in the blood of people with scleroderma:

- Anti-topoisomerase-1 or Anti-Scl-70 antibodies appear in the blood of up to 30 percent of people with diffuse systemic sclerosis.

- Anticentromere antibodies are found in the blood of as many as 50 percent of people with limited systemic sclerosis.

A number of other scleroderma-specific antibodies can occur in people with scleroderma, although less frequently. When present, however, they are helpful in clinical diagnosis and may give additional information as to the risks for specific organ problems.

Because not all people with scleroderma have these antibodies and because not all people with the antibodies have scleroderma, lab test results alone cannot confirm the diagnosis.

In some cases, your doctor may order a skin biopsy (the surgical removal of a small sample of skin for microscopic examination) to aid in or help confirm a diagnosis. However, skin biopsies also have their limitations: biopsy results cannot distinguish between localized and systemic disease, for example.

Diagnosing scleroderma is easiest when a person has typical symptoms and rapid skin thickening. In other cases, a diagnosis may take months, or even years, as the disease unfolds and reveals itself and as the doctor is able to rule out some other potential causes of the symptoms. In some cases, a diagnosis is never made, because the symptoms that prompted the visit to the doctor go away on their own.

Some patients have some symptoms related to scleroderma and may fit into one of the following groups:

- **Undifferentiated connective tissue disease (UCTD):** This is a term for patients who have some signs and symptoms of various related diseases, but not enough symptoms of any one disease to make a definitive diagnosis. In other words, their condition hasn't "differentiated" into a particular connective tissue disease. In time, UCTD can go in one of three directions: it can change into a systemic disease such as systemic sclerosis, systemic lupus erythematosus, or rheumatoid arthritis; it can remain undifferentiated; or it can improve spontaneously.

- **Overlap syndromes:** This is a disease combination in which patients have symptoms and lab findings characteristic of two or more conditions.

How is scleroderma treated?

Because scleroderma can affect many different organs and organ systems, you may have several different doctors involved in your care. Typically, care will be managed by a rheumatologist (a doctor specializing in treatment of musculoskeletal disorders and rheumatic diseases). Your rheumatologist may refer you to other specialists, depending on the specific problems you are having. For example, you may see a dermatologist for the treatment of skin symptoms, a nephrologist for kidney complications, a cardiologist for heart complications, a gastroenterologist for problems of the digestive tract, and a pulmonary specialist for lung involvement.

In addition to doctors, professionals such as nurse practitioners, physician assistants, physical or occupational therapists, psychologists, and social workers may play a role in your care. Dentists, orthodontists, and even speech therapists can treat oral complications that arise from thickening of tissues in and around the mouth and on the face.

Currently, there is no treatment that controls or stops the underlying problem—the overproduction of collagen—in all forms of scleroderma. Thus, treatment and management focus on relieving symptoms and limiting damage. Your treatment will depend on the particular problems you are having. Some treatments will be prescribed or given by your doctor. Others are things you can do on your own.

Here is a listing of the potential problems that can occur in systemic scleroderma and the medical and nonmedical treatments for them. These problems do not occur as a result or complication of localized scleroderma. This listing is not complete because different people experience different problems with scleroderma and not all treatments work equally well for all people. Work with your doctor to find the best treatment for your specific symptoms.

Raynaud phenomenon: More than 90 percent of people with scleroderma have this condition, in which the fingers and sometimes other extremities change color in response to cold temperature or anxiety. For many, Raynaud phenomenon precedes other manifestations of the disease. In other people, however, Raynaud phenomenon is unrelated to scleroderma, but may signal damage to the blood vessels supplying the hands arising from occupational injuries (from using jackhammers, for example), trauma, excessive smoking, circulatory problems, drug use, or exposure to toxic substances. For some people, cold fingers and toes are the extent of the problem and are little more than a nuisance. For others, the condition can worsen and lead to puffy fingers, finger ulcers, and other complications that require aggressive treatment.

If you have Raynaud phenomenon, the following measures may make you more comfortable and help prevent problems:

- Don't smoke! Smoking narrows the blood vessels even more and makes Raynaud phenomenon worse.

- Dress warmly, with special attention to hands and feet. Dress in layers and try to stay indoors during cold weather.

- Use biofeedback, which governs various body processes that are not normally thought of as being under conscious control, and relaxation exercises.

- For severe cases, speak to your doctor about prescribing drugs called calcium channel blockers, such as nifedipine (Procardia), which can open up small blood vessels and improve circulation. Other drugs are in development and may become available.

- If Raynaud phenomenon leads to skin sores or ulcers, increasing your dose of calcium channel blockers (under the direction of your doctor only) may help.

- You can also protect skin ulcers from further injury or infection by applying nitroglycerin paste or antibiotic cream. Severe ulcerations on the fingertips can be treated with bioengineered skin.

Stiff, painful joints: In diffuse systemic sclerosis, hand joints can stiffen due to hardened skin around the joints or inflammation within them. Other joints can also become stiff and swollen.

- Stretching exercises under the direction of a physical or occupational therapist are extremely important to prevent loss of joint motion. These should be started as soon as scleroderma is diagnosed.

- Exercise regularly. Ask your doctor or physical therapist about an exercise plan that will help you increase and maintain range of motion in affected joints. Swimming can help maintain muscle strength, flexibility, and joint mobility.

- Use acetaminophen or an over-the-counter or prescription nonsteroidal anti-inflammatory drug, as recommended by your doctor, to help relieve joint or muscle pain. If pain is severe, speak to a rheumatologist about the possibility of prescription-strength drugs to ease pain and inflammation.

- Learn to do things in a new way. A physical or occupational therapist can help you learn to perform daily tasks, such as lifting and carrying objects or opening doors, in ways that will put less stress on tender joints.

Skin problems: When too much collagen builds up in the skin, it crowds out sweat and oil glands, causing the skin to become dry and stiff. If your skin is affected, try the following:

- Apply oil-based creams and lotions frequently, and always right after bathing.

- Apply sunscreen before you venture outdoors to protect against further damage from the sun's rays.

- Use humidifiers to moisten the air in your home in colder winter climates. Clean humidifiers often to stop bacteria from growing in the water.

- Avoid very hot baths and showers, as hot water dries the skin. Avoid harsh soaps, household cleaners, and caustic chemicals, if at all possible. Otherwise, be sure to wear rubber gloves when you use such products.

- Exercise regularly. Exercise, especially swimming, stimulates blood circulation to affected areas.

Dry mouth and dental problems: Dental problems are common in people with scleroderma for a number of reasons. Tightening facial skin can make the mouth opening smaller and narrower, which makes it hard to care for teeth; dry mouth due to salivary gland damage speeds up tooth decay; and damage to connective tissues in the mouth can lead to loose teeth. You can avoid tooth and gum problems in several ways:

- Brush and floss your teeth regularly. If hand pain and stiffness make this difficult, consult your doctor or an occupational therapist about specially made toothbrush handles and devices to make flossing easier.

- Have regular dental checkups. Contact your dentist immediately if you experience mouth sores, mouth pain, or loose teeth.

- If decay is a problem, ask your dentist about fluoride rinses or prescription toothpastes that remineralize and harden tooth enamel.

- Consult a physical therapist about facial exercises to help keep your mouth and face more flexible.

- Keep your mouth moist by drinking plenty of water, sucking ice chips, using sugarless gum and hard candy, and avoiding mouthwashes with alcohol. If dry mouth still bothers you, ask your doctor about a saliva substitute—or prescription medications such as pilocarpine hydrochloride (Salagen) or cevimeline hydrochloride (Evoxac)—that can stimulate the flow of saliva.

Gastrointestinal (GI) problems: Systemic sclerosis can affect any part of the digestive system. As a result, you may experience problems such as heartburn, difficulty swallowing, early satiety (the feeling of being full after you've barely started eating), or intestinal complaints such as diarrhea, constipation, and gas. In cases where the intestines are damaged, your body may have difficulty absorbing nutrients from food. Although GI problems are diverse, here are some things that might help at least some of the problems you have:

- Eat small, frequent meals.

- To keep stomach contents from backing up into the esophagus, stand or sit for at least an hour (preferably 2 or 3 hours) after eating. When it is time to sleep, keep the head of your bed raised using blocks.

- Avoid late-night meals, spicy or fatty foods, alcohol, and caffeine, which can aggravate GI distress.

- Eat moist, soft foods, and chew them well. If you have difficulty swallowing or if your body doesn't absorb nutrients properly, your doctor may prescribe a special diet.

- Ask your doctor about prescription medications for problems such as diarrhea, constipation, and heartburn. Some drugs called proton pump inhibitors are highly effective against heartburn. Oral antibiotics may stop bacterial overgrowth in the bowel, which can be a cause of diarrhea in some people with systemic sclerosis.

Lung damage: Virtually all people with systemic sclerosis have some loss of lung function. Some develop severe lung disease, which comes in two forms: pulmonary fibrosis (hardening or scarring of lung tissue because of excess collagen) and pulmonary hypertension (high blood pressure in the artery that carries blood from the heart to the lungs). Treatment for the two conditions is different:

- Pulmonary fibrosis may be treated with drugs that suppress the immune system, such as cyclophosphamide (Cytoxan) or azathioprine (Imuran), along with low doses of corticosteroids.

281

- Pulmonary hypertension may be treated with drugs that dilate the blood vessels, such as prostacyclin (Iloprost), or with newer medications that are prescribed specifically for treating pulmonary hypertension.

Regardless of your particular lung problem or its medical treatment, your role in the treatment process is essentially the same. To minimize lung complications, work closely with your medical team. Do the following:

- Watch for signs of lung disease, including fatigue, shortness of breath or difficulty breathing, and swollen feet. Report these symptoms to your doctor.

- Have your lungs closely checked, using standard lung-function tests, during the early stages of skin thickening. These tests, which can find problems at the earliest and most treatable stages, are needed because lung damage can occur even before you notice any symptoms.

- Get regular flu and pneumonia vaccines as recommended by your doctor. Contracting either illness could be dangerous for a person with lung disease.

Heart problems: Common among people with scleroderma, heart problems include scarring and weakening of the heart (cardiomyopathy), inflamed heart muscle (myocarditis), and abnormal heartbeat (arrhythmia). All of these problems can be treated. Treatment ranges from drugs to surgery and varies depending on the nature of the condition.

Kidney problems: Renal crisis occurs in about 10 percent of all patients with scleroderma, primarily those with early diffuse scleroderma. Renal crisis results in severe uncontrolled high blood pressure, which can quickly lead to kidney failure. It's very important that you take measures to identify and treat the hypertension as soon as it occurs. These are things you can do:

- Check your blood pressure regularly. You should also check it if you have any new or different symptoms such as a headache or shortness of breath. If your blood pressure is higher than usual, call your doctor right away.

- If you have kidney problems, take your prescribed medications faithfully. In the past two decades, drugs known as ACE (angiotensin-converting enzyme) inhibitors, including captopril (Capoten), enalapril (Vasotec), and lisinopril, have made scleroderma-related kidney failure a less threatening problem than it used to be. But for these drugs to work, you must take them as soon as the hypertension is present.

Cosmetic problems: Even if scleroderma doesn't cause any lasting physical disability, its effects on the skin's appearance—particularly on the face—can take their toll on your self-esteem. Fortunately, there are procedures to correct some of the cosmetic problems scleroderma causes:

- The appearance of telangiectasias—small red spots on the hands and face caused by swelling of tiny blood vessels beneath the skin—may be reduced or even eliminated with the use of guided lasers.

- Facial changes of localized scleroderma—such as the en coup de sabre that may run down the forehead in people with linear scleroderma—may be corrected through cosmetic surgery. (However, such surgery is not appropriate for areas of the skin where the disease is active.)

How can scleroderma affect my life?

Having a chronic disease can affect almost every aspect of your life, from family relationships to holding a job. For people with scleroderma, there may be other concerns about appearance or even the ability to dress, bathe, or handle the most basic daily tasks. Here are some areas in which scleroderma could intrude.

Appearance and self-esteem: Aside from the initial concerns about health and longevity, people with scleroderma quickly become concerned with how the disease will affect their appearance. Thick, hardened skin can be difficult to accept, particularly on the face. Systemic scleroderma may result in facial changes that eventually cause the opening to the mouth to become smaller and the upper lip to virtually disappear. Linear scleroderma may leave its mark on the forehead. Although these problems can't always be prevented, their effects may be minimized with proper treatment. Also, special cosmetics—and in some cases plastic surgery—can help conceal scleroderma's damage.

Caring for yourself: Tight, hard connective tissue in the hands can make it difficult to do what were once simple tasks, such as brushing your teeth and hair, pouring a cup of coffee, using a knife and fork, unlocking a door, or buttoning a jacket. If you have trouble using your hands, consult an occupational therapist, who can recommend new ways of doing things or devices to make tasks easier. Devices as simple as Velcro fasteners and built-up brush handles can help you be more independent.

Family relationships: Spouses, children, parents, and siblings may have trouble understanding why you don't have the energy to keep house, drive to soccer practice, prepare meals, or hold a job the way you used to. If your condition isn't that visible, they may even suggest you are just being lazy. On the other hand, they may be overly concerned and eager to help you, not allowing you to do the things you are able to do or giving up their own interests and activities to be with you. It's important to learn as much about your form of the disease as you can and to share any information you have with your family. Involving them in counseling or a support group may also help them better understand the disease and how they can help you.

Sexual relations: Sexual relationships can be affected when systemic scleroderma enters the picture. For men, the disease's effects on the blood vessels can lead to problems achieving an erection. For women, damage to the moisture-producing glands can cause vaginal dryness that makes intercourse painful. People of either sex may find they have difficulty moving the way they once did. They may be self-conscious about their appearance or afraid that their sexual partner will no longer find them attractive. With communication between partners, good medical care, and perhaps counseling, many of these changes can be overcome or at least worked around.

Pregnancy and childbearing: In the past, women with systemic scleroderma were often advised not to have children. But thanks to better medical treatments and a better understanding of the disease itself, that advice is changing. (Pregnancy, for example, is not likely to be a problem for women with localized scleroderma.) Although blood vessel involvement in the placenta may cause babies of women with systemic scleroderma to be born early, many women with the disease can have safe pregnancies and healthy babies if they follow some precautions.

One of the most important pieces of advice is to wait a few years after the disease starts before attempting a pregnancy. During the first 3 years, you are at the highest risk of developing severe problems of the heart, lungs, or kidneys that could be harmful to you and your unborn baby.

If you haven't developed severe organ problems within 3 years of the disease's onset, your chances of such problems are less and pregnancy would be safer. But it is important to have both your disease and your pregnancy monitored regularly. You'll probably need to stay in close touch with both the doctor you typically see for your scleroderma and an obstetrician who is experienced in guiding high-risk pregnancies.

Chapter 23

Sjögren Syndrome

What is Sjögren syndrome?

Sjögren syndrome is an autoimmune disease—that is, a disease in which the immune system turns against the body's own cells. Normally, the immune system works to protect us from disease by destroying harmful invading organisms like viruses and bacteria. In the case of Sjögren syndrome, disease-fighting cells attack various organs, most notably the glands that produce tears and saliva (the lacrimal and salivary glands). Damage to these glands causes a reduction in both the quantity and quality of their secretions. This results in symptoms that include dry eyes and dry mouth. In technical terms, the form of eye dryness associated with Sjögren syndrome is called keratoconjunctivitis sicca, or KCS, and the symptoms of dry mouth are called xerostomia. Your doctor may use these terms when talking to you about Sjögren syndrome.

When organs other than the lacrimal and salivary glands are affected, this is known as "extraglandular involvement." Usually, this occurs in patients with primary Sjögren syndrome. Manifestations include joint inflammation; particular forms of autoimmune thyroid, kidney, liver, lung, and skin disease; and changes in nerve function of the upper or lower limbs. A small proportion of patients may progress to a form of malignant lymphoma.

Excerpted from "Questions and Answers about Sjögren's Syndrome," by the National Institute of Arthritis and Musculoskeletal and Skin Diseases (NIAMS, www.niams.nih.gov), part of the National Institutes of Health, December 2006.

You might hear Sjögren syndrome called a rheumatic disease. This means it causes inflammation in joints, muscles, skin, and other organs. Like rheumatoid arthritis and systemic lupus erythematosus, it is also considered one of the autoimmune connective tissue diseases. These conditions affect the framework of the body (joints, muscles, and skin).

What are the symptoms of Sjögren syndrome?

Sjögren syndrome can cause many symptoms. The main ones include the following:

- **Dry eyes:** Eyes affected by Sjögren syndrome may burn or itch. Some people say it feels like they have sand in their eyes. Others have trouble with blurry vision, or are bothered by bright light, especially fluorescent lighting.

- **Dry mouth:** Dry mouth may feel chalky or like your mouth is full of cotton. It may be difficult to swallow, speak, or taste. Because you lack the protective effects of saliva, you may develop more dental decay (cavities) and mouth infections.

As noted in the preceding text, both primary and secondary Sjögren syndrome can also affect other parts of the body, causing symptoms such as the following:

- Multiple sites of joint and muscle pain
- Prolonged dry skin
- Skin rashes on the extremities
- Chronic dry cough
- Vaginal dryness
- Numbness or tingling in the extremities
- Prolonged fatigue that interferes with daily life

What causes dryness in Sjögren syndrome?

Often in the autoimmune attack causing Sjögren syndrome, white blood cells called lymphocytes initially will target and damage the glands that produce tears and saliva. Although no one knows exactly how this occurs, the damaged glands produce tears and saliva that are diminished in both quantity and quality, leading to the symptoms of dryness of the eyes and mouth.

Who gets Sjögren syndrome?

Sjögren syndrome can affect people of either sex and of any age, but most cases occur in women. The average age for onset is late 40s, but in rare cases, Sjögren syndrome is diagnosed in children.

What causes Sjögren syndrome?

Researchers think Sjögren syndrome is caused by a combination of genetic and environmental factors. Several different genes appear to be involved, but scientists are not certain exactly which ones are linked to the disease, since different genes seem to play a role in different people. For example, there is one gene that predisposes Caucasians to the disease. Other genes are linked to Sjögren syndrome in people of Japanese, Chinese, and African American descent. Simply having one of these genes will not cause a person to develop the disease. Some sort of trigger must activate the immune system.

Scientists think that the trigger may be a viral or bacterial infection. It might work like this: A person who has a Sjögren-associated gene gets a viral infection. The virus stimulates the immune system to act, but the gene alters the attack, sending fighter cells (lymphocytes) to the glands of the eyes and mouth. Once there, the lymphocytes attack healthy cells, causing the inflammation that damages the glands and keeps them from working properly. This is an example of autoimmunity. These fighter cells are supposed to die after their attack in a natural process called apoptosis, but in people with Sjögren syndrome, they continue to attack, causing further damage. Scientists think that resistance to apoptosis may be genetic.

The possibility that the endocrine and nervous systems play a role in the disease is also under investigation.

How is Sjögren syndrome diagnosed?

Your doctor will diagnose Sjögren syndrome based on your medical history, a physical exam, and results from clinical or laboratory tests. While reviewing your medical history, your doctor will ask questions about your general health, specific symptoms you are experiencing, and medical problems you and your family members have or have had. Your doctor will also ask about any medications you are taking and about lifestyle habits such as smoking or alcohol consumption. During the exam, your doctor will check for clinical signs of Sjögren syndrome, such as indications of mouth dryness, or signs of other connective tissue diseases.

Depending on what your doctor finds during the history and exam, he or she may want to perform some tests or refer you to a specialist to establish the diagnosis of Sjögren syndrome and/or to see how severe the problem is and whether the disease is affecting other parts of the body as well.

Some common eye and mouth tests include the following:

- **Schirmer test:** This test measures tears to see how the lacrimal (tear) glands are working. The doctor puts thin paper strips under the lower eyelids and measures the amount of wetness on the paper after 5 minutes. People with Sjögren syndrome usually produce less than 8 millimeters of tears.

- **Slit lamp examination:** This test, in which an ophthalmologist uses equipment to magnify and carefully examine the eye, shows how severe the dryness is and whether the outside of the eye is inflamed.

- **Staining with vital dyes (rose bengal or lissamine green):** These tests show the extent to which dryness has damaged the surface of the eye. To perform one of these tests, the doctor puts a drop of a liquid containing a dye into the lower eyelid. The dye stains the surface of the eye, highlighting any areas of injury, thereby allowing the doctor to see with the slit lamp how much damage has occurred on the surface of the eye.

- **Mouth exam:** The doctor will look outside the mouth for signs of major salivary gland swelling and inside the mouth for signs of dryness. Signs of dry mouth include a dry, sticky lining (called oral mucosa); dental caries (cavities) in characteristic locations; thick saliva, or none at all coming out of the major salivary ducts; redness of the mouth lining, often associated with a smooth, burning tongue; and sores at the corners of the lips. The doctor might also try to get a sample of saliva, to check its quality and see how much of it the glands are producing.

- **Lip biopsy:** This test is the best way to find out whether dry mouth is caused by Sjögren syndrome. To perform this test the doctor removes tiny minor salivary glands from the inside of the lower lip and examines them under the microscope. If the glands contain white blood cells in a particular pattern, the test is positive for the salivary component of Sjögren syndrome.

Because there are many causes of dry eyes and dry mouth (including many common medications, other diseases, or previous treatment such as radiation of the head or neck), the doctor needs a thorough history from the patient, and additional tests to see whether other parts of the body are affected. These tests may include:

- **Routine blood tests:** The doctor will take a blood sample to look for levels of different types of blood cells, check blood sugar level, and see how the liver and kidneys are working.

- **Other blood tests:** Various blood tests may be performed to check for antibodies and other immunological substances often found in the blood of people with Sjögren syndrome. Antibodies are gamma globulin molecules, called immunoglobulins, which are important for fighting infection. Everyone has these in their blood, but people with Sjögren syndrome usually have too many of them. Antibodies that are directed against the individual making them are called auto antibodies. Antibodies that may be present in people with Sjögren syndrome include the following.

  - **Immunoglobulins:** The three main classes of immunoglobulins can be measured to see if there is a general increase in antibodies.

  - **Anti-thyroid antibodies:** Auto antibodies against the thyroid gland are created when white blood cells (lymphocytes) migrate into the thyroid gland, causing thyroiditis (inflammation of the thyroid), a common problem in people with Sjögren syndrome.

  - **Rheumatoid factors (RF):** These are auto antibodies commonly found in the blood of people with rheumatoid arthritis as well as in people with Sjögren syndrome and other autoimmune connective tissue diseases.

  - **Antinuclear antibodies (ANAs):** These are auto antibodies directed at the cells' nuclei. The presence of ANAs in the blood can indicate an autoimmune disorder, including Sjögren syndrome.

  - **Sjögren antibodies, anti-SS-A (or -Ro) and anti-SS-B (or -La):** These are specific antinuclear antibodies that occur commonly, but not always, in people with Sjögren syndrome.

- **Chest x-ray:** Sjögren syndrome can cause inflammation in the lungs, so the doctor may want to take an x-ray to check them.

- **Urinalysis:** The doctor will probably test a sample of your urine to see how well the kidneys are working.

What type of doctor diagnoses and treats Sjögren syndrome?

Because the symptoms of Sjögren syndrome develop gradually and are similar to those of many other diseases, getting a diagnosis can take time; in fact, it may take years to diagnose Sjögren syndrome. During those years, depending on the symptoms, a person could see a number of doctors, any of whom could diagnose the disease and be involved in its treatment. Usually, a rheumatologist (a doctor who specializes in diseases of the joints, muscles, and bones) will coordinate treatment among a number of specialists. In a recent survey of a large number of Sjögren syndrome patients, the doctors making their first diagnoses were identified as follows, in order of decreasing frequency.

- Rheumatologist
- Primary care physician/internist
- Ophthalmologist (eye specialist)
- Otolaryngologist (ear, nose, and throat specialist)
- Dentist (oral care specialist)
- Neurologist (nerve and brain specialist)
- Allergist (allergic disease specialist)
- Endocrinologist (endocrine disease specialist)
- Oncologist (cancer specialist)

How is Sjögren syndrome treated?

Treatment can vary from person to person, depending on what parts of the body are affected. But in all cases, the doctor will help relieve your symptoms, especially dryness. For example, you can use artificial tears to help with dry eyes and saliva stimulants and mouth lubricants for dry mouth. Treatment for both mouth and eye dryness is described in more detail in the following text.

If you have extraglandular involvement (that is, a problem that extends beyond the moisture-producing glands of your eyes and mouth), your doctor—or the appropriate specialist—will also treat those problems. Treatment may include the following:

- Nonsteroidal anti-inflammatory drugs, such as ibuprofen (Motrin, Advil) for joint or muscle pain, may be used.
- Corticosteroid medications, such as prednisone, can be used to suppress inflammation that threatens the lungs, kidneys, blood vessels, or nervous system.

- Immune-modifying drugs such as hydroxychloroquine (Plaquenil), methotrexate (Rheumatrex), and cyclophosphamide (Cytoxan) to control the overactivity of the immune system that, in severe cases, can lead to organ damage.

What can I do about dry eyes?

Artificial tears: Available by prescription or over the counter under many brand names, these products keep eyes moist by replacing natural tears. Artificial tears come in different thicknesses, so you may have to experiment to find the right one. Some drops contain preservatives that might irritate your eyes. Drops without preservatives usually don't bother the eyes. These drops typically come in single-dose packages to prevent contamination with bacteria.

Ointments: Ointments are thicker than artificial tears. Because they moisturize and protect the eye for several hours, and may blur your vision, they are most effective during sleep.

Hydroxypropyl methylcellulose (Lacrisert): This is a chemical that lubricates the surface of the eye and slows the evaporation of natural tears. It comes in a small pellet that you put in your lower eyelid. When you add artificial tears, the pellet dissolves and forms a film over your own tears that traps the moisture.

Topical anti-inflammatory agents: Topical steroids and cyclosporin A (Restasis) are used if the surface of the eye is inflamed. Topical steroids can increase the pressure in the eye, so your eye pressure must be monitored regularly.

Punctal occlusion: A surgical procedure used to close the tear ducts that drain tears from the eye, helping to keep more natural tears on the eye's surface. For a temporary closure, the doctor inserts collagen or silicone plugs into the ducts. Collagen plugs eventually dissolve, and silicone plugs are "permanent" until they are removed or fall out. For a longer lasting effect, the doctor can use a laser or a heating device called a cautery to seal the ducts.

What can I do about dry mouth?

There are many remedies for dry mouth. You can try some of them on your own. Your doctor may prescribe others. Here are some many people find useful.

Chewing gum and hard candy: If your salivary glands still produce some saliva, you can stimulate them to make more by chewing gum or sucking on hard candy. However, gum and candy must be sugar-free, because dry mouth makes you extremely prone to progressive dental decay (cavities).

Water: Take sips of water or another sugar-free, noncarbonated drink throughout the day to wet your mouth, especially when you are eating or talking. Note that drinking large amounts of liquid throughout the day will not make your mouth any less dry and will make you urinate more often. You should only take small sips of liquid, but not too often. If you sip liquids every few minutes, it may reduce or remove the mucus coating inside your mouth, increasing the feeling of dryness.

Lip balm: You can soothe dry, cracked lips by using oil- or petroleum-based lip balm or lipstick. If your mouth hurts, your doctor may give you medicine in a mouth rinse, ointment, or gel to apply to the sore areas to control pain and inflammation.

Saliva substitutes: If you produce very little saliva or none at all, your doctor might recommend a saliva substitute. These products mimic some of the properties of saliva, which means they make the mouth feel wet. Gel-based saliva substitutes tend to give the longest relief, but as with all saliva products, their effectiveness is limited by the fact that you eventually swallow them. It is best to use these products rather than water when awakening from sleep: They reduce oral symptoms more effectively, and they do not cause excessive urine formation.

Prescription medications: At least two prescription drugs stimulate the salivary glands to produce saliva. These are pilocarpine (Salagen) and cevimeline (Evoxac). The effects last for a few hours, and you can take them three or four times a day. However, they are not suitable for everyone, so talk to your doctor about whether they might help you. In trials of these drugs, patients have also experienced some reduction in their dry eye symptoms.

In addition to treatments for dry mouth itself, some people need treatment for its complications. For example, people with dry mouth can easily get a mouth infection from a common yeast called *Candida*. About one-third of people with Sjögren syndrome experience this infection, which is called candidiasis. Most often, it causes red patches to appear, along with a burning sensation. This occurs particularly on the tongue and corners of the lips. Candidiasis is treated with prescription antifungal drugs.

What other parts of the body are involved in Sjögren syndrome?

The autoimmune response that causes dry eyes and mouth can cause inflammation throughout the body. People with Sjögren syndrome may have extraglandular problems, as noted above. Following are examples of extraglandular problems and how they are treated.

Skin problems: People who have Sjögren syndrome may have dry skin. Some experience only itching, but it can be severe. Others develop cracked, split skin that can easily become infected. Infection is a risk for people with itchy skin, too, particularly if they scratch vigorously. The skin may darken in infected areas, but it returns to normal when the infection clears up and the scratching stops.

To treat dry skin, apply heavy moisturizing creams and ointments three or four times a day to trap moisture in the skin. Lotions, which are lighter than creams and ointments, aren't recommended because they evaporate quickly and can contribute to dry skin. Also, doctors suggest that you take only short showers (less than 5 minutes), use a moisturizing soap, pat your skin almost dry, and then cover it with a cream or ointment. If you take baths, it's a good idea to soak for 10 to 15 minutes to give your skin time to absorb moisture. Having a humidifier in the bedroom can help hydrate your skin, too. If these steps don't help the itching, your doctor might recommend that you use a skin cream or ointment containing steroids.

Some patients who have Sjögren syndrome, particularly those with lupus, are sensitive to sunlight and can get painful burns from even a little sun exposure, such as through a window. So, if you're sensitive to sunlight, you need to wear sunscreen (at least SPF [sun protection factor] 15) whenever you go outdoors and try to avoid being in the sun for long periods of time.

Vaginal dryness: Common in postmenopausal women with or without Sjögren syndrome, vaginal dryness causes painful intercourse. A vaginal moisturizer and a vaginal lubricant can help. Vaginal moisturizers can attract liquid to the dry tissues, helping to maintain moisture, and are designed for regular use. Vaginal lubricants can make intercourse more comfortable, but they don't moisturize, and therefore aren't appropriate for regular use. Oil-based lubricants, such as petroleum jelly, should be avoided, because they trap moisture and can cause sores and hinder the vagina's natural cleaning process. Regular skin creams and ointments relieve dry skin on the outer surface of the vagina (the vulva).

Lung problems: People with Sjögren syndrome tend to have lung problems caused by inflammation. These conditions include bronchitis (affecting the bronchial tubes) and tracheobronchitis (affecting the windpipe and bronchial tubes). Lung problems are usually caused by white blood cells (lymphocytes) migrating into the lungs and causing a disease called lymphocytic interstitial pneumonitis. Depending on your condition, the doctor may recommend using a humidifier, taking medicines to open the bronchial tubes, or taking corticosteroids to relieve inflammation.

Pleurisy, another Sjögren-related problem, is inflammation of the lining of the lungs. It is treated with corticosteroids and nonsteroidal anti-inflammatory drugs.

Kidney problems: The kidneys filter waste products from the blood and remove them from the body through urine. The most common kidney problem in people with Sjögren syndrome is interstitial nephritis, or inflammation of the tissue around the kidney's filters, which can occur even before dry eyes and dry mouth. Inflammation of the filters themselves, called glomerulonephritis, is less common. Some people develop renal tubular acidosis, which means they can't get rid of certain acids through urine. The amount of potassium in their blood drops, causing an imbalance in blood chemicals that can affect the heart, muscles, and nerves.

Often, doctors do not treat these problems unless they start to affect kidney function or cause other health problems. However, they keep a close eye on the problem through regular exams, and will prescribe medicines called alkaline agents to balance blood chemicals when necessary. Corticosteroids or immunosuppressants are used to treat more severe cases.

Nerve problems: In some patients with Sjögren syndrome, the nervous system may be affected. Most often it affects the peripheral nervous system, which contains the nerves that control sensation and movement. Peripheral nervous system changes occurring in Sjögren syndrome include the following:

- Peripheral neuropathy: A problem that occurs when an immune system attack damages nerves in the legs or arms, causing pain, numbness, tingling, and possibly muscle weakness. Sometimes nerves are damaged because inflamed blood vessels cut off their blood supply.

- Cranial neuropathy: A problem in which nerve damage causes face pain; loss of feeling in the face, tongue, eyes, ears, or throat; and loss of taste and smell.

Nerve problems are treated with medicines to control pain and, if necessary, with corticosteroids or other drugs to control inflammation.

Digestive problems: Inflammation in the liver can cause hepatitis and cirrhosis (hardening of the liver). Sjögren syndrome is closely linked to a liver disease called primary biliary cirrhosis (PBC), which causes itching, fatigue, and, eventually, cirrhosis. Many patients with PBC have Sjögren syndrome. Treatment varies, depending on the problem, but may include pain medicine, anti-inflammatory drugs, steroids, and immunosuppressants.

Thyroid disorders: There is a group of autoimmune thyroid disorders that can appear as either the overactive thyroid of Graves disease or the underactive thyroid of Hashimoto thyroiditis. Many people with these autoimmune thyroid disorders also have Sjögren syndrome and many people with Sjögren syndrome show evidence of thyroid disease.

Raynaud phenomenon: This is a condition in which the blood vessels in the hands, arms, feet, and legs constrict (narrow) when exposed to cold. The result is pain, tingling, and numbness. When vessels constrict, fingers turn white. Shortly after that, they turn blue because of blood that remained in the tissue pools. When new blood rushes in, the fingers turn red. The problem is treated with medicines that dilate blood vessels. Raynaud phenomenon usually occurs before dryness of the eyes or mouth.

Vasculitis: This is an inflammation of the blood vessels, which then become scarred and too narrow for blood to get through to reach the organs. For people with Sjögren syndrome, vasculitis tends to occur in those who also have Raynaud phenomenon and lung and liver problems. It can affect different organs at the same time and have gradually developing systemic (e.g., fever, weight loss, arthritis) or localized (e.g., raised rash) clinical presentations.

What are other autoimmune connective tissue diseases?

Patients who have an autoimmune connective tissue diseases other than Sjögren syndrome may subsequently develop the dry eyes and or dry mouth of Sjögren syndrome. They would then be diagnosed as having secondary Sjögren syndrome, along with their primary connective tissue disease. These other autoimmune connective tissue diseases include:

Polymyositis: An inflammation of the muscles that causes weakness and pain, difficulty moving, and, in some cases, problems breathing and swallowing. If the skin is inflamed too, it's called dermatomyositis. The disease is treated with corticosteroids and immunosuppressants.

Rheumatoid arthritis (RA): A form of arthritis that is characterized by severe inflammation of the joints. This inflammation can eventually damage the surrounding bones (fingers, hands, knees, etc.). RA can also damage muscles, blood vessels, and major organs. Treatment depends on the severity of the pain and swelling and which body parts are involved. It may include physical therapy, aspirin, rest, nonsteroidal anti-inflammatory agents, steroids, or immunosuppressants.

Scleroderma: A disease in which the body accumulates too much collagen, a protein commonly found in the skin. The result is thick, tight skin and possibly damage to muscles, joints, and internal organs such as the esophagus, intestines, lungs, heart, kidneys, and blood vessels. Treatment is aimed at relieving pain and includes drugs, skin softeners, and physical therapy.

Systemic lupus erythematosus (SLE): A disease that causes joint and muscle pain, weakness, skin rashes, and, in more severe cases, heart, lung, kidney, and nervous system problems. As with RA, treatment for SLE depends on the symptoms and may include aspirin, rest, steroids, and anti-inflammatory and other drugs, as well as dialysis and high blood pressure medicine.

Does Sjögren syndrome cause lymphoma?

A small percentage of people with Sjögren syndrome develop lymphoma, which involves salivary glands, lymph nodes, the gastrointestinal tract, or the lungs.

Persistent enlargement of a major salivary gland should be carefully and regularly observed by your doctor and investigated further if it changes in size in a short period of time. Other symptoms may include the following: (Note that many of these can be symptoms of other problems, including Sjögren syndrome itself. Nevertheless, it is important to see your doctor if you have any of these symptoms so that any problem can be diagnosed and treated as early as possible.)

- Unexplained fever
- Night sweats
- Constant fatigue
- Unexplained weight loss
- Itchy skin
- Reddened patches on the skin

If you're worried that you might develop lymphoma, talk to your doctor to learn more about the disease, the symptoms to watch for, any special medical care you might need, and what you can do to relieve your worry.

What research is being done on Sjögren syndrome?

Through basic research on the immune system, autoimmunity, genetics, and connective tissue diseases, researchers continue to learn more about Sjögren syndrome. The hope is that a better understanding of the disease and its causes will lead to better treatments and perhaps even prevention.

Some of the areas of recent research into Sjögren syndrome include the following:

Hormonal factors: Because Sjögren syndrome affects mostly women, female reproductive hormones may play a role. Although studies have shown that levels of estrogen and progesterone differ little between women with Sjögren syndrome and those without, higher levels of prolactin (a hormone that stimulates the production of milk after childbirth and the production of progesterone in the ovary) are found in women with Sjögren syndrome. Research is also looking at how the disease affects men and women differently.

Medication treatment: Recent studies have shown that cevimeline (Evoxac) is effective at easing dry eyes, as well as dry mouth, and that the immunosuppressive drug cyclophosphamide (Cytoxan) is effective for treating some of the nervous system effects of Sjögren syndrome. In a mouse model of this disorder, eye drops of an anti-CD4 antibody were effective at promoting moisture. On the other hand, at least two other therapies under investigation for Sjögren syndrome—the biologic response modifier etanercept (Enbrel) and the mild male hormone dehydroepiandrosterone (DHEA)—have not proven to be effective.

Prevalence of extraglandular involvement: Studies have shown that neurological involvement and Sjögren-related problems with the skin—including alopecia (a condition characterized by hair loss), vitiligo (a condition in which areas of the skin lose their pigment and become white), and vasculitis (a raised rash)—may be more common than previously thought. Studies also indicate that identifying and treating these problems in people with Sjögren syndrome is an important part of managing the disease. Another study shows that clinical depression is also common among Sjögren syndrome patients, and may warrant treatment.

Predicting lung involvement: Knowing who is at highest risk of certain complications can enable doctors to identify and treat these problems earlier and more appropriately. One study showed that serum levels of beta-2 microglobulin (a protein made by plasma cells and associated with inflammation) were higher in people who later developed lung problems with primary Sjögren syndrome.

Role of infection: Doctors believe that infections may trigger Sjögren syndrome in people genetically predisposed to the disease. Viral infection is under investigation as a possible trigger for Sjögren syndrome and other autoimmune diseases. Epstein-Barr virus, hepatitis C virus, and Coxsackie virus are being studied.

Long-term relief for dry mouth: Gene therapy studies suggest that we may someday be able to insert molecules into salivary glands that will control inflammation and prevent their destruction. Scientists also envision a day when they will be able to transplant salivary glands from one person to another. Development of a safe and effective artificial salivary gland is already underway.

Chapter 24

Arthritis Related to Other Disorders

Chapter Contents

Section 24.1

Arthritis and Human Immunodeficiency Virus

"HIV-Related Rheumatic Disease Syndrome," © Johns Hopkins Medicine Office of Corporate Communications. Reprinted with permission. Reviewed by David A. Cooke, MD, FACP, June 29, 2009.

What Is It?

Acquired immune deficiency syndrome, AIDS, is an infectious disease that has reached epidemic proportions both in this country and worldwide. The current estimate is that approximately 39.5 million people worldwide are infected with HIV; about 2.3 million of these are children. As of 2003, approximately 1.2 million persons in the United States were living with HIV/AIDS, with as many as 24–27 percent unaware they have HIV infection.

AIDS is caused by a virus called human immunodeficiency virus (HIV), which is transmitted primarily through sexual contact, through blood and blood products, and from infected mothers to their infants either in utero or through breast milk. AIDS produces a spectrum of symptoms, including several arthritic-related conditions.

Although HIV resembles a variety of autoimmune diseases, there is no evidence that HIV-infected individuals have an increase in two of the more common autoimmune diseases: systemic lupus erythematosus and rheumatoid arthritis. In fact, it has been observed that, in some cases, these two conditions may be alleviated by the presence of HIV.

Approximately 33 percent of HIV-infected individuals experience joint pain at some time during the course of the disease. Between 5 percent and 10 percent are diagnosed as having some form of reactive arthritis, such as Reiter's syndrome or psoriatic arthritis. As the virus progresses and the immune system declines, arthritic symptoms are more likely to take hold.

If you are infected with HIV, you may also experience a variety of joint problems that seem to have no apparent cause. This syndrome is called HIV- or AIDS-associated arthropathy. Characterized by discomfort and stiffness that develop over one to six weeks and lasting six weeks to six months, this syndrome generally involves the large joints—the hips, knees, or ankles. Usually, the condition does not cause long-term damage and only mild inflammation. Anti-inflammatory drugs are only mildly effective; injections of steroids seem to provide greater relief.

Another form of arthritis that seems to be related to HIV is called painful articular syndrome. Present in about 10 percent of AIDS patients, this form is characterized by acute, severe, sharp pain in the knees, elbows, and shoulders. Although research is inconclusive, it is generally thought that this form of arthritis occurs when HIV directly affects the joint.

Signs and Symptoms

- Joint pain
- Achiness
- Swelling
- Stiffness

Diagnosis

If you have already tested positive for HIV, your doctor will likely consider any joint and muscle pain and stiffness you report as reactive to the virus. He or she will therefore make any treatment and preventive recommendations within the overall context of your condition.

Treatment

Generally, HIV-related arthritic symptoms respond well to standard treatment. Nonsteroidal anti-inflammatory drugs, such as aspirin and ibuprofen (Advil, Nuprin, Motrin), reduce pain and swelling. Moderate exercises and a healthy, balanced diet are also important. The pain of painful articular syndrome usually lasts anywhere from two to 24 hours and may be severe enough to require narcotic analgesics—codeine, for example. When the arthritic symptoms are more severe or persistent, your doctor may recommend short courses of corticosteroids or immunosuppressant agents, although the use of these, especially methotrexate, can lead to infection with an already compromised immune system. As a result, they should be used with caution and only in the most severe cases.

Section 24.2

Arthritis and Inflammatory Bowel Disease

Overview

Enteropathic (en-ter-o-path-ic) arthritis is a form of chronic, inflammatory arthritis associated with the occurrence of an inflammatory bowel disease (IBD), the two best-known types of which are ulcerative colitis and Crohn disease. About one in five people with Crohn or ulcerative colitis will develop enteropathic arthritis.

The most common areas affected by enteropathic arthritis are inflammation of the peripheral (limb) joints, as well as the abdominal pain and possibly bloody diarrhea associated with the IBD component of the disease. In some cases, the entire spine can become involved as well.

Is There a Cure?

Currently, there is no known cure for enteropathic arthritis but there are medications and therapies available to manage the symptoms of both the arthritis and bowel components of the disease.

Causes of Enteropathic Arthritis

Many people don't realize that the gastrointestinal tract contains the largest immune system in the body. The immune system is the body's natural defense against foreign invaders, and it is somehow altered in people who have these conditions. Some researchers believe that the long-lasting inflammation found in the intestines of people with IBD damages the bowel, which in turn may allow bacteria to enter the damaged bowel wall and circulate through the blood stream. The body's reaction to these bacteria may cause other problems including inflammation in the joints and/or spine, skin sores, and inflammation of the eyes. Currently this hypothesis is neither fully understood nor confirmed by rigorous scientific study.

Ankylosing spondylitis and related diseases tend to run in families, so there is a genetic factor involved as well. Those who test positive for the HLA-B27 genetic marker are much more likely to have spinal involvement with enteropathic arthritis than those who test negative.

Disease Course/Prognosis

The course and severity of enteropathic arthritis varies from person to person. The disease "flares"—the times when the disease is most active and inflammation is occurring—tend to be self-limiting, often subsiding after 6 weeks, but reoccurrences are common. In some cases the arthritis may become chronic and destructive.

Symptoms of Enteropathic Arthritis

The symptoms for enteropathic arthritis can basically be divided in two groups:

1. The symptoms of inflammatory bowel disease (IBD)

2. The arthritic symptoms in the joints and possibly elsewhere in the body

IBD Symptoms

Ulcerative colitis and Crohn disease are the two types of IBD most commonly associated with enteropathic arthritis in spondylitis. Abdominal pain and bloody diarrhea are the most common symptoms of IBD.

Arthritis Symptoms

Note that the arthritis symptoms may precede the IBD symptoms.

About one in five people with enteropathic arthritis will have inflammatory arthritis in one or more peripheral (limb) joints such as an arm or leg, although the lower limbs are more commonly affected. The severity of the peripheral arthritis normally coincides with the severity of the IBD, thus when diarrhea and abdominal pain are flaring, the peripheral arthritis tends to flare as well.

About one in six people with IBD also has spinal inflammation, although this inflammation is independent of the severity of the bowel disease symptoms. In many, this may just be arthritis in the sacroiliac (SI) joints, but in about five percent of people, the entire spine is involved, as it is in AS.

Part Three

Medical and Surgical Treatments for Arthritis

Chapter 25

Your Arthritis
Health Care Provider

Chapter Contents

Section 25.1

What Is a Rheumatologist?

A rheumatologist is an internist or pediatrician who is qualified by additional training and experience in the diagnosis and treatment of arthritis and other diseases of the joints, muscles, and bones. Many rheumatologists conduct research to determine the cause and better treatments for these disabling and sometimes fatal diseases.

What kind of training do rheumatologists have?

After four years of medical school and three years of training in either internal medicine or pediatrics, rheumatologists devote an additional two to three years in specialized rheumatology training. Most rheumatologists who plan to treat patients choose to become board certified. Upon completion of their training, they must pass a rigorous exam conducted by the American Board of Internal Medicine to become certified.

What do rheumatologists treat?

Rheumatologists treat arthritis, certain autoimmune diseases, musculoskeletal pain disorders, and osteoporosis. There are more than 100 types of these diseases, including rheumatoid arthritis, osteoarthritis, gout, lupus, back pain, osteoporosis, fibromyalgia, and tendonitis. Some of these are very serious diseases that can be difficult to diagnose and treat.

When should you see a rheumatologist?

If musculoskeletal pains are not severe or disabling and last just a few days, it makes sense to give the problem a reasonable chance to be resolved. But sometimes, pain in the joints, muscles, or bones is severe or persists for more than a few days. At that point, you should see your physician.

Many types of rheumatic diseases are not easily identified in the early stages. Rheumatologists are specially trained to do the detective work necessary to discover the cause of swelling and pain. It's important to determine a correct diagnosis early so that appropriate treatment can begin early. Some musculoskeletal disorders respond best to treatment in the early stages of the disease.

Because some rheumatic diseases are complex, one visit to a rheumatologist may not be enough to determine a diagnosis and course of treatment. These diseases often change or evolve over time. Rheumatologists work closely with patients to identify the problem and design an individualized treatment program.

How does the rheumatologist work with other health care professionals?

The role the rheumatologist plays in health care depends on several factors and needs. Typically the rheumatologist works with other physicians, sometimes acting as a consultant to advise another physician about a specific diagnosis and treatment plan. In other situations, the rheumatologist acts as a manager, relying upon the help of many skilled professionals including nurses, physical and occupational therapists, psychologists, and social workers. Team work is important, since musculoskeletal disorders are chronic. Health care professionals can help people with musculoskeletal diseases and their families cope with the changes the diseases cause in their lives.

Is specialty care more expensive?

You may be surprised to learn that specialized care may save time and money and reduce the severity of disease. A rheumatologist is specially trained to spot clues in the medical history and physical examination. The proper tests done early may save money in the long run. Prompt diagnosis and specially tailored treatment often save money and buy time in treating the disease.

Section 25.2

Choosing a Doctor

Excerpted from "Choosing a Doctor," by the National Institute on
Aging (NIA, www.nia.nih.gov), part of the National Institutes of Health,
March 2009.

There are many reasons why you might be looking for a new doctor. Maybe you've moved to another city or perhaps your doctor is retiring. If you need a new doctor, the following ideas can help you find
one who is right for you.

People and Places to Help with Your Search

Ask people you trust, for example, friends, family, and coworkers,
about doctors they use and like. You might ask questions such as the
following:

- Do you know a good doctor?

- Would you recommend your doctor?

- What do you like about your doctor?

- How long does it take to get an appointment?

- Can you usually see your doctor right away if you need to, like
  on the same day if you get sick?

In addition to talking to friends, family, and coworkers, you can talk
with other health professionals you see, for example, your heart doctor or the doctor you see for your lung problems, and ask for recommendations. If your doctor is retiring or leaving the practice, you might
ask if he or she has picked a replacement. You can check with your
insurance plan for a list of doctors in your area. Another idea is to
contact a local hospital, medical center, medical society, physician referral service, or nearby medical school. Online resources, like the
website www.healthfinder.gov, may be useful too.

After talking with people, checking with local resources, and looking online, you may find a few names keep coming up. These might be

the doctors you want to consider. Make a list of several names of doctors to pick from in case your first choice is not taking new patients or does not participate in your health insurance plan.

Calling the Doctors on Your List

After you pick two or three doctors, call their offices. The office staff can give you information about the doctor's education and training. They can also tell you about office policies, what insurance the office takes, if they file the insurance claims for you, what types of payment they accept, and to what hospitals the doctor sends patients.

You might say, "Before I make an appointment, I have some questions about the office and the practice." Some questions you might want to ask include the following:

- What type of health insurance does the office take? You want to find out if the doctor accepts Medicare or any other health insurance you have.

- Where is the doctor's office located? Is there parking? You want to make sure that it will be easy for you to get there.

- How long is the usual office visit? You want a doctor who will take time to listen carefully to your concerns, answer your questions, and explain things clearly and fully in a way that you can understand. Good doctor-patient communication is important for developing treatment plans that address your specific health needs.

- Is the doctor part of a group practice? If the doctor is part of a group, you may want to find out who the other doctors are and their specialties.

- Who sees patients if the doctor is out of town or not available? If the doctor is not part of a group practice, you want to make sure that the doctor has a plan when he or she is not there.

- Can I get lab work or x-rays done in the office or nearby? You want to find out if you will need to go to another location for tests or if most lab tests are done in the doctor's office.

- Is the doctor Board certified? Board-certified doctors have extra training and pass special exams after medical school to become specialists in a field of medicine such as family practice, internal medicine, or geriatrics.

Other Helpful Questions

It might be helpful to learn about the doctor's experience treating older patients or people with a medical history similar to yours. Here are more questions you might want to ask the office staff:

- Does the doctor see many older patients?

- Does the doctor treat many patients with the same chronic health problem that I have (for example, diabetes or heart problems)?

- If I have to go to the hospital, will the doctor take care of me or will a hospital doctor?

The First Appointment

After choosing a doctor, make your first appointment. This visit is a time for you to get to know the doctor and for the doctor to get to know you.

You will probably be asked to fill out a new-patient form. To help you, bring a list of your past medical problems and all the medicines you take. Include both prescription and over-the-counter drugs, even vitamins, supplements, and eye drops. Write down the dosage you take, such as 20 mg once a day. You might even put all your drugs in a bag and bring them with you to the appointment. Also, write down any drug allergies or serious drug reactions you've had. You will need to give all your drug information to the doctor to include in your medical record.

During the visit, take time to ask the doctor any questions you have about your health. You might want to write these questions down before your visit so you don't forget them. Some questions you may want to ask include the following:

- Will you give me written instructions about my care?

- May I bring a family member (spouse, daughter, or son) to my office visits?

- Are you willing to talk with my family about my condition if I give my permission?

During your first appointment, the doctor or nurse will likely ask you questions about your current health and the medical history of your family. This information will also be added to your medical record.

After your first visit, think about if you felt comfortable and confident with this doctor. For example, were you at ease asking questions? Did the doctor clearly answer your questions? Were you treated with respect? Did you feel that your questions were considered thoughtfully? Did you feel the doctor hurried or did not address all your concerns? If you are still not sure the doctor is right for you, schedule a visit with one of the other doctors on your list.

Once you find a doctor you like, your job is not finished. Make sure to have your medical records sent to your new doctor. Your former doctor may charge you for mailing your records.

Remember that a good doctor-patient relationship is a partnership. Regular office visits and open communication with the doctor and office staff are key to maintaining this partnership, treating your medical problems effectively, and keeping you in good health.

Section 25.3

Physician-Patient Partnership Improves Physical Functioning

Excerpted from "Managing Osteoarthritis: Helping the Elderly Maintain Function and Mobility." *Research in Action,* Issue 4. AHRQ Publication No. 02-0023, May 2002. Agency for Health Care Policy and Research, Rockville, MD, www.ahrq.gov. Reviewed by David A. Cooke, MD, FACP, July 26, 2009.

Physician-Patient Partnership Improves Physical Functioning

AHRQ research shows that patients have better outcomes when they receive education and training about their condition because they become more involved in their care. Two ways to achieve improved outcomes are through self-management and occupational therapy.

Self-Management of Osteoarthritis

AHRQ researchers indicate that the key to good management of osteoarthritis is an effective physician-patient partnership. This partnership should accomplish the following:

• Promote proper use of medications

- Encourage patients to change their behavior to improve symptoms or slow disease progression

- Instruct patients on how to interpret and report symptoms accurately

- Help patients adjust to new social and economic circumstances and cope with emotional consequences

- Support patients' efforts to participate in treatment decisions and maintain normal activities

Creating patient education programs helps patients achieve this role by giving them the knowledge and skills they need for self-management. AHRQ funded the development of the Chronic Disease Self-Management Program, which is based on changes in diet, exercise, and compliance with treatment regimens. The CDSMP has been shown to improve health status and reduce costs. Specifically, the CDSMP helps patients interpret and report symptoms accurately and has led to substantial reductions in pain, depression, and the use of health services in patients with chronic disease.

Changing the patient's health behaviors and perception of symptoms can improve the symptoms or slow the progression of osteoarthritis.

Regular exercise helps patients retain mobility and counteracts loss of muscle strength. Exercise such as walking or aquatics improves aerobic capacity and stamina while decreasing depression and anxiety. If patients attribute pain to the progression of osteoarthritis, then they may avoid activities that increase pain. However, if patients attribute pain to loss of muscle tone and strength, then they may increase physical activity.

Patients can be referred to organizations in their community that offer exercise programs, swimming facilities, information meetings, social activities, self-help education, support groups, and mobile services for transportation and meals. Finally, research sponsored by AHRQ indicates that patients can be supported from the physician's office by telephone with no significant increase in costs to either the patients or physicians. These telephone conversations can be used to discuss joint pain, medications, treatment compliance, drug toxicities, date of next scheduled visit, and barriers to receiving care.

Occupational Therapy

Occupational therapists can evaluate a person's ability to perform daily living activities and recommend devices such as elevated toilet seats or wall bars for bathtubs. They also teach joint protection and energy conservation. For example, living on one floor of the home helps to avoid painful step climbing and avoiding kneeling or squatting helps to protect the joints.

AHRQ cofunded the Well Elderly Study with the National Institute on Aging and the National Center for Medical Rehabilitation Research. This study evaluated the effectiveness of preventive occupational therapy as a way to avoid functional disability in people age 60 and over. During a 9-month period, one group of participants received weekly group and individual occupational therapy. This therapy focused on home and community safety, shopping, mastering the public transportation system, joint protection, adaptive equipment, energy conservation, exercise, and nutrition. A second group of patients attended a program that focused only on social activities, such as community outings, craft projects, films, games, and dances.

At the end of the study, those who were in the occupational therapy study group reported the following:

- Better quality of interaction with other people
- Improved health status
- More satisfaction with life
- Improved mental health, physical functioning, role functioning, vitality, and social functioning
- Less pain
- Fewer emotional problems

Six months after the initial study, the patients who received preventive occupational therapy were reassessed. These elderly participants continued to experience the following:

- Better quality of interaction with other people
- Improved mental health, physical functioning, role functioning, vitality, and social functioning
- Less pain
- Fewer emotional problems

Section 25.4

Tips for Talking to Your Doctor

"Quick Tips—When Talking with Your Doctor." Agency for Healthcare
Research and Quality (AHRQ) Publication No. 01-0040a, www.ahrq.gov,
May 2002. Reviewed by David A. Cooke, MD, FACP, June 29, 2009.

Research has shown that patients who have good relationships
with their doctors tend to be more satisfied with their care—and to
have better results. Here are some tips to help you and your doctor
become partners in improving your health care.

Give Information—Don't Wait to Be Asked!

- You know important things about your symptoms and your
  health history. Tell your doctor what you think he or she needs
  to know.

- It is important to tell your doctor personal information—even if
  it makes you feel embarrassed or uncomfortable.

- Bring a "health history" list with you, and keep it up to date.
  You might want to make a copy of the form for each member of
  your family.

- Always bring any medicines you are taking, or a list of those
  medicines (include when and how often you take them) and what
  strength. Talk about any allergies or reactions you have had to
  your medicines.

- Tell your doctor about any herbal products you use or alternative medicines or treatments you receive.

- Bring other medical information, such as x-ray films, test results, and medical records.

Get Information

- Ask questions. If you don't, your doctor may think you understand everything that was said.

- Write down your questions before your visit. List the most important ones first to make sure they get asked and answered.

- You might want to bring someone along to help you ask questions.

- This person can also help you understand and/or remember the answers.

- Ask your doctor to draw pictures if that might help to explain something.

- Take notes.

- Some doctors do not mind if you bring a tape recorder to help you remember things. But always ask first.

- Let your doctor know if you need more time. If there is not time that day, perhaps you can speak to a nurse or physician assistant on staff. Or, ask if you can call later to speak with someone.

- Ask if your doctor has washed his or her hands before starting to examine you. Research shows that handwashing can prevent the spread of infections. If you're uncomfortable asking this question directly, you might ask, "I've noticed that some doctors and nurses wash their hands or wear gloves before touching people. Why is that?"

Take Information Home

- Ask for written instructions.

- Your doctor also may have brochures and audio tapes and videotapes that can help you. If not, ask how you can get such materials.

Once You Leave the Doctor's Office, Follow Up

- If you have questions, call.

- If your symptoms get worse, or if you have problems with your medicine, call.

- If you had tests and do not hear from your doctor, call for your test results.

- If your doctor said you need to have certain tests, make appointments at the lab or other offices to get them done.

319

- If your doctor said you should see a specialist, make an appointment.

Remember, quality matters, especially when it comes to your health.

Chapter 26

Diagnosing and Treating Arthritis

How are rheumatic diseases diagnosed?

Diagnosing rheumatic diseases can be difficult because some symptoms and signs are common to many different diseases. A general practitioner or family doctor may be able to evaluate a patient or refer him or her to a rheumatologist (a doctor who specializes in treating arthritis and other rheumatic diseases).

The doctor will review the patient's medical history, conduct a physical examination, and obtain laboratory tests and x-rays or other imaging tests. The doctor may need to see the patient more than once and possibly a number of times to make an accurate diagnosis.

It is vital for people with joint pain to give the doctor a complete medical history. Answers to the following questions will help the doctor make an accurate diagnosis:

- Is the pain in one or more joints?
- When does the pain occur?
- How long does the pain last?
- When did you first notice the pain?
- What were you doing when you first noticed the pain?

Excerpted from "Questions and Answers about Arthritis and Rheumatic Diseases," by the National Institute of Arthritis and Musculoskeletal and Skin Diseases (NIAMS, www.niams.nih.gov), part of the National Institutes of Health, October 2008.

- Does activity make the pain better or worse?

- Have you had any illnesses or accidents that may account for the pain?

- Are you experiencing any other symptoms besides pain?

- Is there a family history of arthritis or other rheumatic disease?

- What medicine(s) are you taking?

- Have you had any recent infections?

Because rheumatic diseases are so diverse and sometimes involve several parts of the body, the doctor may ask many other questions.

It may be helpful for people to keep a daily journal that describes the pain. Patients should write down what the affected joint looks like, how it feels, how long the pain lasts, and what they were doing when the pain started.

The doctor will examine the patient's joints for redness, warmth, damage, ease of movement, and tenderness. Because some forms of arthritis, such as lupus, may affect internal organs, a complete physical examination that includes the heart, lungs, abdomen, nervous system, eyes, ears, mouth, and throat may be necessary. The doctor may order some laboratory tests to help confirm a diagnosis. Samples of blood, urine, or synovial fluid (lubricating fluid found in the joint) may be needed for the tests. Many of these same tests may be useful later for monitoring the disease or the effectiveness of treatments.

Common laboratory tests and procedures include the following:

- **Antinuclear antibody (ANA):** This test checks blood levels of antibodies that are often present in people who have connective tissue diseases or other autoimmune disorders, such as lupus. Because the antibodies react with material in the cell's nucleus (control center), they are referred to as antinuclear antibodies. There are also tests for individual types of ANAs that may be more specific to people with certain autoimmune disorders. ANAs are also sometimes found in people who do not have an autoimmune disorder. (In such cases, the result is referred to as a "false positive.") Therefore, having ANAs in the blood does not necessarily mean that a person has a disease.

- **CCP (or anti-CCP):** This test checks blood levels of antibodies to citrulline, a protein that can be detected in up to 70 percent of people in the early stages of rheumatoid arthritis. Because the presence of anti-CCPs is associated with more aggressive disease, the test can also be useful in helping doctors plan treatment.

- **C-reactive protein test:** This nonspecific test is used to detect generalized inflammation. Levels of the protein are often increased in patients with active disease such as rheumatoid arthritis or any other disease that causes inflammation.

- **Complement:** This test measures the level of complement, a group of proteins in the blood. Complement helps destroy germs and other foreign substances that enter the body. A low blood level of complement is common in people who have active lupus.

- **Complete blood count (CBC):** This test determines the number of white blood cells, red blood cells, and platelets present in a sample of blood. Some rheumatic conditions or drugs used to treat arthritis are associated with a low white blood count (leukopenia), low red blood count (anemia), or low platelet count (thrombocytopenia).

- **Creatinine:** This blood test measures the level of creatinine, a breakdown product of creatine, which is an important component of muscle. Creatinine is excreted from the body entirely by the kidneys, and the level remains constant and normal when kidney function is normal. This test is commonly used to diagnose and monitor kidney disease in patients who have a rheumatic condition such as lupus.

- **Erythrocyte sedimentation rate (sed rate or ESR):** This blood test is used to detect inflammation in the body. Higher sed rates, indicating the presence of inflammation, are typical of many forms of arthritis, such as rheumatoid arthritis and ankylosing spondylitis. Higher sed rates are also typical of many of the immunologic connective tissue diseases, such as lupus and scleroderma.

- **Hematocrit (PCV, packed cell volume):** This test and the test for hemoglobin (a substance in the red blood cells that carries oxygen throughout the body) measure the number of red blood cells present in a sample of blood. A decrease in the number of red blood cells (anemia) is common in people who have inflammatory arthritis or another rheumatic disease.

- **Rheumatoid factor:** This test detects the presence of rheumatoid factor, an antibody found in the blood of most (but not all) people who have rheumatoid arthritis. In rheumatoid arthritis, it is associated with more aggressive disease. Rheumatoid factor may be found in many diseases besides rheumatoid arthritis and sometimes in people without health problems. (In the latter case, the result is referred to as a "false positive.")

- **Synovial fluid examination:** Synovial fluid may be examined for white blood cells (found in patients with rheumatoid arthritis and infections), bacteria or viruses (found in patients with infectious arthritis), or crystals in the joint (found in patients with gout or other types of crystal-induced arthritis). To obtain a specimen, the doctor injects a local anesthetic, then inserts a needle into the joint to withdraw the synovial fluid into a syringe. The procedure is called arthrocentesis or joint aspiration.

- **Urinalysis:** In this test, a urine sample is studied for protein, red blood cells, white blood cells, and bacteria. These abnormalities may indicate kidney disease, which may be seen in lupus as well as several rheumatic conditions. Some medications used to treat arthritis also can cause abnormal findings on urinalysis.

To see what the joint looks like inside, the doctor may order x-rays or other imaging procedures. X-rays provide an image of the bones, but they do not show cartilage, muscles, and ligaments. Other noninvasive imaging methods such as computed tomography (CT or CAT scan), magnetic resonance imaging (MRI), and arthrography show the whole joint. The doctor also may look for damage to a joint by using an arthroscope: a small, flexible tube which is inserted through a small incision at the joint. The arthroscope transmits the image from inside the joint to a video screen.

What are the treatments?

Treatments for rheumatic diseases include rest and relaxation, exercise, proper diet, medication, and instruction about the proper use of joints and ways to conserve energy. Other treatments include the use of pain relief methods and assistive devices, such as splints or braces. In severe cases, surgery may be necessary. The doctor and the patient develop a treatment plan that helps the patient maintain or improve his or her lifestyle. Treatment plans usually combine several types of treatment and vary depending on the rheumatic condition and the patient.

Rest, exercise, and diet: People who have a rheumatic disease should develop a comfortable balance between rest and activity. One sign of many rheumatic conditions is fatigue. Patients must pay attention to signals from their bodies. For example, when experiencing pain or fatigue, it is important to take a break and rest. Too much rest, however, may cause muscles to become weak and joints to become stiff.

People with a rheumatic disease such as arthritis can participate in a variety of sports and exercise programs. Physical exercise can reduce joint pain and stiffness and increase flexibility, muscle strength, and endurance. Exercise also can result in weight loss, which in turn reduces stress on painful joints and contributes to an improved sense of well-being. Before starting any exercise program, people with arthritis should talk with their doctor.

Doctors often recommend getting exercise in each of these three categories. The benefits listed below often reinforce each other.

- Range-of-motion exercises (e.g., stretching, dance) help maintain normal joint movement, maintain or increase flexibility, and relieve stiffness.

- Strengthening exercises (e.g., weight lifting) maintain or increase muscle strength. Strong muscles help support and protect joints affected by arthritis.

- Aerobic or endurance exercises (e.g., walking, bicycle riding, swimming) improve cardiovascular fitness, help control weight, improve strength, and improve overall well-being. Studies show that aerobic exercise can also reduce inflammation in some joints.

Another important part of a treatment program is a well-balanced diet. Along with exercise, a well-balanced diet helps people manage their body weight and stay healthy. Diet is especially important for people who have gout. People with gout should avoid alcohol and foods that are high in purines, such as organ meats (liver, kidney), sardines, anchovies, and gravy.

Medications: A variety of medications are used to treat rheumatic diseases. The type of medication depends on the rheumatic disease and on the individual patient. The medications used to treat most rheumatic diseases do not provide a cure, but rather limit the symptoms of the disease. One exception is infectious arthritis, which can be cured if medications are used properly. Another exception is Lyme disease, which is spread by the bite of certain ticks: If the infection is caught early and treated with antibiotics, symptoms of arthritis may be prevented or may disappear.

Medications commonly used to treat rheumatic diseases provide relief from pain and inflammation. In some cases, especially when a person has rheumatoid arthritis or another type of inflammatory arthritis, the medication may slow the course of the disease and prevent further damage to joints or other parts of the body.

The doctor may delay using medications until a definite diagnosis is made because medications can hide important symptoms or signs (such as fever and swelling) and thereby interfere with diagnosis. Patients taking any medication, either prescription or over the counter, should always follow the doctor's instructions. The doctor should be notified immediately if the medicine is making the symptoms worse or causing other problems, such as upset stomach, nausea, or headache. The doctor may be able to change the dosage or medicine to reduce these side effects.

Following are some of the types of medications commonly used in the treatment of rheumatic diseases.

- **Analgesics:** Analgesics (pain relievers) such as acetaminophen (Tylenol) are often used to reduce the pain caused by many rheumatic conditions. For severe pain or pain following surgery or a fracture, doctors may prescribe stronger prescription or narcotic analgesics.

- **Topical analgesics:** People who cannot take oral pain relievers or who continue to have some pain after taking them may find topical analgesics helpful. These creams or ointments are rubbed into the skin over sore muscles or joints and relieve pain through one or more active ingredients. These are the most common:

  - **Counterirritants:** These ingredients, such as menthol, oil of wintergreen, eucalyptus oil, or camphor, work by irritating the nerve endings in the skin. This distracts the brain from the deeper source of pain. They are found in many products such as Eucalyptamint and Icy Hot.

  - **Salicylates:** This ingredient works like aspirin, by blocking chemicals in the body that contribute to pain. Salicylates are found in Aspercreme, Ben-Gay, Flexall, and several other over-the-counter preparations.

  - **Capsaicin:** This natural ingredient found in cayenne peppers is an effective pain reliever for many. It is available in a number of products, including Zostrix and Capzasin-P.

- **Nonsteroidal anti-inflammatory drugs (NSAIDs):** A large class of medications useful against both pain and inflammation, NSAIDs are staples in arthritis treatment. A number of NSAIDs—such as ibuprofen (Advil, Motrin), naproxen sodium (Aleve), and ketoprofen (Orudis, Oruvail) are available over the counter. More than two dozen others, including a subclass of NSAIDs called COX-2 inhibitors, are available only with a prescription. All NSAIDs work similarly: by blocking substances called prostaglandins that contribute to inflammation and pain. However, each NSAID is a different chemical, and each has a slightly different effect on the body. Warning: NSAIDs can cause stomach irritation or, less often, they can affect kidney function. The longer a person uses NSAIDs, the more likely he or she is to have side effects, ranging from mild to serious. Many other drugs cannot be taken when a patient is being treated with NSAIDs because NSAIDs alter the way the body uses or eliminates these other drugs. Check with your health care provider or pharmacist before you take NSAIDs. Also, NSAIDs sometimes are associated with serious gastrointestinal problems, including ulcers, bleeding, and perforation of the stomach or intestine. People age 65 and older, as well as those with any history of ulcers or gastrointestinal bleeding, should use NSAIDs with caution. The Food and Drug Administration has warned that long-term use of NSAIDs, or use by people who have heart disease, may increase the chance of a heart attack or stroke. So it's important to work with your doctor to choose the one that's safest and most effective for you. Side effects also may include stomach upset and stomach ulcers, heartburn, diarrhea, fluid retention, hypertension, and kidney damage. For unknown reasons, some people seem to respond better to one NSAID than another.

- **Disease-modifying antirheumatic drugs (DMARDs):** A family of medicines that are used to treat inflammatory arthritis like rheumatoid arthritis and ankylosing spondylitis, DMARDs may be able to slow or stop the immune system from attacking the joints. This in turn decreases pain and swelling. DMARDs typically require regular blood tests to monitor side effects, which may include increased risk of infection. In addition to relieving signs and symptoms, DMARDs may help to retard or even stop joint damage from progressing. However, DMARDs cannot fix joint damage that has already occurred. Some of the most commonly prescribed DMARDs are methotrexate, hydroxychloroquine, sulfasalazine, and leflunomide.

- **Biologic response modifiers:** Biologic response modifiers, or biologics, are a new family of genetically engineered drugs that block specific molecular pathways of the immune system that are involved in the inflammatory process. They are often prescribed in combination with DMARDs such as methotrexate. Because biologics work by suppressing the immune system, they could be problematic for patients who are prone to frequent infection. They are typically administered by injection at home or by intravenous infusion at a clinic. Some commonly prescribed biologics include etanercept, adalimumab, infliximab, abatacept, and rituximab.

- **Corticosteroids:** Corticosteroids, such as prednisone, cortisone, Solu-Medrol, and hydrocortisone, are used to treat many rheumatic conditions because they decrease inflammation and suppress the immune system. The dosage of these medications as well as their method of administration will vary depending on the diagnosis and the patient. Again, the patient and doctor must work together to determine the right amount of medication. Corticosteroids can be given by mouth, in creams applied to the skin, intravenously, or by injection directly into the affected joint(s). Short-term side effects of corticosteroids include swelling, increased appetite, weight gain, and emotional ups and downs. These side effects generally stop when the drug is stopped. It can be dangerous to stop taking corticosteroids suddenly, so it is very important that the doctor and patient work together when changing the corticosteroid dose. Side effects that may occur after long-term use of corticosteroids include stretch marks, excessive hair growth, osteoporosis, high blood pressure, damage to the arteries, high blood glucose, infections, and cataracts.

- **Hyaluronic acid substitutes:** Hyaluronic acid products, such as Hyalgan and Synvisc, mimic a naturally occurring body substance that serves to lubricate joints and is believed to be deficient in joints with osteoarthritis. Depending on the particular product, patients receive a series of three to five injections, which are administered directly into the affected knee(s) or hip(s) to help provide temporary relief of pain and flexible joint movement.

Medical devices: A number of devices may be used to treat some rheumatic diseases. For example, transcutaneous electrical nerve stimulation (TENS) has been found effective in modifying pain perception. TENS blocks pain messages to the brain with a small device that directs mild electric pulses to nerve endings that lie beneath the painful area of the skin.

Some health care facilities use a blood-filtering device called the Prosorba Column to filter out harmful antibodies in people with severe rheumatoid arthritis.

Hydrotherapy, mobilization therapy, and relaxation therapy: Hydrotherapy involves exercising or relaxing in warm water. The water takes some weight off painful joints, making it easier to exercise. It helps relax tense muscles and relieve pain.

Mobilization therapies include traction (gentle, steady pulling), massage, and manipulation. (Someone other than the patient moves stiff joints through their normal range of motion.) When done by a trained professional, these methods can help control pain, increase joint motion, and improve muscle and tendon flexibility.

Relaxation therapy helps reduce pain by teaching people various ways to release muscle tension throughout the body. In one method of relaxation therapy, known as progressive relaxation, the patient tightens a muscle group and then slowly releases the tension. Doctors and physical therapists can teach patients a variety of relaxation techniques.

Splints and braces: Splints and braces are used to support weakened joints or allow them to rest. Some prevent the joint from moving; others allow some movement. A splint or brace should be used only when recommended by a doctor or therapist, who will explain to the patient when and for how long the device should be worn. The doctor or therapist also will demonstrate the correct way to put it on and will ensure that it fits properly. The incorrect use of a splint or brace can cause joint damage, stiffness, and pain.

Assistive devices: A person with arthritis can use many kinds of devices to ease the pain. For example, using a cane when walking can reduce some of the weight placed on a knee or hip affected by arthritis. A shoe insert (orthotic) can ease the pain of walking caused by arthritis of the foot or knee. Other devices can help with activities such as opening jars, closing zippers, and holding pencils.

Surgery: Surgery may be required to repair damage to a joint after injury or to restore function or relieve pain in a joint damaged by arthritis. Many types of surgery are performed for arthritis. These include the following:

- **Arthroscopic surgery:** Surgery to view the joint using a thin lighted scope inserted through a small incision over the joint. If repair is needed, tools may be inserted through additional small incisions.

- **Bone fusion:** Surgery in which joint surfaces are removed from the ends of two bones that form a joint. The bones are then held together with screws until they grow together forming one rigid unit.

- **Osteotomy:** A surgery in which a section of bone is removed to improve the positioning of a joint.

- **Arthroplasty:** Also known as total joint replacement. This procedure removes and replaces the damaged joint with an artificial one.

Nutritional supplements: Nutritional supplements are sometimes helpful in treating rheumatic diseases. These include products such as S-adenosylmethionine (SAM-e) for osteoarthritis and fibromyalgia, dehydroepiandrosterone (DHEA) for lupus, and glucosamine and chondroitin sulfate for osteoarthritis.

The Glucosamine/Chondroitin Arthritis Intervention Trial (the results of which were published in 2006) assessed the effectiveness and safety of glucosamine and chondroitin sulfate when taken together or separately. The trial was cosponsored by the National Center for Complementary and Alternative Medicine and NIAMS. The trial found that the combination of glucosamine and chondroitin sulfate did not provide significant relief from osteoarthritis pain among all participants. However, a smaller subgroup of study participants with moderate to severe pain received significant relief from the combined supplements.

Generally speaking, reports on the safety and effectiveness of any nutritional supplement should be viewed with caution because the Food and Drug Administration does not regulate supplements the way it monitors medications, and many have not been proven helpful in formal studies.

What are some myths about treating arthritis?

At this time, the only type of arthritis that can be cured is that caused by infections. Although symptoms of other types of arthritis can be effectively managed with rest, exercise, and medication, there are no cures. Some people claim to have been cured by treatment with herbs, oils, chemicals, special diets, radiation, or other products. However, there is no scientific evidence that such treatments cure arthritis. Moreover, some may lead to serious side effects. Patients should talk to their doctor before using any therapy that has not been prescribed or recommended by their health care team.

How can you work with your doctor to limit your pain?

The role you play in planning your treatment is very important. It is vital for you to have a good relationship with your doctor in order to work together. You should not be afraid to ask questions about your condition or treatment. You must understand the treatment plan and tell the doctor whether or not it is helping you. Research has shown that well-informed patients who participate actively in their own care experience less pain and make fewer visits to the doctor.

What can be done to help?

Many people find that having arthritis or another rheumatic disease limits their activities. When people can no longer participate in some of their favorite activities, their overall well-being can be affected. Even when arthritis impairs only one joint, a person may have to change many daily activities to reduce pain and protect that joint from further damage. When a condition affects the entire body, as it often does with rheumatoid arthritis, lupus, or fibromyalgia, many daily activities have to be changed to deal with pain, fatigue, and other symptoms.

Changes in the home may help a person with chronic arthritis continue to live safely, productively, and with less pain. People with arthritis may become weak, lose their balance, or fall. In the bathroom, installing grab bars in the tub or shower and by the toilet, placing a secure seat in the tub, and raising the height of the toilet seat can help. Special kitchen utensils can accommodate hands affected by arthritis to make meal preparation easier. An occupational therapist can help people who have rheumatic conditions to identify and make adjustments in their homes to create a safer, more comfortable, and more efficient environment.

Friends and family members can help a patient with a rheumatic condition by learning about that condition and understanding how it affects the patient's life. Friends and family can provide emotional and physical assistance. Their support, as well as support from other people who have the same disease, can make it easier to cope.

Chapter 27

Overview of Pain Medicines for Rheumatic Diseases

Medications are agents that help counteract the condition's effect on the body. Many categories of medication are used for arthritis pain management. Following are descriptions of the pain medications typically used to treat the most common types of arthritis.

Osteoarthritis

A variety of medications are available to treat osteoarthritis pain.

Nonsteroidal Anti-Inflammatory Drugs (NSAIDs)

These are among the most common treatments for osteoarthritis pain. Purchased over-the-counter or by prescription, NSAIDs—such as aspirin, ibuprofen (Advil or Motrin), and diclofenac (Cataflam, Voltaren)—act quickly to relieve pain. There are more than 30 drugs classified as NSAIDs and each has a slightly different chemical structure, is metabolized differently, and seems to work differently among patients. (Other drugs, such as methotrexate, chloroquine, penicillamine, and gold salts, work through the immune system and have some anti-inflammatory effects.) For severe osteoarthritis pain, the NSAID ketorolac (Toradol) can be given as an injection for speedy, although brief, pain relief.

Excerpted from "Arthritis Pain Medications," © 2009 National Pain Foundation (www.nationalpainfoundation.org). Reprinted with permission.

- Aspirin is probably the least expensive NSAID available. Its active ingredient is synthesized from salicin, a natural substance found in willow bark and other plants. American take more than 30 billion aspirin tablets a year at a cost of $1 billion. However, aspirin has multiple side effects—so many, in fact, that the drug probably would not receive modern-day U.S. Food and Drug Administration approval. While low does of aspirin appear to help prevent heart attacks and may help prevent colon cancer and Alzheimer's Disease, aspirin can cause gastrointestinal problems and trigger life-threatening allergic reactions in some people.

- Long-term use of NSAIDs can cause complications in arthritis patients. These can range from minor bleeding in the gastrointestinal tract, to liver or kidney toxicity (poisoning). In fact, stomach irritation is so common with frequent NSAID use that some doctors also prescribe misoprostol (Cytotec), a drug that protects the stomach lining. Misoprostol has its own potential side effects, including nausea, gas, headaches, and vomiting; it can cause miscarriage and should never be given to pregnant women). One prescription product, approved in just the past few years, combines the NSAID diclofenac sodium with misoprostol and is marketed under the name Arthrotec. One of the newest NSAIDs, celecoxib (Celebrex), is reported to be easier on the stomach than older NSAIDs.

- NSAIDs also can interact with other drugs, even over-the-counter preparations. Antacids, for example, can decrease the absorption of NSAIDs, reducing their pain-fighting effect. Prescription medicines also can have adverse effects when mixed with NSAIDs. NSAIDs can augment the action of diuretics, lithium, oral hypoglycemic agents, and phenytoin (Dilantin).

- It is extremely important to follow all the label instructions and cautions when taking NSAIDs and to consult with your health care provider if you have any concerns.

Oral Tramadol (Ultram)

Available for moderate to severe pain. When introduced to the United States in 1966, the U.S. Food and Drug Administration classified tramadol as a nonnarcotic drug. However, some cases of addiction have been reported. Tramadol also has been linked to seizures in susceptible individuals, especially when the drug is given at high doses. The risk of seizure is higher in patients who are also taking antidepressant drugs such as desipramine (Norpramin) or doxepin (Sinequan). Caution also has been advised with well-known antidepressants fluoxetine hydrochloride (Prozac), sertraline hydrochloride (Zoloft), and paroxetine (Paxil).

Narcotic Drugs (Opioids)

When pain is extreme, narcotic drugs derived from opium may prescribed. For arthritis, the most common narcotics prescribed are propoxyphene (Darvon), codeine (Tylenol #3 or #4) or hydrocodone (Vicodin and Lorcet), although oxycodone (Percodan and Percocet) is being prescribed more often now. These narcotic drugs bring swift pain relief, allowing the patient more activity during the day and better sleep at night.

Opioids can have side effects and may lead to dependency, but rarely addiction. Prescribing them should be done only when more conservative treatment has failed, and a patient understands the risks and rewards involved in their use. Opioids are being used more often in advanced arthritis.

Mixed Agonists/Antagonists (Synthetic Narcotics)

This class of drugs is used at times for arthritis pain. They include pentazocine (Talwin-NX or Talacen), nalbuphine (Nubain), butorphanol (Stadol or Stadol NS), and buprenorphine (Buprenex). Only pentazocine is available in oral form and likely to be useful in some cases of advanced arthritis.

This group of drugs has what is called a "low ceiling effect," meaning a small dose may be helpful, but more can cause complications. They also cannot be mixed with strong natural opioids.

Viscosupplements

Two agents have been approved by the FDA [U.S. Food and Drug Administration] for osteoarthritis of the knee. They are injected into the knee to replace the hyaluronic acid, a substance that gives the knee joint viscosity, and which appears to break down in osteoarthritis.

The two viscosupplements currently on the market are Hyalgan and Synvisc. For Hyalgan, five injections over 6–10 weeks are needed, and for Synvisc, only three injections are needed.

Glucosamine Sulfate

One of the most exciting recent developments in arthritis treatment, glucosamine has been shown to relieve pain and potentially rebuild damaged cartilage. Available without a prescription, glucosamine is found in high concentrations in seashells, from which glucosamine is harvested. Glucosamines are used by the body to manufacture proteoglycans, substances that hold collagen threads together. Collagen is an element of cartilage. Some studies have shown that glucosamine sulfate actually "feeds" the joints and stimulates regrowth at the cellular level. Glucosamine sulfate also matches NSAIDs in providing long-lasting pain relief, researchers have found—and without NSAIDs' side effects.

A powdered form of glucosamine sulfate, which can be mixed into juice, is expected to be available soon. Glucosamine sulfate is used to treat patients of all ages and all stages of osteoarthritis.

Rheumatoid Arthritis

NSAIDs

These are among the most common treatments for rheumatoid arthritis (RA) pain.

For more information about NSAIDs, see text under the Osteoarthritis heading.

Non-NSAIDs

Pain relievers that are **not** anti-inflammatories—such as acetaminophen (Tylenol), aspirin plus oxycodone (Percodan), propoxyphene (Darvon), pentazocine (Talwin), meperidine hydrochloride (Demerol), and codeine—can actually cause damage in rheumatoid arthritis patients. If pain is suppressed, but inflammation isn't, movement can worsen the inflammation by releasing more of the enzymes that damage bones and ligaments.

Glucosamine Sulfate

This over-the-counter supplement is found in high concentrations in seashells, from which glucosamine is harvested. While glucosamine has been shown to relieve pain and possibly rebuild cartilage in the joints of osteoarthritis patients, it does not appear to have the same pain-relieving effect for rheumatoid arthritis patients. Still, some doctors recommend that rheumatoid patients take a standard dose of glucosamine sulfate—three 500-milligram capsules daily—because it may help prevent some of RA's degenerative effects.

Cortisone

The most powerful anti-inflammatory drugs are the cortisone-type drugs, or corticosteroids. They can be lifesavers when given for asthma attacks or an adrenal crisis. They may provide complete pain relief when given in high doses on a short-term basis for patients with rheumatoid arthritis flare-ups or when injected into a painful, red-hot, swollen joint. Doctors try to avoid side effects by giving as low a dose as possible and injecting the drugs only at the site of the inflammation.

Corticosteroids should be considered a last resort treatment. Their side effects from long-term use include osteoporosis (brittle bones), cataracts, glaucoma, high blood pressure, stomach bleeding or irritation, weight gain, frequent infections, and worsening of diabetes mellitus.

Antibiotics

Doctors sometimes find there is a bacterial component in some kinds of inflammatory arthritis, which can be treated by antibiotics.

Because antibiotics can throw off the body's natural balance, it is recommended that patients also take prebiotic supplements, such as insulin, fructooligosaccharides (FOS), take probiotics, or eat organic yogurt with various friendly bacterial cultures.

Biologic Response Modifiers (BRMs)

These substances target specific parts of the immune system, but leave other parts alone. For rheumatoid arthritis, the BRM etanercept interferes with a chemical called TNF [tumor necrosis factor], which is believed to play a major role in inflammation and joint damage. Another biologic agent, infliximab, blocks TNF through another pathway and has been approved for use in rheumatoid arthritis and Crohn disease. Oral proteolytic enzymes also are considered biologic response modifiers; they act like biological "vacuum cleaners" to rid the body of harmful proteins that can lodge in the joints.

Disease-Modifying Anti-Rheumatic Drugs (DMARDs)

These agents are used primarily to treat rheumatoid arthritis, but also help people with ankylosing spondylitis, psoriatic arthritis, and a few other arthritis-related diseases. DMARDs can slow the advance of disease. The group includes leflunomide and cyclosporine (originally developed to prevent organ transplant rejection).

Narcotic Drugs (Opioids)

When pain is extreme, narcotic drugs derived from opium may be prescribed. For arthritis, the most common narcotics prescribed are propoxyphene (Darvon), codeine (Tylenol #3 or #4) or hydrocodone (Vicodin and Lorcet), although oxycodone (Percodan and Percocet) is being prescribed more often now. These opioids bring swift pain relief, allowing the patient more activity during the day and better sleep at night.

Opioids can have side effects and may lead to dependency, but rarely addiction. Prescribing them should be done only when more conservative treatment has failed, and a patient understands the risks and rewards involved in their use. Opioids are being used more often in advanced arthritis.

Mixed Agonists/Antagonists (Synthetic Narcotics)

This class of drugs is used at times for arthritis pain. They include pentazocine (Talwin-NX or Talacen), nalbuphine (Nubain), butorphanol (Stadol or Stadol NS), and buprenorphine (Buprenex). Only pentazocine is available in oral form and likely to be useful on in some cases of advanced arthritis.

This group of drugs has what is called a "low ceiling effect," meaning a small dose may be helpful, but more can cause complications. They also cannot be mixed with strong natural narcotic drugs.

Ankylosing Spondylitis

Early diagnosis and treatment of this condition is critical to controlling pain and stiffness, and perhaps plays a part in preventing the bones in the neck and back from fusing. In women, ankylosing spondylitis (AS), or spinal arthritis, often is mild and difficult to diagnose. Treatment is tailored to the individual.

DMARDs or Slow-Acting Anti-Rheumatic Drugs (SAARDs)

While these agents typically are used more frequently to treat other forms of arthritis, they can provide relief. However, they may take several months to become effective. The group includes leflunomide, sulfasalazine, and cyclosporine (originally developed to prevent organ transplant rejection).

NSAIDs

More than 30 drugs are classified as NSAIDs, which can help relieve pain and stiffness, but do not affect the advance of ankylosing spondylitis.

For more information about NSAIDs, see text under the Osteoarthritis heading.

Oral Tramadol (Ultram)

Available for moderate to severe pain. For more information about oral tramadol, see text under the Osteoarthritis heading.

Narcotic Drugs

When pain is extreme, narcotic drugs, derived from opium, may be prescribed. For more information about narcotic drugs, see text under the Rheumatoid arthritis heading.

Gout

To control the pain and inflammation of acute gout episodes, doctors usually prescribe NSAIDs, colchicine, or corticosteroids.

NSAIDs

These are among the most common treatments for gout pain.

For more information about NSAIDs, see text under the Osteoarthritis heading.

Colchicine

Once a traditional gout treatment, this agent often is replaced by NSAIDs. Colchicine usually is given orally, but can be given intravenously if it upsets the stomach.

This drug often causes diarrhea and can prompt more serious side effects including damage to bone marrow.

Corticosteroids

These potent drugs, such as prednisone, act quickly to relieve pain and swelling. If only one of two joints is affected by gout, doctors sometimes inject a corticosteroid crystal solution through the same needle used to remove fluid from the joint.

Long-term corticosteroid use can cause side effects, including osteoporosis (brittle bones), cataracts, glaucoma, high blood pressure, stomach bleeding or irritation, weight gain, frequent infections, and worsening of diabetes mellitus.

Other Gout Drugs

Once the pain and swelling is controlled, further treatment of gout depends on finding out the cause of the body's overabundance of uric acid. If the body produces too much uric acid, doctors typically prescribe a drug called allopurinol. If the body cannot excrete uric acid well, probenecid or sulfinpyrazone is prescribed.

Systemic Lupus Erythematosus (SLE)

The more severe the disease, the more aggressive the treatment. Pain relievers and NSAIDs usually are effective for fever, stiffness, headaches, and rash. More aggressive treatment is needed if there is serious disease progression, evidenced by such developments as hemolytic anemia, major involvement of the heart or lungs, significant kidney damage, or severe central nervous system symptoms.

NSAIDs

These are the most common treatments for SLE pain.

For more information about NSAIDs, see text under the Osteoarthritis heading.

Steroid Creams

These creams often are used for skin rashes, although a non-steroid cream derived from vitamin A called Tegison has helped some patients. Always protect your skin from the sun by using sunblock creams and wearing hats and tightly woven fabrics.

Antimalarial Drugs

These drugs are most often prescribed if the main symptoms are skin and joint pain. The most common drugs are hydroxychloroquine (Plaquenil), chloroquine (Aralen), and quinacrine (Atabrine). Researchers aren't sure why these drugs work; they may inhibit the immune response and or somehow interfere with inflammation. Antimalarials may also be used in combination with other anti-SLE drugs, including immunosuppressants and corticosteroids. Hydroxychloroquine may reduce the risk of blood clots as well as reduce cholesterol levels, which sometimes become elevated in patients who must take corticosteroids.

Side effects of antimalarials can include skin rash, change in skin color, gastrointestinal problems, headache, hair loss, muscle aches, and damage to the retina (although the latter is very uncommon when low doses are used).

Corticosteroids

Severe SLE is treated with corticosteroids, also called steroids, which suppress the inflammatory process, and help relieve may of the complications and symptoms, including anemia and kidney involvement. Steroids include prednisone (Deltasone, Orasone), methylprednisolone (Medrol, Solu-Medrol), hydrocortisone, and dexamethasone (Decadron). Your doctor will tailor your prescriptions to the severity and location of your disease. The drugs may be administered orally or as an injection. An intravenous administration of methylprednisolone using "pulse" therapy for three days is proving useful for flare-ups in the joints.

Long-term use of steroids can cause weight gain, high blood pressure, acne, and susceptibility to infection, insomnia, and bone damage. To counter bone loss, the American College of Rheumatology recommends that patients take 1,500 mg of calcium a day; vitamin D supplements may also be warranted.

Immunosuppressant Drugs

In severe, active SLE cases, particularly when kidney or central nervous system involvement or acute blood vessel inflammation is present, drugs known as immunosuppressants often are used, either alone or with corticosteroids. These drugs suppress the immune system. The most common immunosuppressants are azathioprine (Imuran), methotrexate (Rheumatrex), and cyclophosphamide (Cytoxan). Other drugs commonly used include chlorambucil (Leukeran), nitrogen mustard (Mustargen), and cyclosporine (Sandimmune). Mycophenolate mofetil is a promising new immunosuppressant, which may help patients who do not respond to other immunosuppressants. About a third of patients take immunosuppressants at some point in the course of the disease, most commonly for serious kidney problems and also for neurologic and arthritis symptoms and when flares are widespread.

These drugs can cause stomach and intestinal distress, skin rashes, mouth sores, and hair loss. If the immune system is suppressed too much, serious side effects—anemia, menstrual irregularities, possible infertility, shingles, and liver and bladder toxicity—can occur.

Hormones

SLE patients typically have abnormally low levels of the hormone dehydroepiandrosterone (DHEA). Some studies show that taking DHEA may be modestly effective in treating SLE, especially in helping to prevent the bone loss that can accompany steroids.

Side effects include acne and hair growth.

Chapter 28

Osteoarthritis Medicines

This information can help you work with your doctor or nurse to choose pain relief medicine for osteoarthritis.

Each of the medicines in this text comes with benefits and risks.

- On the up side, they reduce pain and swelling. They can also help you stay active.

- On the down side, they may cause stomach bleeding or raise your chance for a heart attack.

People are different in how they weigh benefits and risks. Some people feel that a small increased chance of heart attack would be okay if they could get the pain relief they need. Other people would not want this kind of trade-off.

This text can help you learn about the benefits and risks of pain-relief medicines for osteoarthritis. Knowing about the benefits and risks can help you decide what is right for you.

Over-the-Counter (OTC) Pain Relievers

Acetaminophen (Tylenol®)

- Most people can take acetaminophen (Tylenol®) without problems as long as they follow the directions on the bottle.

Excerpted from "Choosing Pain Medicine for Osteoarthritis" Consumer Summary Guide, by the Agency for Healthcare Research and Quality (AHRQ, effectivehealthcare.ahrq.gov), January 10, 2007.

- Research shows that acetaminophen (Tylenol®) reduces mild pain. It probably does not help with inflammation or swelling.

OTC NSAIDs

- Non-steroidal anti-inflammatory drugs are called NSAIDs. They include aspirin, ibuprofen (Advil®, Motrin®), and naproxen (Aleve®). These pills work by blocking pain enzymes.

- Research shows that NSAIDs reduce pain caused by swelling. They also give general pain relief.

- Aspirin is also an NSAID, but there is not much research about using aspirin for osteoarthritis pain.

Glucosamine and Chondroitin

- Glucosamine and chondroitin are supplements. They are not regulated as drugs in the United States, so their quality may vary. There is no way to be sure that the supplements you get in the store are as good as the ones used in the research studies.

- Research shows that the combination of glucosamine hydrochloride plus chondroitin sulfate may reduce moderate to severe pain without causing serious problems.

Skin Creams

- Capsaicin cream, like Zostrix® or Theragen®, is made from chili peppers. Research shows that it reduces mild pain. Five out of 10 people using it will have warm, stinging, or burning feelings. The burning feelings fade away over time.

- Salicylate cream includes Aspercreme® and Ben-Gay Arthritis®. Research shows that salicylate cream does not work for osteoarthritis pain.

Prescription (Rx) Pain Relief Pills

Rx pain pills include prescription-strength NSAIDs and opiates (morphine, Tylenol-3®, Vicodin®). This text does not cover opiates. There are three kinds of Rx NSAID pills.

Traditional Rx NSAID Pills

- These are Rx pills like ibuprofen (Motrin®), diclofenac (Voltaren®), and indomethacin (Indocin®).

- Rx NSAID pills are stronger and often cost more than OTC NSAIDs.
- Research shows that they relieve pain and swelling.

Cyclooxygenase-2 (COX-2) Inhibitors

- Celecoxib (Celebrex®) is a kind of NSAID called a COX-2 inhibitor. It relieves pain as well as other NSAIDs do.
- Short-term research studies found that celecoxib (Celebrex®) is safer on the stomach than other NSAID pills.
- Two other COX-2 inhibitors (Vioxx® and Bextra®) were taken off the market in 2005 because they have a high risk of causing heart attacks.

Salicylates

- Salicylates are Rx NSAID pills like salsalate (Disalcid®).
- We do not know how salicylates compare to other osteoarthritis pain relievers because there is very little research.
- Warning: If you have ever had stomach bleeding, high blood pressure, heart attack, liver or kidney problems, you have higher risk for serious problems. Talk to your doctor or nurse before taking any pain pills.

Understanding the Risk of Problems

The Risk of Stomach Bleeding with NSAID Pills

All NSAID pills, including aspirin, block enzymes that protect the stomach. This can cause stomach bleeding. It is not possible to predict any one person's risk. Research can't tell how long you can use NSAID pills without bleeding. In general, stomach bleeding is more likely for people taking NSAIDs who:

- are older, especially more than 75 years old;
- take higher doses;
- use NSAIDs for a longer time;
- also take medicine to help prevent blood clots, like aspirin or warfarin (Coumadin®).

Older people taking NSAID pills have higher risk of stomach bleeding.

345

- For people age 16–44, five out of 10,000 people taking NSAIDs will have a serious bleed.

- For people age 16–44, one out of 10,000 people taking NSAIDs will die from a bleed.

- For people age 45–64, 15 out of 10,000 people taking NSAIDs will have a serious bleed.

- For people age 45–64, two out of 10,000 people taking NSAIDs will die from a bleed.

- For people age 65–74, 17 out of 10,000 people taking NSAIDs will have a serious bleed.

- For people age 65–74, three out of 10,000 people taking NSAIDs will die from a bleed.

- For people age 75 or older, 91 out of 10,000 people taking NSAIDs will have a serious bleed.

- For people age 75 or older, 15 out of 10,000 people taking NSAIDs will die from a bleed.

Signs of Stomach Bleeding

Call your doctor or nurse right away if you:

- vomit blood;

- see blood in your bowel movement, or your bowel movement is black and sticky like tar;

- feel very weak.

If you have ever had stomach bleeding, do not take any of the NSAID pills, including aspirin. If your doctor or nurse recommends NSAID pills, be sure to tell him or her that you had stomach bleeding in the past.

Risk of Heart Attack

NSAIDs can increase the chance of a heart attack. For every 10,000 people taking NSAIDs, 30 of them will have a heart attack that they would not have had if they were not taking NSAIDs. Recent research has found the following about NSAIDs.

- Some NSAIDs increase the chance of a heart attack:
    - Celecoxib (Celebrex®)

- Ibuprofen (Motrin®) in high doses (800 mg three times a day)
- Diclofenac (Voltaren®) in high doses (75 mg twice a day)
- Naproxen (Aleve®, Naprosyn®) does not increase the chance of a heart attack.
- We do not know how other NSAIDs compare when it comes to the chance of a heart attack.

Risk to the Liver

Liver problems are rare with acetaminophen (Tylenol®) and the other pain pills described in this text. However, taking too much acetaminophen (Tylenol®) can lead to liver problems. Be sure to follow the directions on the bottle. Keep in mind that other medicines contain acetaminophen (Tylenol®). Be sure to check the labels so that you do not take too much.

Risk to the Kidneys

The risk is low, but all NSAID pills and acetaminophen (Tylenol®) can cause or worsen high blood pressure and kidney problems. Two out of 1,000 people stop their medicine because of kidney problems.

Sorting It Out

Benefit

The first step in choosing pain medicine is to sort out what kind of pain relief you need. Do you want to be more active? Pain relief medicine can help you keep moving. Start low. Use lower strength and lower dose pills for mild pain. Try capsaicin skin cream (Theragen®, Zostrix®) or acetaminophen (Tylenol®), because they have fewer risks than other pain relievers.

Do you want to reduce swelling or inflammation? Try NSAID pills such as naproxen (Aleve®) or ibuprofen (Advil®, Motrin®). You can lower your risk of problems by using the lowest dose you can for the shortest time you can.

Risk

The second step is to know your risks for problems, like stomach bleeding and heart problems. Have you ever had stomach bleeding or were told you are at high risk for bleeding? Do not use NSAID pills, including aspirin, unless they are recommended by your doctor or nurse. The best way to avoid stomach bleeding is to use acetaminophen (Tylenol®) as your pain pill, or use capsaicin skin cream (Zostrix®, Theragen®).

Have you ever had a heart attack or were told you are at high risk for one? Most people can take acetaminophen (Tylenol®), aspirin, or naproxen (Aleve®, Naprosyn®). There is a chance of heart problems with other pain relief pills, so talk to your doctor or nurse before trying them.

Do you take low-dose aspirin? Aspirin, even at low doses, can cause stomach bleeding. If you want to take low-dose aspirin, consider a pain reliever that is not an NSAID pill, like capsaicin skin cream (Theragen®, Zostrix®), acetaminophen (Tylenol®), or glucosamine and chondroitin.

Warning: Combining aspirin and other NSAID pills makes bleeding more likely.

Cost

The third step is to find out about the cost. Is cost an issue for you? Compare the prices of different drugs. If Rx drugs are included in your health insurance plan, check with your plan about the cost to you.

Chapter 29

Rheumatoid Arthritis Medicines

This information can help you work with your doctor or nurse to find a medicine for rheumatoid arthritis (RA). It is a lifelong condition. RA causes inflammation (swelling, redness, and pain) that can damage the joints. No treatment can cure RA. But the drugs in this text can slow down the disease and help you feel better.

Besides helping you learn about what happens with RA, this text explains the benefits and risks of RA drugs.

Learning about Medicines for RA

Medicines are the main treatment for RA. They reduce joint swelling and relieve pain. Most people need to keep taking RA medicines for life. This text talks about two kinds of RA medicines, DMARDs and steroids.

DMARDs

The drugs that work best for RA are called DMARDs. DMARD stands for disease-modifying anti-rheumatic drug. These medicines don't just relieve pain. They slow or stop the changes in your joints.

DMARDs come in two groups. Some are pills. The others are given by shot or IV [intravenous, or into the vein]. Both suppress the

Excerpted from "Rheumatoid Arthritis Medicines: A Guide for Adults," by the Agency for Healthcare Research and Quality (AHRQ, effectivehealthcare.ahrq.gov), April 9, 2008.

immune system. That means they slow down the body's attack on itself.

Steroids

Steroids help with joint pain and swelling, but it is not known if they can slow down the disease. Prednisone is the name of a steroid often used for RA.

Learning about the Benefits

Research shows that DMARDs work. They can slow down the disease and relieve pain. But it's hard to predict which drug will work best for any one person. About 65 out of 100 people need to change their RA drug. Some people switch because their drug isn't working well enough. Others switch because of side effects.

Some of the medicines have been compared with each other in research studies. Here's what we know from this research.

Starting Your First RA Drug

- Methotrexate (Rheumatrex®, Trexall®) is a DMARD pill that is often used. It works as well as a DMARD given by shot or IV.

- Two other DMARD pills, leflunomide (Arava®) and sulfasalazine (Azulfidine®, Sulfazine®), work as well as methotrexate (Rheumatrex®, Trexall®).

- Adalimumab (Humira®), etanercept (Enbrel®), and infliximab (Remicade®) all work about the same.

Changing and Combining RA Drugs

- If methotrexate (Rheumatrex®, Trexall®) isn't working well enough, you have options. Adding a DMARD given by shot or IV works better than methotrexate by itself.

- Combining prednisone with hydroxychloroquine (Plaquenil®), methotrexate (Rheumatrex®, Trexall®), or sulfasalazine (Azulfidine®, Sulfazine®), works better than any of these DMARD pills by themselves.

Some do not work as well.

- Anakinra (Kineret®) is a DMARD shot that does not work as well as the other shots.

- Combining methotrexate (Rheumatrex®, Trexall®) and sulfasalazine (Azulfidine®, Sulfazine®) does not work any better than either DMARD pill by itself.

Talking with Your Doctor or Nurse about RA Drugs

Benefits

DMARDs reduce swelling and make it easier to do everyday tasks. They also help prevent joint damage and long-term disability. Most people can find a DMARD that works for them. Ask your doctor or nurse these questions.

Most people can start with a DMARD pill. Many people get good results when they start with methotrexate (Rheumatrex®, Trexall®). It can work as well as the DMARDs given by shot or IV.

DMARDs do not start working right away. They can take weeks or months to start working. Your doctor or nurse may prescribe a pain reliever until the DMARD starts to work.

If the first drug does not work or stops working, switching to another DMARD can help. Adding a second kind of DMARD may work for you. If you are taking methotrexate (Rheumatrex®, Trexall®), adding a DMARD given by shot or IV can help. Adding prednisone to a DMARD pill is also an option.

Risks

Infections: RA drugs weaken the body's defenses. That means that serious infections, like pneumonia, are more likely with these drugs. A serious infection needs antibiotics and often must be treated in a hospital.

Other serious problems: Methotrexate (Rheumatrex®, Trexall®) can cause liver and kidney problems. It can also cause low red blood cell counts and painful mouth sores. Steroids like prednisone can weaken bones, raise blood sugar, and cause weight gain. That is why steroids are often prescribed in low doses and for a short time.

Needle reactions: DMARD shots can cause redness, itching, rash, and pain at the spot where the shot is given. More people taking anakinra (Kineret®) have these reactions than people taking other DMARD shots. About half of the people getting DMARDs by IV have a reaction. They get chills, dizzy, or sick to the stomach. But only about two out of 100 people stop their medicine because of reactions. It's rare, but DMARDs given by IV can also cause a serious reaction, like a seizure.

Risks of serious birth defects: Methotrexate (Rheumatrex®, Trexall®) and leflunomide (Arava®) can cause serious birth defects. Both men and women taking these DMARD pills should talk with their doctor or nurse before planning a pregnancy.

Be sure to use two forms of birth control while taking these DMARD pills. For example, you could use birth control pills and a condom each time you have sex.

Reducing Your Risks

- See your doctor or nurse for regular checkups and blood tests. Checkups and blood tests will help catch infections and other problems early.

- Stay away from people who are sick.

- Call your doctor or nurse right away if you have signs of infection, like fever or cough.

- Make sure your flu shot and pneumonia shot are up to date. These shots can help you fight off infections. Check with your doctor or nurse before getting any other vaccines.

- Be sure to get enough calcium and vitamin D. RA weakens the bones. You can help keep your bones healthy by getting enough calcium and vitamin D. Milk, yogurt, and green leafy vegetables are high in calcium. You can also take calcium and vitamin D pills.

Still Unknown

Research can't tell us yet how DMARD pills, other than methotrexate (Rheumatrex®, Trexall®), compare with the DMARDs given by shot or IV. Research can't tell us yet how abatacept (Orencia®) and rituximab (Rituxan®) compare with other DMARDs.

Chapter 30

Injections to Treat Arthritis Pain and Inflammation

Chapter Contents

Section 30.1

Viscosupplementation and Corticosteroid Injection

"Injections to Treat Knee Pain Caused by Arthritis," reprinted with permission from www.allaboutarthritis.com, an informational website from DePuy Orthopaedics, Inc., a Johnson & Johnson company. © 2006 DePuy Orthopaedics, Inc. All rights reserved.

If your knee pain is severe, your physician may elect to inject preparations for the treatment of knee pain directly into your arthritic knee. Knee injections may take several forms:

Viscosupplementation

Hyaluronic acid (HA) injections are designed to restore the cushioning and lubricating properties of synovial fluid, reduce the pain of knee osteoarthritis, improve joint mobility, and enhance a patient's range of motion. Hyaluronic acid remains in the knee post-injection for only a few days.

The method of action of HA is unknown. Experiments have shown that adding hyaluronic acid to the cells in human synovial membrane stimulates them to produce hyaluronic acid themselves.[1] The half life of hyaluronan injected into the joint is short at 24–48 hours.[2] During that time, it may be that hyaluronan promotes long-lasting changes by stimulating the lining of cells of the joint to synthesize more hyaluronan.[3] Another theory is that the injection has possible anti-inflammatory properties.[4]

HA injections create a shock absorber between bones and ease the pain associated with weight bearing and joint movement. Viscosupplementation injections will not cure osteoarthritis or repair damaged cartilage in the knee, but they may relieve joint pain for a period of time.

Corticosteroid Injection

Corticosteroids, also known as glucocorticoids, refer to a group of naturally occurring human hormones. These hormones, commonly referred to as "cortisone," can be artificially produced in the laboratory and purified for injection into inflamed or arthritic joints, due to rheumatoid arthritis, osteoarthritis, or trauma. For knee arthritis, cortisone injections into the joint can often help reduce the inflammation for two to three months.

Before administering the cortisone injection, your doctor may insert a needle into the knee joint and remove or pull excess fluid from the joint. Doctors normally give less than three cortisone injections a year because of the possibility that excessive steroid injections may actually speed the process of joint deterioration.

Possible Complications of Knee Injections

Following the injection of cortisone or hyaluronic acid into the knee, there may occasionally be increased pain or an inflammatory reaction to the injected medication. These reactions usually occur within the first 24 to 48 hours after the injection and ice, elevation, and medications such as analgesic can help.

Injections into a joint must always be done under sterile conditions to minimize the possibility of infection. If an infection does occur after the knee has been injected, it must be dealt with promptly to avoid irreversible destruction of the joint cartilage. Pain greater than expected, swelling, and/or redness of the knee joint or the development of a fever should raise concerns about an infection and be reported immediately to your doctor. Rapid diagnosis, intravenous antibiotic therapy, followed by surgical drainage of pus, removal of any infected debris, and washing the joint with sterile fluids is essential to the effective management of an infected knee.

1. http://www.thephysiotherapysite.co.uk/arthritis/visco-supplementation.html

2. http://www.thedoctorwillseeyounow.com/articles/arthritis

3. http://www.thedoctorwillseeyounow.com/articles/arthritis

4. http://www.aafp.org/afp/20000801/565.html

Section 30.2

Botulinum Toxin Injections and Osteoarthritis

Do Botox injections offer a satisfactory non-surgical alternative for patients suffering with painful knee osteoarthritis? Trials are underway, so stay tuned.

No longer the secret potion of women and men interested in hiding facial wrinkles between the eyebrows, around the eyes, on the forehead, and around the lips, injections of Botox are now thought to be useful for more than 50 medical conditions, including excessive sweating, constipation, headache, clubfoot, and even hiccups. We may be able to add severe knee pain from osteoarthritis to the list if the results from a small preliminary study—in which patients had a 50% or greater improvement in knee pain with Botox injections—can be replicated.

Botox, derived from *Clostridium botulinum*, the bacterium that causes botulism, acts by binding to the nerve endings of muscles, blocking the release of the chemical that causes muscles to contract. When Botox is injected into a specific muscle, that muscle becomes paralyzed or weakened, but surrounding muscles are unaffected, allowing for normal function. The long-term effects of repeated Botox injections are unknown. When it comes to osteoarthritis, it's thought that Botox injections to the knee disrupt pain nerve function and Botox may reduce nerve-related inflammation in the knee.

As you age, your knees need all the help they can get. Swivel, bend, slide, glide. Swivel, bend, slide, glide: It's what your knees do in endless repetitions every day of your life as you go about your daily activities. No fabricated machine comes close to the capabilities of this joint. However, after years of use (and abuse), the knee eventually starts to show signs of wear and tear—and the pain of osteoarthritis or degenerative joint disease sets in, making your 3,000 or so daily steps an extremely difficult proposition.

As you read this, 50 million Americans currently suffering from knee osteoarthritis are wincing, gulping down ibuprofen, grimacing, slathering on strong-smelling liniments, limping, and wondering how they are going to make it through another day. Each year, millions of Americans hobble into the offices of orthopedic surgeons in search of relief for their non-stop knee distress. Some will need additional prescription medication for pain relief. Many will be prescribed specific muscle-strengthening exercises to perform daily to ease the load on their delicate and damaged knees. For tens of thousands, however, the extensive damage caused by osteoarthritis will be so severe that their only remaining option is a knee arthroplasty, more commonly known as a total knee replacement.

To determine the potential benefits of injecting Botox directly into the knee joint cavity, researchers embarked on a six-month study of Botox versus placebo in 37 patients with moderate to severe refractory knee pain due to osteoarthritis. The participants (36 men and one woman) received either 100 units of Botox with lidocaine (a short-acting anesthetic) or a saline placebo with lidocaine. Double-blind assessments were scheduled for baseline, one-month, three-month, and six-month time points. Study investigators measured self-reported total pain scores and a physical function score. Scores for walking pain, day pain severity, night pain severity, and an observed timed-stands test were also factored in.

At the one-month point in this study, two placebo patients had dropped out from lack of benefit. Of the 18 patients in the severe pain group (half on Botox and half on placebo), there was a significant decrease in pain and improvement in physical function for those who received the Botox injection. Those injected with the placebo experienced minimal improvement. In the moderate pain group, neither injection produced significant changes in the primary outcome measures. Interestingly, in the moderate pain group, there was a 25% reduction in daytime pain severity after the placebo injections.

Three-month measurements were completed by January 2007, and the trial is scheduled for completion in August 2007. To date, however, thanks to Botox, researchers point to clinically and statistically significant decreases in severe osteoarthritis knee pain and improvements in physical function. "If Botox injections for refractory joint pain continue to prove beneficial, it offers a very welcome solution for fragile patients," says Maren L. Mahowald, MD, the Rheumatology Section Chief at the Minneapolis VA Medical Center. Dr. Mahowald, a Professor of Medicine at the University of Minnesota, Minneapolis, was principal investigator in the Botox study. "Local joint treatment with Botox injections could replace oral medications that carry the risk of systemic side effects, and Botox injections may negate or delay the need for joint surgery." Much more research will be needed to determine the most effective and safe dose of Botox for the joint injections and the most appropriate dosing intervals.

Chapter 31

Tools and Devices Help Arthritis Patients Do Everyday Tasks

Lisa Bielstein knows that arthritis can make simple things, such as opening a jar or pruning a rose, a painful experience.

Diagnosed at age 29 with rheumatoid arthritis 10 years ago, the Dacula [Georgia] mom of three was racked with pain and fatigue for almost a year before doctors diagnosed her condition. But she wasn't about to give up on the things she loved to do. On medication to prevent joint damage, she has learned to look for tools that help her adapt to her daily tasks.

"I look for everyday little things that can make life easier," she said.

To help her continue gardening, she has sought a bench with wheels; pruning shears and trowels that have big handles with soft grips; and soft-sided buckets that are easier to carry. In the kitchen, she uses lightweight pans, lever-style bottle and jar openers; and soft-handled utensils for cooking. "I invested in a signature stamp at work because I sign a lot of checks," she said. When she does write, she uses a large-barreled pen with a cushion grip.

Braces help reduce the stiffness and pain in her wrists and shore up her knees. She can't afford to be sedentary, even with the stiffness, she said. She owns a business and keeps up with her three active sons.

"I have always been an extremely active person. I've been on the go since I was young," Bielstein said. Active in the Arthritis Foundation,

Georgia chapter, she walked in the inaugural Gwinnett Arthritis Walk in May.

"Arthritis can just be so devastating—daily activities like getting a jar open can be painful. I want to get out and enjoy life," Bielstein said.

Dr. Hayes Wilson, chief of rheumatology at Piedmont Hospital, estimates that 1.7 million Georgians—about one in five—have some arthritic illness, causing their joints to become inflamed and painful. Of that 1.7 million, 9,200 are children with juvenile arthritis, according to the Arthritis Foundation, Georgia chapter.

Many of Wilson's patients are women like Bielstein. "Rheumatoid arthritis is a disease of young women of child-bearing years—one of the biggest misconceptions is it is a disease of older people," Wilson said.

People with arthritis often have to learn to use their body power in a different way to tackle projects and hobbies, he said. Avid walkers can switch to bikes; golfers with hand arthritis can use clubs with a bigger grip.

These days, ergonomic tools for everyday tasks are more readily available for people sidelined with injuries or those whose physical conditions, such as arthritis, limit mobility, said Debi Hinerfeld, president of the Georgia Occupational Therapy Association. (Occupational therapists help people become as independent as possible after an injury, disease, developmental delay, or social/emotional crisis, she said.)

Hinerfeld remembers when adaptive tools were available only through her professional catalogs.

"When I started doing this, anything you bought [to aid patients] was out of a therapy catalog," she said. "Now you can buy these practically anywhere, even Wal-Mart."

Hinerfeld said, "The best tools for any job include those that allow a person to perform the work easily; being able to conserve energy, prevent injury and to do whatever that person wants to do in his or her life to live life to the fullest degree possible."

Think about Comfort, Simplicity

- Be selective. Think about the tasks that are difficult for you on a regular basis and look for products that can make them easier.

- Select products with texture. For example, when selecting glassware, drinking glasses with bumpy exteriors are easier to grasp than glasses with smooth exteriors.

- Seek lightweight products that require minimal upkeep and are safe to use.

- Avoid products that are difficult to grasp or require twisting with your fingers to open and close. Instead, look for flip-top caps, zippers and larger, easy-to-open lids.

- Look for items that are comfortable to wear, carry, or operate. Products that can be carried close to your body may alleviate pressure on arms, hands, and back.

- Avoid the bells and whistles. Look for products that are simple and practical, rather than fancy gadgets with intricate pieces.

Look for the Arthritis Foundation's blue and white Ease-of-Use commendation logo. The Atlanta-based Arthritis Foundation sponsors a research lab at Georgia Tech where these products are tested by an independent panel of health professionals and people with arthritis.

Look for Well-Designed Equipment

Anyone can look for tools to make their everyday lives easier, occupational therapist Debi Hinerfeld notes. Although there is no "adaptive tools" aisle in stores, look for specific designs in everything from cooking utensils to gardening tools. They include:

- those with built-up handles to allow someone with a poor grasp to have a better grip;

- tools that have extended reach and possibly an adjustable angle at the bottom to prevent back injury from having to bend down too far and to prevent twisting of the back;

- tools that are made of lightweight materials that conserve energy and allow users to get the job done without too many rest breaks.

Chapter 32

Help Your Arthritis Treatment Work

Chapter Contents

Section 32.1

How Patients Can Prevent Arthritis Damage

Excerpted from "Help Your Arthritis Treatment Work,"
by the U.S. Food and Drug Administration (FDA, www.fda.gov), 2005.

Ease the Pain, Help Prevent More Damage

Arthritis can strike at any age. It hurts the joints, where two bones meet. It damages the joints and makes them stiff and painful. Sometimes it's so bad it can cripple a person.

Correct treatment can ease the pain and help prevent more damage. You can help your treatment work.

If Your Joints Have Signs of Arthritis, Talk to Your Doctor

If you have arthritis, the doctor may prescribe a medicine for you or tell you to use a medicine you buy without a prescription, such as aspirin. You may need to take more than one medicine.

Joints with arthritis may have the following symptoms:

- Swelling
- Warmth
- Redness
- Pain

Before Taking New Medicine

Ask your doctor the following questions:

- How should I take this medicine?
- Are there any special instructions?
- What side effects could there be?
- If I have any side effects, what should I do?
- What should I do if I forget to take a dose?

If you took the medicine before and it caused problems, tell the doctor.

Also tell the doctor if you are taking other medicines. And ask if you should keep taking them.

Read the Label of Medicine You Buy without a Prescription

Like arthritis medicine, many medicines for headaches or colds or flu have pain relievers in them.

Some common pain relievers are aspirin, acetaminophen, ibuprofen, ketoprofen, and naproxen.

So before you buy any medicine, read the label to see what's in it.

Does it have a pain reliever? If it does, ask your doctor or pharmacist if it's OK for you to take it.

Too much of the same type of medicine can hurt you.

Be Careful with Medicine

- Never take any medicine for arthritis without your doctor's advice.
- Never take someone else's medicine.
- Keep all medicine away from children.
- Throw out medicine that reaches its "Discard" or "Exp" (expiration) date.

Remember: There can be problems with any medicine, even those you can buy without a prescription.

Rest and Exercise

You may need extra rest when your arthritis gets worse, or flares up. But even then, it's good to gently exercise the joints that hurt.

Gentle exercise can ease the pain and help you sleep better. Ask your doctor how to exercise your joints.

Learn about Your Arthritis

It helps to learn about your arthritis. Many people do this by joining a group with other people who have the disease.

To find a group, look in the newspaper. Or ask your doctor or the hospital. The local Arthritis Foundation office has information, too.

Watch out for Cures That Don't Work

Some people with arthritis can't find any treatment that helps very much. That's why there are so many ads for gadgets, health foods, and supplements to treat arthritis.

Many of these have never been tested. They're just a waste of money.

Protect Yourself with the Facts

- Pain and stiffness often come and go by themselves, for no known reason. You may use an untested product and then feel better. But you may have felt better even without the product.

- There is no cure for arthritis. But correct treatment can ease pain and stiffness.

- If you use worthless products, you delay real help. So the damage gets worse.

Remember: If it sounds too good to be true, it probably isn't true.

What If Correct Treatment Doesn't Help?

If all else fails, an operation might help. Talk about this with your doctor.

Section 32.2

Heat and Cold Therapies for Arthritis

Excerpted from "Questions and Answers about Arthritis and Rheumatic Diseases," by the National Institute of Arthritis and Musculoskeletal and Skin Diseases (NIAMS, www.niams.nih.gov), part of the National Institutes of Health, October 2008.

Heat and cold can both be used to reduce the pain and inflammation of arthritis. The patient and doctor can determine which one works best.

Heat Therapy

Heat therapy increases blood flow, tolerance for pain, and flexibility. Heat therapy can involve treatment with paraffin wax, microwaves, ultrasound, or moist heat. Physical therapists are needed for some of these therapies, such as microwave or ultrasound therapy, but patients can apply moist heat themselves. Some ways to apply moist heat include placing warm towels or hot packs on the inflamed joint or taking a warm bath or shower.

Cold Therapy

Cold therapy numbs the nerves around the joint (which reduces pain) and may relieve inflammation and muscle spasms. Cold therapy can involve cold packs, ice massage, soaking in cold water, or over-the-counter sprays and ointments that cool the skin and joints.

Chapter 33

Surgical Procedures Used to Treat Arthritis

Chapter Contents

Section 33.1

Orthopedic Procedures Increase Dramatically

Excerpted from "Orthopedic Procedures Increase Dramatically
in Seven Years," by the Agency for Healthcare Research and Quality
(AHRQ, www.ahrq.gov), July 18, 2007.

Orthopedic procedures, including knee reconstruction or replacement (knee arthroplasty), total and partial hip replacement, and spinal fusion, increased by nearly 25 percent between 1997 and 2005, climbing from 822,000 to 1.3 million, according to the latest *News and Numbers* summary from the Agency for Healthcare Research and Quality.

The data indicate that that between 1997 and 2005:

- The number of knee surgeries climbed by 69 percent, from 328,800 in 1997 to 555,800. Hip replacements rose 32 percent from 290,700 to 383,500 procedures, and spinal fusion operations rose 73 percent, from 202,100 to 349,400 procedures.

- Women were 60 percent more likely than men to have hip replacement procedures and 70 percent more likely to have knee surgery. Spinal fusions were equally likely in men and women.

- Costs related to hospital stays for orthopedic procedures totaled $31.5 billion—11 percent of all hospital patient-care costs.

- Medicare paid the largest share of hospital costs for knee surgery and hip replacements (covering nearly 60 percent of all knee surgeries and 64 percent of all hip replacements). On the other hand, private insurance was billed for more than half (52 percent) of spinal fusion procedures.

Section 33.2

Arthroscopic Surgery

"Arthroscopy," © 2009 A.D.A.M., Inc. Reprinted with permission.

Definition

Arthroscopy is a method of viewing a joint, and, if needed, to perform surgery on a joint. An arthroscope consists of a tiny tube, a lens, and a light source.

How the Test Is Performed

This procedure is typically performed on the knee, shoulder, elbow, or wrist. The type of anesthesia depends on the particular joint and other factors. A regional anesthetic numbs the affected area, but the patient may remain awake, depending on whether other medications are used. For more extensive surgery, general anesthesia may be used. In this case the patient is asleep and pain-free.

The area is cleaned and a pressure band (tourniquet) may be applied to restrict blood flow. The health care provider then makes a surgical cut into the joint. Sterile fluid is passed through the joint space to provide a better view.

Next, a tool called an arthroscope is inserted into the area. An arthroscope consists of a tiny tube, a lens, and a light source. It allows a surgeon to look for joint damage or disease. The device also allows the surgeon to perform reconstructive procedures on the joint, if needed.

Images of the inside of the joint are displayed on a monitor.

One or two small additional surgical cuts may be needed, in order to use other instruments. These instruments can be used to remove bits of cartilage or bone, take a tissue biopsy, or perform other minor surgery. In addition, ligament reconstruction can be performed using the arthroscope in many cases.

How to Prepare for the Test

You should not eat or drink anything for 12 hours before the procedure. You may be told to shave your joint area. You may be given a sedative before leaving for the hospital.

You will be asked to wear a hospital gown during the procedure so the body part for surgery is accessible.

You must sign a consent form. Make arrangements for transportation from the hospital after the procedure.

How the Test Will Feel

You may feel a slight sting when the local anesthetic is injected. After this medicine starts to work, you should feel no pain.

The joint may need to be manipulated to provide a better view, so there may be some tugging on the leg (or arm, if done on the shoulder).

After the test, the joint will probably be stiff and sore for a few days. Ice is commonly recommended after arthroscopy to help relieve swelling and pain.

Slight activity such as walking can be resumed immediately, however excessive use of the joint may cause swelling and pain and may increase the chance of injury. Normal activity should not be resumed for several days or longer. Special preparations may need to be made concerning work and other responsibilities. Physical therapy may also be recommended.

Depending on your diagnosis, there may be other exercises or restrictions.

Why the Test Is Performed

Your doctor may order this test if you have:

- a need for joint surgery;
- damaged meniscus (the piece of cartilage that cushions the knee joint area);
- joint pain from an injury;
- joint disease;
- lesions or other problems detected by x-rays;
- signs of bone fragments from a fracture;
- signs of a torn ligament;
- unexplainable joint pain.

Arthroscopy can also help see if a disease is getting better or worse (this is called monitoring the disease) or determine whether a treatment is working.

What Abnormal Results Mean

Abnormal results may be due to:

- bleeding;
- bone fragments;
- damaged meniscus cartilage;
- dislocation;
- lesions;
- rotator cuff tendonitis;
- torn ligaments.

Risks

- Joint stiffness
- Increased pain
- Infection (fever)
- Inflammation
- Swelling

Considerations

The diagnostic accuracy of an arthroscopy is about 98%, although x-rays and sometimes MRI [magnetic resonance imaging] scans are taken first because they are noninvasive.

Section 33.3

Bone Fusion Surgery

Definition

Spinal fusion is surgery to fuse spine bones (vertebrae) that cause you to have back problems.

Fusing means two bones are permanently placed together so there is no longer movement between them. Spinal fusion is usually done along with other surgical procedures of the spine.

Description

You will be asleep and feel no pain (general anesthesia).

Your surgeon has several choices about where to make the incision (cut).

- The surgeon may make an incision on your back or neck over the spine. You will be lying face-down on a special table. Muscles and tissue are separated to expose the spine.

- The surgeon may make a cut through one side of your belly (for surgery on your lower back). The surgeon will use tools called retractors to gently separate, hold the soft tissues and blood vessels apart, and have room to work.

- The surgeon may make the cut on the front of the neck, toward the side.

Other surgery, such as a diskectomy, laminectomy, or a foraminotomy, is almost always done first.

The surgeon will use a graft (such as bone) to hold (or fuse) the bones together permanently. There are several different ways of fusing vertebrae together:

- Strips of bone graft material may be placed over the back part of the spine.

- Bone graft material may be placed between the vertebrae.
- Special cages may be placed between the vertebrae. These cages are packed with bone graft material.

The surgeon may get the graft from different places:

- From another part of your body (usually around your pelvic bone). This is called an autograft. Your surgeon will make a small cut over your hip and remove some bone from the back of the rim of the pelvis.
- From a bone bank, called allograft.
- A synthetic bone substitute can also be used, but this is not common yet.

The vertebrae are often also fixed together with screws, plates, or cages. They are used to keep the vertebrae from moving until the bone grafts are fully healed.

Surgery can take 3 to 4 hours.

Why the Procedure Is Performed

Spinal fusion may be recommended for:

- treatment for spinal stenosis;
- after diskectomy in the neck;
- injury or fractures to the bones in the spine;
- weak or unstable spine caused by infections or tumors;
- spondylolisthesis, a condition in which one vertebra slips forward on top of another;
- abnormal curvatures, such as those from scoliosis or kyphosis.

Risks

Risks for any surgery are:

- blood clots in the legs that may travel to the lungs;
- breathing problems;
- infection, including in the lungs (pneumonia), or bladder or kidney;
- blood loss;

- heart attack or stroke during surgery;
- reactions to medications.

Risks for spine surgery are:

- infection in the wound or vertebral bones;
- damage to a spinal nerve, causing weakness, pain, loss of sensation, problems with your bowels or bladder;
- the spinal column above and below the fusion are more likely to cause other back problems later.

Before the Procedure

Always tell your doctor or nurse what drugs you are taking, even drugs or herbs you bought without a prescription.

During the days before the surgery:

- If you are a smoker, you need to stop. Patients who have spinal fusion and continue to smoke may not heal as well. Ask your doctor for help.
- Two weeks before surgery, your doctor or nurse may ask you to stop taking drugs that make it harder for your blood to clot. These include aspirin, ibuprofen (Advil, Motrin), naproxen (Aleve, Naprosyn), and other drugs like these.
- If you have diabetes, heart disease, or other medical problems, your surgeon will ask you to see your regular doctor.
- Talk with your doctor if you have been drinking a lot of alcohol.
- Ask your doctor which drugs you should still take on the day of the surgery.
- Always let your doctor know about any cold, flu, fever, herpes breakout, or other illnesses you may have.

On the day of the surgery:

- You will usually be asked not to drink or eat anything for 6 to 12 hours before the procedure.
- Take your drugs your doctor told you to take with a small sip of water.
- Your doctor or nurse will tell you when to arrive at the hospital.

After the Procedure

You will need to stay in the hospital for 3 to 4 days after surgery. The repaired spine should be kept in the right position to maintain alignment.

If the surgery involved a surgical cut in the chest, a chest tube may be used to drain fluid build-up. The tube is usually removed after 24 to 72 hours.

You will receive pain medicines in the hospital. You may have a pump where you control how much pain medicine you get, you may get shots or intravenous (IV) injections, or you may take pain pills.

You will be taught how to move properly and how to sit, stand, and walk. You'll be told to use a "log-rolling" technique when getting out of bed. This means that you move your entire body at once, without twisting your spine.

You may not be able to eat for 2 to 3 days and will be fed through an IV. When you leave the hospital, you may need to wear a back brace or cast.

Outlook (Prognosis)

Spine surgery will often provide full or partial relief of symptoms.

Future spine problems are possible for all patients after spine surgery. After spinal fusion, the area that was fused together can no longer move. Therefore, the spinal column above and below the fusion are more likely to be stressed when the spine moves, and have problems later. Also, if you needed more than one kind of back surgery (such as laminectomy and spinal fusion), you may have more of a chance of future problems.

Chapter 34

Understanding Joint Replacement Surgery

What is joint replacement surgery?

Joint replacement surgery is removing a damaged joint and putting in a new one. A joint is where two or more bones come together, like the knee, hip, and shoulder. The surgery is usually done by a doctor called an orthopedic surgeon. Sometimes, the surgeon will not remove the whole joint, but will only replace or fix the damaged parts.

The doctor may suggest a joint replacement to improve how you live. Replacing a joint can relieve pain and help you move and feel better. Hips and knees are replaced most often. Other joints that can be replaced include the shoulders, fingers, ankles, and elbows.

What can happen to my joints?

Joints can be damaged by arthritis and other diseases, injuries, or other causes. Arthritis or simply years of use may cause the joint to wear away. This can cause pain, stiffness, and swelling. Bones are alive, and they need blood to be healthy, grow, and repair themselves. Diseases and damage inside a joint can limit blood flow, causing problems.

Excerpted from "Joint Replacement Surgery: Information for Multicultural Communities," by the National Institute of Arthritis and Musculoskeletal and Skin Diseases (NIAMS, www.niams.nih.gov), part of the National Institutes of Health, updated April 2009.

What is a new joint like?

A new joint, called a prosthesis, can be made of plastic, metal, or both. It may be cemented into place or not cemented, so that your bone will grow into it. Both methods may be combined to keep the new joint in place.

A cemented joint is used more often in older people who do not move around as much and in people with "weak" bones. The cement holds the new joint to the bone. An uncemented joint is often recommended for younger, more active people and those with good bone quality. It may take longer to heal, because it takes longer for bone to grow and attach to it.

New joints generally last at least 10 to 15 years. Therefore, younger patients may need to have the same damaged joint replaced more than once.

Do many people have joints replaced?

Joint replacement is becoming more common. About 773,000 Americans have a hip or knee replaced each year. Research has shown that even if you are older, joint replacement can help you move around and feel better.

Any surgery has risks. Risks of joint surgery will depend on your health before surgery, how severe your arthritis is, and the type of surgery done. Many hospitals and doctors have been replacing joints for several decades, and this experience results in better patient outcomes. For answers to their questions, some people talk with their doctor or someone who has had the surgery. A doctor specializing in joints will probably work with you before, during, and after surgery to make sure you heal quickly and recover successfully.

Do I need to have my joint replaced?

Only a doctor can tell if you need a joint replaced. He or she will look at your joint with an x-ray machine or another machine. The doctor may put a small, lighted tube (arthroscope) into your joint to look for damage. A small sample of your tissue could also be tested.

After looking at your joint, the doctor may say that you should consider exercise, walking aids such as braces or canes, physical therapy, or medicines and vitamin supplements. Medicines for arthritis include drugs that reduce inflammation. Depending on the type of arthritis, the doctor may prescribe corticosteroids or other drugs.

However, all drugs may cause side effects, including bone loss.

If these treatments do not work, the doctor may suggest an operation called an osteotomy, where the surgeon "aligns" the joint. Here, the surgeon cuts the bone or bones around the joint to improve alignment. This may be simpler than replacing a joint, but it may take longer to recover. However, this operation is not commonly done today.

Joint replacement is often the answer if you have constant pain and can't move the joint well—for example, if you have trouble with things such as walking, climbing stairs, and taking a bath.

What happens during surgery?

First, the surgical team will give you medicine so you won't feel pain (anesthesia). The medicine may block the pain only in one part of the body (regional), or it may put your whole body to sleep (general). The team will then replace the damaged joint with a prosthesis.

Each surgery is different. How long it takes depends on how badly the joint is damaged and how the surgery is done. To replace a knee or a hip takes about 2 hours or less, unless there are complicating factors. After surgery, you will be moved to a recovery room for 1 to 2 hours until you are fully awake or the numbness goes away.

What happens after surgery?

With knee or hip surgery, you may be able to go home in 3 to 5 days. If you are elderly or have additional disabilities, you may then need to spend several weeks in an intermediate-care facility before going home. You and your team of doctors will determine how long you stay in the hospital.

After hip or knee replacement, you will often stand or begin walking the day of surgery. At first, you will walk with a walker or crutches. You may have some temporary pain in the new joint because your muscles are weak from not being used. Also, your body is healing. The pain can be helped with medicines and should end in a few weeks or months.

Physical therapy can begin the day after surgery to help strengthen the muscles around the new joint and help you regain motion in the joint. If you have your shoulder joint replaced, you can usually begin exercising the same day of your surgery. A physical therapist will help you with gentle, range-of-motion exercises. Before you leave the hospital (usually 2 or 3 days after surgery), your therapist will show you how to use a pulley device to help bend and extend your arm.

Will my surgery be successful?

The success of your surgery depends a lot on what you do when you go home. Follow your doctor's advice about what you eat, what medicines to take, and how to exercise. Talk with your doctor about any pain or trouble moving.

Joint replacement is usually a success in more than 90 percent of people who have it. When problems do occur, most are treatable. Possible problems include the following:

- **Infection:** Areas in the wound or around the new joint may get infected. It may happen while you're still in the hospital or after you go home. It may even occur years later. Minor infections in the wound are usually treated with drugs. Deep infections may need a second operation to treat the infection or replace the joint.

- **Blood clots:** If your blood moves too slowly, it may begin to form lumps of blood parts called clots. If pain and swelling develop in your legs after hip or knee surgery, blood clots may be the cause. The doctor may suggest drugs to make your blood thin or special stockings, exercises, or boots to help your blood move faster. If swelling, redness, or pain occurs in your leg after you leave the hospital, contact your doctor right away.

- **Loosening:** The new joint may loosen, causing pain. If the loosening is bad, you may need another operation. New ways to attach the joint to the bone should help.

- **Dislocation:** Sometimes after hip or other joint replacement, the ball of the prosthesis can come out of its socket. In most cases, the hip can be corrected without surgery. A brace may be worn for a while if a dislocation occurs.

- **Wear:** Some wear can be found in all joint replacements. Too much wear may help cause loosening. The doctor may need to operate again if the prosthesis comes loose. Sometimes, the plastic can wear thin, and the doctor may just replace the plastic and not the whole joint.

- **Nerve and blood vessel injury:** Nerves near the replaced joint may be damaged during surgery, but this does not happen often. Over time, the damage often improves and may disappear. Blood vessels may also be injured.

As you move your new joint and let your muscles grow strong again, pain will lessen, flexibility will increase, and movement will improve.

What research is being done?

Scientists are studying replacement joints to find out which are best to improve movement and flexibility. They are also looking at new joint materials and ways to improve surgery. Other researchers are working to find out what causes joint damage, how to prevent it, and how to treat it.

Some scientists are studying a condition called osteolysis, a condition where bone is lost around the implant in response to inflammation. This can cause the prosthesis to loosen and may require a second surgery. In 2008, scientists found that cells called fibroblasts trigger the inflammation that results in osteolysis. This finding could help scientists develop new drugs that prevent osteolysis in joint replacements.

Other scientists are also trying to find out why some people who need surgery don't choose it. They want to know what things make a difference in choosing treatment, in recovery, and in well-being.

Chapter 35

Knee Replacement

Chapter Contents

Section 35.1

All about Total Knee Replacement

From "Total Knee Replacement," by the National Guideline
Clearinghouse (www.guideline.gov), December 2008.

Primary total knee replacement (TKR) is most commonly performed for knee joint failure caused by osteoarthritis (OA); other indications include rheumatoid arthritis (RA), juvenile rheumatoid arthritis, osteonecrosis, and other types of inflammatory arthritis. The aims of TKR are relief of pain and improvement in function. Candidates for elective TKR should have radiographic evidence of joint damage, moderate-to-severe persistent pain not adequately relieved by an extended course of nonsurgical management, and clinically significant functional limitation resulting in diminished quality of life.

The success of primary TKR in most patients is strongly supported by more than 20 years of follow-up data. There appears to be rapid and substantial improvement in the patient's pain, functional status, and overall health-related quality of life in about 90 percent of patients; about 85 percent of patients are satisfied with the results of surgery.

Short-term outcomes, as documented by functional outcome scales, are generally substantially improved after TKR. Functional outcome is improved after TKR for people across the spectrum of disability status. In general, prostheses are durable, but failure does occur.

Age younger than 55 at the time of TKR, male gender, diagnosis of osteoarthritis, obesity, and presence of comorbid conditions are risk factors for revision.

Factors related to a surgeon's case volume, technique, and choice of prosthesis may have important influences on surgical outcomes. One of the clearest associations with better outcomes appears to be the procedure volume of the individual surgeon and the hospital.

Technical factors in performing surgery may influence both the short- and long-term success rate. Proper alignment of the prosthesis appears to be critical. Many design features, such as use of mobile bearings or designs sparing cruciate ligaments, have theoretical advantages, but durability and success rates appear roughly similar with most commonly used designs.

There is consensus regarding the following perioperative interventions that improve TKR outcomes: systemic antibiotic prophylaxis, aggressive postoperative pain management, perioperative risk assessment and management of medical conditions, and preoperative education.

The effectiveness of anticoagulation for the prevention of pulmonary emboli is unclear. There are insufficient data to support specific perioperative rehabilitation strategies, methods to reduce postoperative anemia, postoperative physical activity recommendations, and the site of postacute care.

Revision TKR is done to alleviate pain and improve function. Fracture or dislocation of the patella, instability of the components or aseptic loosening, infection, and periprosthetic fractures are common reasons for total knee revision. A painful knee without an identifiable cause is a controversial indication. Contraindications for revision TKR include persistent infection, poor bone quality, highly limited quadriceps or extensor function, poor skin coverage, and poor vascular status. Results are not as good as with primary TKR; outcomes are better for aseptic loosening than for infections. When infection is involved, successful results occur with a two-stage revision. Failed revisions require a salvage procedure (resection of arthroplasty, arthrodesis, or amputation), with inferior results compared with revision TKR.

There is clear evidence of racial/ethnic and gender disparities in the provision of TKR in the United States. Racial or ethnic differences in the provision of care are not limited to joint replacements. The limited role of economic and other access factors in these racial or ethnic disparities can be demonstrated by significant differences in the rate of procedures in the Veterans Administration (VA) system, where cost and access are assumed equivalent across race or ethnic groups.

Patients' acceptance of physician recommendations varies greatly. Among persons with a potential need for TKR, only 12.7 percent of women and 8.8 percent of men were "definitely willing" to have the procedure. The interaction between the patient and physician affects the final recommendations and the patient's acceptance of those recommendations. Physicians' beliefs about their patients, the limited familiarity with these procedures in minority communities, patients' mistrust of the health care system, and personal beliefs about the most effective treatment of joint problems may all have a role in these racial or ethnic disparities.

Section 35.2

Knee Replacement Rates Vary by Ethnicity

From "Patient preference may underlie ethnic variation in knee replacement surgery," by the Agency for Healthcare Research and Quality (AHRQ, www.ahrq.gov), September 2005.

Knee osteoarthritis (OA) is a major cause of knee pain and disability. Individuals who obtain no relief from medication often undergo total knee replacement (TKR). Whites are twice as likely as blacks or Hispanics to undergo TKR, a difference that persists even after controlling for health insurance.

Patient preferences appear to underlie much of the variation in TKR, concludes a study supported in part by the Agency for Healthcare Research and Quality. Researchers surveyed an ethnically diverse group of 198 patients with knee OA about whether their doctor recommended TKR, their thoughts about the procedure, and their trust in physicians and the health system.

Regardless of severity of OA, white patients were more likely than minority patients to have considered undergoing TKR. In addition, white patients were more likely to consider TKR if their OA worsened and their physician recommended the procedure. They also were more likely than minority patients to view TKR as a beneficial procedure.

Blacks had a higher physician recommendation rate than whites, and, although the rate was not statistically significant, it suggested that physician bias was not a factor in TKR in this group. Yet, many minority patients surveyed would not be willing to consider surgery even if their physicians recommended it. Major determinants of preferences were patients' beliefs about the efficacy of the procedure and knowing individuals in their close social environment who had undergone TKR. Improved physician-patient communication to provide more information and reassurance about the procedure could help more eligible patients benefit from TKR, note the researchers.

Source: "Ethnic variation in knee replacement: Patient preferences or uninformed disparity?" by Maria E. Suarez-Almazor, MD, PhD, Julianne

Souchek, PhD, P. Adam Kelly, PhD, and others, in the May 23, 2005, *Archives of Internal Medicine* 165, pp. 1117–1124.

Section 35.3

Experience Is Key for Knee Replacement Outcomes

From "Experience Is Key for Total Knee Replacement Outcomes," by the National Institute of Arthritis and Musculoskeletal and Skin Diseases (NIAMS, www.niams.nih.gov), part of the National Institutes of Health, January 2005.

A study funded by the National Institute of Arthritis and Musculoskeletal and Skin Diseases suggests a positive relationship between surgeons and hospitals performing a high volume of total knee replacements (TKR) and the outcomes for these interventions. The study found that patients of surgeons who perform 50 or more TKRs per year had a lower incidence of morbidity and postoperative complications than those whose doctors do 12 or less. Also, hospitals with 200 or more TKRs per year demonstrated similar positive outcomes in contrast to facilities that do less than 25 procedures per year.

The study research team, headed by Jeffrey N. Katz, MD, MS, analyzed 80,904 claims of Medicare patients who had primary or revision TKR between January 1 and August 31, 2000. The team determined the rates for mortality and complications for the first 90 days after the surgery. Complications included: deep wound infection requiring surgical attention or removal of prosthesis, pulmonary embolus, acute myocardial infarction, or pneumonia requiring hospitalization. The data were adjusted for age, gender, comorbid conditions, Medicaid eligibility (a marker of low income), and arthritis diagnosis.

TKR is a relatively low-risk surgical procedure in terms of 90-day rates of mortality and adverse events, when performed by an experienced surgeon in an experienced hospital. Most of the findings in this study are consistent with those reported in literature on associations between procedure volume and outcome for hip replacements and other surgical procedures. Of the 80,904 patients in the sample, 0.6

percent died, 0.8 percent had an acute myocardial infarction, 0.8 percent had a pulmonary embolus, 0.4 percent had a deep wound infection, and 1.4 percent were hospitalized for pneumonia.

Source: Katz JN, et al. Association between hospital and surgeon procedure volume and outcome of total knee replacement. *Journal of Bone and Joint Surgery* 2004;86-A(9): 1909–1916.

Chapter 36

Other Types of Joint Surgery

Chapter Contents

Section 36.1

Hip Replacement

Excerpted from "Questions and Answers about Hip Replacement," by the National Institute of Arthritis and Musculoskeletal and Skin Diseases (NIAMS, www.niams.nih.gov), part of the National Institutes of Health, May 2006.

What is a hip replacement?

Hip replacement, or arthroplasty, is a surgical procedure in which the diseased parts of the hip joint are removed and replaced with new, artificial parts. These artificial parts are called the prosthesis. The goals of hip replacement surgery include increasing mobility, improving the function of the hip joint, and relieving pain.

What does hip replacement surgery involve?

The hip joint is located where the upper end of the femur, or thigh bone, meets the pelvis, or hip bone. A ball at the end of the femur, called the femoral head, fits in a socket (the acetabulum) in the pelvis to allow a wide range of motion.

During a traditional hip replacement, which lasts from 1 to 2 hours, the surgeon makes a 6- to 8-inch incision over the side of the hip through the muscles and removes the diseased bone tissue and cartilage from the hip joint, while leaving the healthy parts of the joint intact. Then the surgeon replaces the head of the femur and acetabulum with new, artificial parts. The new hip is made of materials that allow a natural gliding motion of the joint.

In recent years, some surgeons have begun performing what is called a minimally invasive, or mini-incision, hip replacement, which requires smaller incisions and a shorter recovery time than traditional hip replacement. Candidates for this type of surgery are usually age 50 or younger, of normal weight based on body mass index, and healthier than candidates for traditional surgery. Joint resurfacing is also being used.

Regardless of whether you have traditional or minimally invasive surgery, the parts used to replace the joint are the same and come in two general varieties: cemented and uncemented.

Cemented parts are fastened to existing, healthy bone with a special glue or cement. Hip replacement using these parts is referred to as a "cemented" procedure. Uncemented parts rely on a process called biologic fixation, which holds them in place. This means that the parts are made with a porous surface that allows your own bone to grow into the pores and hold the new parts in place. Sometimes a doctor will use a cemented femur part and uncemented acetabular part. This combination is referred to as a hybrid replacement.

In the past, doctors reserved hip replacement surgery primarily for people over 60 years of age. The thinking was that older people typically are less active and put less stress on the artificial hip than do younger people. In more recent years, however, doctors have found that hip replacement surgery can be very successful in younger people as well. New technology has improved the artificial parts, allowing them to withstand more stress and strain and last longer.

Today, a person's overall health and activity level are more important than age in predicting a hip replacement's success. Hip replacement may be problematic for people with some health problems, regardless of their age. For example, people who have chronic disorders such as Parkinson disease, or conditions that result in severe muscle weakness, are more likely than people without chronic diseases to damage or dislocate an artificial hip. People who are at high risk for infections or in poor health are less likely to recover successfully. Therefore they may not be good candidates for this surgery. Recent studies also suggest that people who elect to have surgery before advanced joint deterioration occurs tend to recover more easily and have better outcomes.

Is a cemented or uncemented prosthesis better?

The answer to this question is different for different people. Because each person's condition is unique, the doctor and you must weigh the advantages and disadvantages.

Cemented replacements are more frequently used for older, less active people and people with weak bones, such as those who have osteoporosis, while uncemented replacements are more frequently used for younger, more active people.

Studies show that cemented and uncemented prostheses have comparable rates of success. Studies also indicate that if you need an additional hip replacement, or revision, the rates of success for cemented and uncemented prostheses are comparable. However, more long-term data are available in the United States for hip replacements with cemented prostheses, because doctors have been using them here since the late 1960s, whereas uncemented prostheses were not introduced until the late 1970s.

The primary disadvantage of an uncemented prosthesis is the extended recovery period. Because it takes a long time for the natural bone to grow and attach to the prosthesis, a person with uncemented replacements must limit activities for up to 3 months to protect the hip joint. Also, it is more common for someone with an uncemented prosthesis to experience thigh pain in the months following the surgery, while the bone is growing into the prosthesis.

What can be expected immediately after surgery?

You will be allowed only limited movement immediately after hip replacement surgery. When you are in bed, pillows or a special device are usually used to brace the hip in the correct position. You may receive fluids through an intravenous tube to replace fluids lost during surgery. There also may be a tube located near the incision to drain fluid, and a type of tube called a catheter may be used to drain urine until you are able to use the bathroom. The doctor will prescribe medicine for pain or discomfort.

On the day after surgery or sometimes on the day of surgery, therapists will teach you exercises to improve recovery. A respiratory therapist may ask you to breathe deeply, cough, or blow into a simple device that measures lung capacity. These exercises reduce the collection of fluid in the lungs after surgery.

As early as 1 to 2 days after surgery, you may be able to sit on the edge of the bed, stand, and even walk with assistance.

While you are still in the hospital, a physical therapist may teach you exercises such as contracting and relaxing certain muscles, which can strengthen the hip. Because the new, artificial hip has a more limited range of movement than a natural, healthy hip, the physical therapist also will teach you the proper techniques for simple activities of daily living, such as bending and sitting, to prevent injury to your new hip.

How long are recovery and rehabilitation?

Usually, people do not spend more than 3 to 5 days in the hospital after hip replacement surgery. Full recovery from the surgery takes about 3 to 6 months, depending on the type of surgery, your overall health, and the success of your rehabilitation.

What are possible complications of hip replacement surgery?

According to the American Academy of Orthopaedic Surgeons, more than 193,000 total hip replacements are performed each year in the United States and more than 90 percent of these do not require revision.

New technology and advances in surgical techniques have greatly reduced the risks involved with hip replacements.

The most common problem that may arise soon after hip replacement surgery is hip dislocation. Because the artificial ball and socket are smaller than the normal ones, the ball can become dislodged from the socket if the hip is placed in certain positions. The most dangerous position usually is pulling the knees up to the chest.

The most common later complication of hip replacement surgery is an inflammatory reaction to tiny particles that gradually wear off of the artificial joint surfaces and are absorbed by the surrounding tissues. The inflammation may trigger the action of special cells that eat away some of the bone, causing the implant to loosen. To treat this complication, the doctor may use anti-inflammatory medications or recommend revision surgery (replacement of an artificial joint). Medical scientists are experimenting with new materials that last longer and cause less inflammation. Less common complications of hip replacement surgery include infection, blood clots, and heterotopic bone formation (bone growth beyond the normal edges of bone). Studies are also looking at the use of bisphosphonates, ciprofloxacin, pentoxifylline, and other medications to prevent this bone resorption around the implants.

When is revision surgery necessary?

Hip replacement is one of the most successful orthopedic surgeries performed. Studies have shown that more than 90 percent of people who have hip replacement surgery will never need to replace an artificial joint. However, because more people are having hip replacements at a younger age, and wearing away of the joint surface becomes a problem after 15 to 20 years, replacement of an artificial joint, which is also known as revision surgery, is becoming more common. It is more difficult than first-time hip replacement surgery, and the outcome is generally not as good, so it is important to explore all available options before having additional surgery.

Doctors consider revision surgery for two reasons: if medication and lifestyle changes do not relieve pain and disability, or if x-rays of the hip show damage to the bone around the artificial hip that must be corrected before it is too late for a successful revision. This surgery is usually considered only when bone loss, wearing of the joint surfaces, or joint loosening shows up on an x-ray. Other possible reasons for revision surgery include fracture, dislocation of the artificial parts, and infection.

What types of exercise are most suitable for someone with a total hip replacement?

Proper exercise can reduce stiffness and increase flexibility and muscle strength. People who have an artificial hip should talk to their doctor or physical therapist about developing an appropriate exercise program. Most of these programs begin with safe range-of-motion activities and muscle-strengthening exercises. The doctor or therapist will decide when you can move on to more demanding activities. Many doctors recommend avoiding high-impact activities, such as basketball, jogging, and tennis. These activities can damage the new hip or cause loosening of its parts. Some recommended exercises are walking, stationary bicycling, swimming, and cross-country skiing. These exercises can increase muscle strength and cardiovascular fitness without injuring the new hip.

What hip replacement research is being done?

To increase the chance of surgical success and decrease the risk of complications and prosthesis failure, researchers are working to develop new surgical techniques, more stress-resistant materials, and improved prosthesis designs. They are also studying ways to reduce the body's inflammatory response to the artificial joint components.

Researchers are also studying gender and ethnic discrepancies in those who have the procedure, and characteristics that make some people more likely to have successful surgery.

Other areas of research address issues of recovery and rehabilitation, such as appropriate postsurgical analgesia for older people, and home-health and outpatient programs.

Section 36.2

Shoulder Replacement

After 15 years of shooting high-power rifles in his job as a police department SWAT [special weapons and tactics] team member—as well as working as a building contractor in his spare time—Stephen Blemings had developed painful arthritis in his shoulder.

"The pain was so bad I could barely move my arm," said Blemings, who was 39 at the time.

Blemings actively researched treatment options and decided on a partial shoulder replacement designed to replace only the damaged "ball" portion of his joint and leave the socket intact.

"This procedure allows the native anatomy to be maintained without losing bone," said orthopaedic surgeon Ethan Wiesler, MD. "The implant should last 20 years or more."

Wiesler said candidates for the procedure are people who have shoulder arthritis involving the ball side of the shoulder joint. Arthritis affects the cartilage, or protective lining, of the joints. As it wears away, bone rubs against bone, causing pain and limiting movement.

"We're seeing more and more of it in active people and it is becoming more common in young people," he said.

Shoulder replacement surgery may be an option when the associated pain and mobility problems cannot be managed with medication. With the traditional total replacement surgery, the natural "ball" at the top of the arm bone is removed and a metal implant that is attached to a stem is inserted down the center of the arm bone. The socket portion of the joint is shaved clean and replaced with a plastic socket.

With partial shoulder replacement, there are many types of implants to choose from. For patients who are young and active, the best option may be a special type of implant designed to restore as closely as possible the native shoulder anatomy. It requires less bone removal, uses a smaller incision, and has a quicker recovery time than total joint replacement and other partial implants. With this option, a metal cap is placed over the damaged "ball" of the upper arm bone.

Blemings said that after the surgery, he was able to return to all of his activities.

"I didn't miss a beat and don't have any limitations," he said. "It has been through a lot of wear and tear, from hammering and sawing to hanging drywall."

Common Causes for Shoulder Replacement

- Although far less common than hip and knee replacements, shoulder joint replacements have been performed since the 1950s.

- The shoulder is a "ball and socket" joint, similar to the hip, that allows you to raise, twist, or bend your arm. The most common reasons for replacing this joint are osteoarthritis, or "wear and tear" arthritis, rheumatoid arthritis, severe fractures, or arthritis that develops after a fracture or dislocation of the shoulder.

- While arthritis has many different causes, in many cases the cause is unknown, according to Dr. Wiesler.

Section 36.3

Joint Revision Surgery

"Joint Revision Surgery—When Do I Need It?" Reproduced
with permission from Your Orthopaedic Connection. Rosemont, IL,
American Academy of Orthopaedic Surgeons, © 2009.

Joint replacement surgery is undoubtedly one of the greatest medical advances of our time. Hip and knee replacements have been performed in millions of Americans over the last four decades. These procedures have improved patients' quality of life by easing pain, improving range of motion, and increasing activity levels.

Currently, over 700,000 hip and knee replacements are performed in the United States annually. Although joint replacement surgery has been amazingly successful, approximately 10% of implants will fail and require a second procedure, called revision, to remove the old implants and replace them with new components.

Joint revision surgery is a complex procedure that requires extensive preoperative planning, specialized implants and tools, and mastery of difficult surgical techniques to achieve a good result.

Most hip and knee replacement[1] procedures will perform well for the remainder of the patient's life. Current hip and knee replacements are expected to function at least 10 to 20 years in 90 percent of patients. This is due to several factors.

- There are more surgeries performed on older individuals. Older individuals tend to put lower demands on their implants.

- Current state-of-the-art materials and techniques have improved the quality of implant fixation to bone. This had historically been a weak link that created a potential site of failure.

- Innovations in implant[2] technology: Innovations have significantly decreased the amount of wear particles that are created by friction on joint surfaces.

As increasing numbers of young patients have these procedures, and as seniors continue to live longer, a growing segment of joint replacement patients will outlast their implants.

399

The decision to perform a revision joint replacement surgery will be based on several factors. The joint may become painful or swollen, due to loosening, wear, or infection. The function of the implant may decline, resulting in a limp, stiffness, or instability. Finally, serial examinations or X-rays may demonstrate a change in the position or condition of the components. All of these factors will determine when joint revision surgery is needed.

Reasons Implants May Fail

The anatomy of the hip and knee is very different after joint replacement as compared with its preoperative state. For example, there are large metallic objects and possibly cement. In addition, there may be scar tissue and bone loss. These factors must be addressed in revision joint surgery.

Implants may fail for any of several physiologic reasons: loosening, infection, dislocation, or patient-related factors. The anatomy and pathophysiology of failed joint replacement implants[3] contribute to the decision to perform revision surgery.

Loosening

Some revisions will be necessary because the implants have loosened. When they were first put in, the large metal and plastic implants were placed with the intention of staying fixed for a long time. They were either cemented into position or bone was expected to grow into the surface of the implant. In either case, the implant was firmly fixed to bone.

However, the friction of the joint surfaces rubbing against each other wears away the surfaces of the implant, creating tiny particles. These particles accumulate around the joint. In a process called aseptic, or non-infected, loosening, the bonds of the implant to the bone are destroyed by the body's attempts to digest the wear particles. When the prosthesis becomes loose, the patient may experience pain, deformity, or instability. In addition, the process of digestion, or lysis, of wear particles also digests normal bone. This can weaken or even fracture the bone, and jeopardize the success of the revision surgery. In this event, surgery will also address the bone stock deficiencies. Aseptic loosening is the most common mode of failure of hip and knee implants.

Infection

Infection is another physiologic cause of implant failure. The large foreign metal and plastic implants can serve as a surface for bacteria to latch onto. In addition, the tissue that has been previously operated on has an altered blood supply, which may not be adequate to fight infection. Even if the implants remain well-fixed, the pain, swelling, and drainage often make revision necessary. Lastly, the chronic fight against an infection can weaken the patient and endanger his or her life. Realistic risk of infection with current surgical techniques and antibiotic regimens is about 0.5%.[4]

Dislocation

Dislocation is yet another mode of failure of joint replacement surgery.[5] (Dislocation is a sudden popping out or migration of the implant from its normal position.) It is more commonly a problem of hips rather than knees. The rate of dislocation after hip replacement ranges from 0 to 10%, but averages about one in 50 patients. Some of these patients will experience multiple dislocations and require revision. The dislocation may be caused by loosening, inadequate soft tissues, bony or scar tissue impingement, incompatible component position, neurologic factors (such as neuropathy or Parkinsonism), or patient noncompliance.

Patient-Related Factors

Younger and more active patients have a higher rate of revision.[6,7] Patients whose primary surgery was performed for inflammatory arthritis, patients with avascular necrosis, and patients with a previous hip fracture are at higher risk for loosening. These anatomic and physiologic conditions lead to the necessity of joint revision surgery.

Diagnosis

Joint replacement surgery has been shown to decrease pain and increase function in the vast majority of patients. Once a patient progresses through the postoperative period, symptoms of pain, as well as the stability and motion of the joint, should remain stable for an extended period of time.

The natural history of failed implant surgery is an increase in pain, a change in the position of the implant, or a decrease in the function of the implant with limp or dislocation. Patients who demonstrate these symptoms and signs may require revision joint surgery. Therefore, a standard assessment[8] is performed, including a history and physical examination, x-rays, laboratory tests, and possibly aspiration or scintigraphic studies.

Physical Examination

The history and physical examination will identify patients who have a change in their pain level. Also, information can be obtained regarding activity levels and use of assistive devices, such as crutches or a cane. Pain of the hip may present as either groin or buttock pain. In addition, pain of the hip can sometimes be perceived of as knee pain, and vice versa. Swelling of the knee can be assessed easily, but swelling of the hip area may be more subtle. Mechanical failure or infection may also present with redness and warmth of the affected joint. A limp or deformity may be identified.

X-Rays

X-rays taken of the area around the joint replacement provide important clues regarding stability of the implant. Failure due to the most common cause, aseptic loosening, can be identified by several findings. For example, the implant may have moved, compared to previous x-rays, or there may be a lucent line between the component and the cement or bone, signifying that the bond between the bone and implant has degraded. Areas of bone loss can be identified. Mechanical failure with broken implants or severe wear is also assessed by comparison to previous x-rays. For these reasons, serial follow-up radiographs are recommended to catch joint failure at an early stage.

Laboratory Tests

Common laboratory tests for possible failed joints include a complete blood count, an erythrocyte sedimentation rate (ESR), and a C-reactive protein test (CRP). These studies are most helpful in the detection of infected joint replacements. The blood count may identify an anemia from chronic disease, and rarely may detect an elevated white blood cell count. The ESR and CRP may be abnormal in the presence of an inflammatory process, such as infection.

Additional Tests

Joint fluid may be removed with a needle and analyzed, a technique called aspiration, to give clues as to a possible infection. The knee joint can usually be reached with a needle in the physician's office, but the hip more commonly requires a setting that has fluoroscopic x-ray capabilities. In addition, scintigraphic studies that use short-acting radioactive isotopes may be used. One scintigraphic study, the Technetium 99 bone scan, can detect abnormal bone activity such as infection, fracture, or irritation from prosthetic motion. Another study, the Indium 111 scan, may be used to detect infection. All of these methods can be used when the natural history of joint replacement changes and revision becomes a possibility.

Treatment Alternatives to Revision Surgery

Although there are some surgical alternatives to revision joint surgery, they are rarely used, due to two main factors: These procedures can sometimes be more complex and lead to worse results than revision surgery and the results of modern revision joint surgery are outstanding.

One alternative to hip revision is called resection arthroplasty. This involves removal of the entire hip joint. This can give some relief of pain but naturally will lead to a decrease in function as compared to modern hip replacement.

Another procedure is called fusion, also known as arthrodesis. It may be used as an alternative to knee revision. Again, pain may be relieved, but at the expense of keeping the knee in a straight, non-bending position. These procedures may have a use in cases of severe joint infections that cannot be eradicated.

Greater than 90% of patients who undergo revision procedures will be expected to have good to excellent results, even considering the higher rate of complications as compared to first-time joint replacement. After weighing the alternatives, most patients and physicians prefer revision to other surgical options.

Nonsurgical Treatment

Benefits and Limits

Revision joint surgery, as previously stated, can be a major procedure that requires complex techniques. It can also have a higher complication rate than primary surgery. In addition, some patients are not medically able to tolerate a long and difficult surgical procedure.

Because of this, nonoperative treatment options are sometimes considered as a first step in the treatment of a failed implant. Obviously, problems that would damage remaining bone quality or make later treatment difficult would eliminate the nonsurgical options. Also, patients treated nonsurgically must realize that they may have significant limits on their function and activity.

Pain that is caused by a failed joint replacement may initially be treated with an increase in pain medications. These treatments may be limited by side effects, such as gastrointestinal upset and ulcers, drowsiness, and constipation. Increased reliance on assistive devices, such as a cane, crutches, or a walker, may be used to postpone revision. Likewise, a brace may decrease episodes of instability or dislocation. These techniques may be cumbersome and a burden to the patient, however. Modification and restriction of activity itself can be used to decrease symptoms. The less active a patient is, the less likely they are to be symptomatic. Finally, some infected joint replacements are treated with suppressive antibiotics to control the infection symptoms. This approach has a variable success rate and would not be expected to eradicate the infection.

Surgical Intervention and Considerations: Hip Surgery

Surgical intervention with joint replacement surgery[9] can be a complex and challenging procedure. Several potentially difficult portions of the surgery must be considered. Common to all joint revisions is an assessment of existing bone quality, removal of the failed components, reconstruction of remaining bone and soft-tissue structures, and successfully fixing the new components to the bone.

Consideration of each of these challenges is essential to produce successful revision joint surgery.

In hip revision surgery, both the femoral (stem and ball) components as well as the acetabular (socket) portion must be addressed.

- The hip bones may have deficiencies due to lysis and loosening, fracture, or shielding of the bone from normal stress. These deficiencies are graded according to several classification methods.

- Once this assessment is performed, a method to remove the existing components is selected. If some parts of the implant are still functioning, efforts may be made to retain them. Specialized removal techniques[7] have been developed, including surgically splitting the femur bone to remove the cement and implants, as well as power and hand instruments, which accurately cut around the prosthesis.

- When the failed components are removed, the remaining bone may require a complex reconstruction, involving larger or longer implants, bone grafting using ground-up bone or large segments of bone, and possibly cement and metal cages.

- Finally, the selected revision hip implant must be firmly fixed to the bone, either through bone growing into small pores in the outer layer of the implant or by cementing the construct into place.

Surgical Intervention and Considerations: Knee Surgery

Knee revision surgery entails consideration of the femur (thighbone), tibia (shinbone), and patella (kneecap) components.

- Bone stock deficiencies are classified according to several grading systems, and lysis, fracture, or stress shielding can lead to bone loss.
- The failed components are removed by a combination of surgical methods and specialized instruments. Reconstruction may require implants with extensions to reach better quality bone and that effectively replace lost ligament stability.
- Ground-up or bulk bone graft may be used.
- An implant is fixed in place through cemented or bone ingrowth techniques.

Surgical Technique

Joint revision surgery is usually performed as a planned surgical procedure. Patient condition and characteristics of the failed and new components will contribute to the planning process. Most surgical methods will proceed along a similar stepwise pattern.[11]

Before Surgery

Preoperatively, blood donation may be required due to the extensive dissection necessary to perform this surgery. Additionally, antibiotics will be given either before or early in the case to aid in prevention of infection. The patient will be brought to the operating room suite and anesthetized.[9]

Considerations

The surgical incision may utilize the site of the previous incision or it may be placed in another location. It is likely that a more extended incision will be used in order to facilitate implant and scar removal as well as simplify the insertion of the new component. Great care is taken during dissection, as the normal position and appearance of nerves and blood vessels can be altered by the previous surgery and wear of the old components. The failed implants and any old cement pieces are removed using specialized techniques.[10] In addition, abnormal bone and scar tissue is removed to achieve a new bed for fixation of the prosthesis.

Techniques

Reconstruction of the hip or knee bones must then be performed. Some procedures will have bone almost equal to a primary procedure. Others will have more severe bone loss. In these cases, revision will require the use of bone graft and/or metallic plates, cages, and screws. Once bone has been reconstructed, the process of implantation can begin.

Several techniques are available to implant the revision joints. Hip implants can be:

• porous-coated to allow bone in-growth;

• fixed close to the joint if bone quality is acceptable, or may have to rely on fixation down the bone if there is poor remaining tissue. Alternatively, the hip can be cemented into position;

• implanted using a combination of bone graft and cement.

Knee revision implants:

• may be about the same size as primary implants, or they can have extensive stems, wedges, and build-ups if bone quality is poor;

• may substitute for damaged or absent ligaments;

• will often use cement for fixation, but occasionally uncemented techniques are selected.[10]

After Surgery

Once the components are in place, the closure of tissue layers is performed. Drains are placed to collect any fluids or blood. The joint may be protected after surgery in a brace or splint. The medical condition of the patient is closely monitored and blood count is assessed. Antibiotics and some method of blood clot prevention will be continued in the postoperative period. This will complete the steps of the surgical procedure.

Potential Surgical Complications

Any surgery can have potential complications. The complexity of revision joint surgery increases the chance of complications. A realistic assessment of these risks is essential prior to a revision procedure.

Infection, bleeding, and trauma to nerves or blood vessels are a possibility with any surgical procedure. These are addressed and minimized by using antibiotics before and after surgery, working in a sterile operating room, use of blood-preserving techniques, and utilizing well-planned surgical exposures. The risk of these complications is higher than primary procedures.

Malpositioning or loosening of the new components is possible. In addition, the revision implants may migrate due to poor bone quality or inadequate fixation to the bone. More severe destructive processes with greater preoperative bone loss are more likely to create this problem.

Deep venous thrombosis and pulmonary embolism, or blood clots in the legs or lungs, can occur in conjunction with a revision procedure. The extensive surgery with subsequent twisting and trauma of the blood vessels can create clotting. In addition, the relative immobility of the patient after surgery increases the chance of clots. A clot in the lungs can become a life-threatening situation if the clot is large.

Dislocation of a hip implant is more common after revision surgery. This is due to the extensive dissection required to remove the failed components, as well as the poorer quality of the surrounding soft tissues after multiple procedures. In order to decrease the chance of dislocation, soft tissues are stretched out, which can lead to a lengthening of the operated leg.

Medical conditions can be aggravated or caused by the extensive revision procedure. Patients may have heart and lung complications, or stroke conditions. Rarely, death can occur. The decision to perform revision joint surgery is made when the benefits of pain relief and functional improvement outweigh the risks of these potential complications.

Rehabilitation and Convalescence

Rehabilitation after joint revision surgery is as aggressive as possible without damaging the new implant construct. In most cases, physical therapy will be initiated within 24 hours of the procedure. Therapy will continue for up to three months following the surgery.

Weight bearing may be restricted at first and a protective brace may be utilized.

Assistive devices, such as a walker or crutches, will be used early in the convalescence period. Patients will progress to a cane or no assistive device. In the hip, as in primary surgery, precautions may be placed regarding sitting, bending, and sleeping positions. For the knee, emphasis will be placed on regaining motion.

Restrictions remain in place for six to 12 weeks. Some patients will begin their rehabilitation in a rehabilitation hospital setting, while others will opt for home and outpatient therapy.

Improvements in strength and limp may continue over one to two years.

Conclusion

The decision to have joint revision surgery is based on many factors. Although joint replacement is successful in many patients, certain signs and symptoms will indicate that the implant has failed. Joint revision surgery is necessary when pain, swelling, limp, stiffness, or instability of a failed prosthesis become too great. Fortunately, modern techniques and materials for revision surgery will yield many more active years for most patients.

Reference List

1. Paprosky WG, Greidanus NV, Antonius J: Minimum 10-year results of extensively-porous-coated stems in revision hip arthroplasty. *Clin Orthop* 1999;369:230–242.

2. Katz RP, Callaghan JJ, Sullivan PM, Johnston RC: Long-term results of revision total hip arthroplasty with improved cementing techniques. *J Bone Joint Surg Br* 1997; 79:322–326.

3. Younger TI, Bradford MS, Magnus RE, Paprosky WG: Extended proximal femoral osteotomy: A new technique for femoral revision arthroplasty. *J Arthroplasty* 1995; 10:329–338.

4. Jiranek WA, Hanssen AD, Greenwald AS: Antibiotic-Loaded Bone Cement For Infection Prophylaxis in Total Joint Replacement. *J Bone Joint Surg Am* 2006, 88:2487–2500.

5. Shinar AA, Harris WH: Bulk structural autogenous grafts and allografts for reconstruction of the acetabulum in total

hip arthroplasty. A sixteen-year average follow-up. *J Bone Joint Surg Am* 1997; 79:159–168.

6. Huo MH, Parvizi J, Gilbert NF. What's New in Hip Arthroplasty. *J Bone Joint Surg Am* 2006, 88:2100–2111.

7. Archibeck MJ, White RE. What's New in Adult Reconstructive Knee Surgery. *J Bone Joint Surg Am* 2005, 87:1656–1665.

8. Leopold SS, Rosenberg AG, Bhatt RD, Sheinkop MD, Quigley LR, Galante JO: Cementless acetabular revision: Evaluation at an average of 10.5 years. *Clin Orthop* 1999; 369:179–186.

9. Schmalzreid TP, Callaghan JJ: Wear in total hip and knee replacements. *J Bone Joint Surg Am* 1999; 81:115–136.

10. Hanssen AD, Rand JA: Evaluation and treatment of infection at the site of a total hip or knee arthroplasty. *Instr Course Lect* 1999; 48:111–122.

11. Haas SB, Insall JN, Montgomery W III, Windsor RE. Revision total knee arthroplasty with use of modular components with stems inserted without cement. *J Bone Joint Surg Am* 1995; 77:1700–1707.

Chapter 37

Before, During, and After Joint Replacement

Home Set-up

It is important to set up your home **before** joint surgery. This will allow you to easily move around your home with a walker or crutches after surgery, reduce the risk of falls, and maintain your hip or knee joint precautions.

- Ensure hallways and rooms are free of clutter and tripping hazards (e.g., scatter rugs, footstools, etc.)

- Add non-slip surfaces to outside stairs and walkways.

- Install stair railings or make sure the existing ones are secure.

- Set up a firm chair with armrests.

- Ensure good lighting in hallways and other well-used areas.

- Arrange for extra help with household tasks if needed (e.g., vacuuming, laundry).

- Move frequently used household items to counter height (e.g., pots and pans). Consider moving items in the lower parts of the fridge/freezer to a higher shelf.

Excerpted from "Before, During, and After Hip and Knee Replacement Surgery: A Patient Guide," © 2008 Vancouver Coastal Health (www.vch.ca). Reprinted with permission. The complete text of this booklet is available at http://vch.eduhealth.ca/PDFs/FB/FB.130.B393.pdf.

- Stock your freezer/pantry with healthy foods and snacks. If needed, private food/meal delivery services are available in many areas.

- Keep an ice pack in your freezer for possible joint swelling after surgery. Alternatively, you can use a bag of frozen peas.

- Have a thermometer at home to check your temperature if needed after surgery.

Bathroom

- Install a raised toilet seat with armrests/toilet safety frame to assist you to sit or stand.

- Remove sliding doors from your bathtub and replace with a shower curtain.

- Set up a tub transfer bench (in the bathtub) or a shower chair (in a shower stall).

- Use a non-slip bath mat both inside and outside the bathtub or shower.

- Install a handheld shower hose in the bathtub.

- Grab bars in the bathtub/shower stall and by the toilet are very useful. Removable grab bars are available. Do **not** use towel racks or toilet paper holders to assist you to stand or sit.

Seating after Hip Surgery

- As you are not able to bend your hip past 90 degrees for 3 months after hip surgery, all surfaces that you sit on must be 2 inches above knee height. This includes chairs, beds, and toilets.

- Use a high-density (firm) foam cushion or bed blocks to increase chair height. The cushion should be firm enough that it will not compress when you sit on it. Plan to take your foam cushion with you to adapt chairs outside of the house.

- Set up a firm chair with armrests (not a rocking chair).

- Set up a table beside your chair for frequently used items as you will not be able to bend forward to the coffee table.

- If your bed is too low, add another mattress or place the frame on bed blocks.

Equipment List (Arrange up to 2 Weeks before Surgery)

Hip Surgery

Equipment you must bring to hospital, unless otherwise told:

- Walker—Standard or 2-wheeled
- Crutches
- High-density (firm) foam cushion (at least 4 inches x 16 inches x 18 inches, needed for going home in the car)
- Dressing equipment (long-handled reacher, long-handled shoe horn, and sock aid)

Knee Surgery

- Walker—Standard or 2-wheeled
- Crutches
- Dressing equipment (long-handled reacher, long-handled shoe horn, and sock aid)

Equipment for Home

For hip surgery, the equipment below is required. For knee surgery, the equipment below is recommended.

- 4-inch raised toilet seat (with or without armrests) or commode chair with wheels
- 26-inch long-handled reacher
- 24-inch long-handled shoehorn
- Sock aid
- 24-inch long-handled sponge
- Non-slip bath mat
- Elastic shoelaces (otherwise use slip-on shoes with an enclosed heel)
- Handheld shower hose

Bathing

- Shower: Use a walk-in shower and shower chair.

- Bathtub: Use a tub transfer bench or raised shower board.
- Removable tub clamp or installed grab bars

Where to Get Equipment

Medical Supply Store

- Equipment for rent and/or purchase
- May deliver to your home and/or install
- Costs may be covered by extended health plans—check your plan.

Friends/Family

- Check with friends and family who may have equipment you can borrow.
- Please ensure that equipment fits in your home and is in good working order before you have your surgery.

Transportation Support

Some transportation support services require application forms to be completed by you and your doctor or health professional. These services include temporary disabled parking passes.

Exercise

Exercising before surgery will help you have a faster and easier recovery. Do activities that put less stress on your joint. Try:

- exercises in water, such as swimming or water walking at a community pool;
- cycling;
- Nordic pole walking;
- gentle stretching and strengthening;
- specific exercises suggested by a physiotherapist;
- balance exercises (valuable in preventing falls).

These activities will make your muscles strong, improve your endurance, and help keep your joint moving. Exercising before surgery will also help you to build up your confidence and knowledge of how to exercise after surgery. Remember: After surgery, daily exercise will be part of your rehabilitation for many months.

Be sure to strengthen your arm muscles. You will need strong arms after your surgery to use walking aids, get in and out of bed, and get on and off a chair. If possible, do strengthening exercises for at least 3 weeks before surgery. For example: Push up through your arms while seated. Work up to 10 repetitions two times each day.

If this exercise causes you discomfort or if you are new to exercise and/or have other health conditions, always talk to your family doctor before starting a new exercise program. If you don't know how to get started, talk to a physiotherapist.

Nutrition

Good nutrition helps you to recover from surgery and reduces the risk of infection. Important nutrients before and after surgery include the following.

Protein

Protein promotes healing after surgery. To meet increased protein needs, try to eat at least three servings from each of these food groups every day. For example, for meat and alternatives, one serving equals 2 3 oz of meat, poultry, or fish; two eggs; 3/4 cup beans; 3/4 cup tofu; and 2 tablespoons peanut butter.

For milk and alternatives, one serving equals 1 cup milk or soy beverage; 2 ounces cheese; and 3/4 cup yogurt.

Multivitamin

While a basic multivitamin is recommended to promote healing, large doses of any nutrient are generally not recommended. If you have a history of anemia, talk to your doctor, pharmacist, or dietitian about supplements.

Calcium and Vitamin D

Calcium and vitamin D are important for strong bones. Adults should have two to three servings of milk or calcium-fortified products a day. A minimum of 400 IU vitamin D supplement is recommended for all people over 50 years old. Talk to your doctor, pharmacist, or dietitian about current supplement recommendations that are right for you.

Fiber and Water

It's important to have a regular bowel habit before joint surgery because constipation can be a complication. Include fiber in your diet, such as whole grains, bran, fruits, vegetables, beans, and lentils. Spread the fiber throughout the day and drink at least eight glasses of water or other low-calorie fluid a day.

Weight Management

Being overweight or underweight can affect your recovery from surgery. If you are overweight, moderate weight loss is a good strategy to reduce hip and/or knee pain and to allow you to do more activities. Every extra pound you carry places 3–6 pounds of force on your knees and hips. If you are trying to lose weight before surgery, aim for a gradual loss of no more than 1 pound per week. Avoid fad diets as they may cause you to be undernourished and prolong recovery.

Being underweight can make it harder for your body to heal after surgery. It is important to eat well before surgery.

Talk to a dietitian if you are worried about being overweight or underweight before surgery.

Preoperative Education

When does it occur? As far in advance as possible. The hospital will call to register you for a Preoperative Education Class. At this session, you will learn more about your surgery, what to expect while you are in hospital, and what you need to prepare at home. It is a good idea to bring a family member or support person with you to this session. Your preop education may be provided at your Preadmission Clinic visit.

Preadmission Clinic (PAC)

When does it occur? A few days before your surgery. The Preadmission Clinic will call you to schedule an appointment. This appointment may last a few hours. The nurse will discuss many points including the following:

- When to stop eating and drinking before surgery
- Medicine management before and after surgery. Some medicines and supplements must be stopped 1–2 weeks before surgery to

avoid problems with bleeding or sleepiness. Talk to your surgeon if you have questions about your medicines.

- Allergies

Bring all of your medicines/supplements to your Preadmission Clinic appointment.
You may have some tests done including the following:

- Blood work
- X-ray
- ECG (electrocardiogram)

You may also be scheduled to meet with an anesthesiologist. This is a medical doctor who is trained to give anesthetic drugs and monitor you throughout your surgery. Bring any questions about your anesthesia to your Preadmission Clinic appointment.

Your surgery may be canceled if you have: an active infection anywhere in your body, a skin infection over the joint, a cold, or the flu. If you are sick before surgery, call your surgeon.

One Day before Surgery: A Final Checklist

By now you should have picked up your medical equipment and set up your home. Here is a final checklist of things you need to do before coming to the hospital:

- Label all of your equipment with your name (e.g., walker, crutches, dressing equipment) if you are bringing these items to the hospital.
- Make arrangements for transportation to and from the hospital.
- Make arrangements for someone to stay with you or be nearby for at least the first 72 hours after you leave the hospital.
- Have a bath or shower using regular soap the night before, or the morning of your surgery (do not shave your legs as any cuts or skin irritation may result in your surgery being canceled).
- Pack your bag for the hospital. Bring:
  - toiletry items (e.g., toothbrush, hair brush etc.);
  - loose fitting clothes to exercise in and to wear home;

- comfortable, closed toe and heel shoes/slippers with nonslip soles (your shoes should be roomy since you will have some swelling in your feet);
- if you wear elastic support stockings, bring them with you;
- eyeglasses and reading materials;
- hearing aids;
- if needed, credit card information for items such as hospital TV rental.

Do not bring valuables to the hospital.

During Your Hospital Stay: Day of Surgery

Before Surgery

- Go to the Admitting Desk in the hospital.
- Bring all of your medicines with you, as directed by the Preadmission Clinic.
- Ask friends or family to bring your labeled equipment to the hospital ward unless otherwise instructed.
- To prepare for surgery, you will change into a hospital gown and a nurse will start an intravenous line (IV) in your arm.

During Surgery: Anesthesia

Each hospital manages your anesthetic differently. Many people who have joint replacement surgery have spinal anesthetic. This is like the freezing you get at the dentist, except this freezing goes into your back and makes you numb from the chest down and stops you from feeling pain. The anesthesiologist will make sure you are comfortable throughout the surgery, giving you medicine through your IV that makes you relaxed and sleepy. If you have a spinal anesthetic, you will not be able to move your legs for up to 4 hours after surgery.

Some people receive general anesthetic. This is a combination of drugs that will make you unconscious during the surgery.

Bring any questions you have about anesthesia to your Preadmission Clinic appointment.

After Surgery: Recovery Room

- You are moved from the operating room to the recovery room.

- You may have oxygen by mask for a short time or nasal oxygen overnight.

- The nurse monitors your vital signs, including your pulse and blood pressure.

- You will have pain medicine on a regular basis. Tell your nurse if you are in pain.

- Some people may have compression devices placed on their lower legs. Compression devices gently squeeze your calf muscle to help with blood circulation.

- The stay in the recovery room is usually 1 to 3 hours.

After Surgery: The Hospital Ward

- Once you are medically stable, you are transferred to the orthopedic ward.

- You will be told how much weight you can put on your new joint (weight bearing status). This can vary for each individual. Often people are told to weight bear as tolerated, but you may have a weight-bearing restriction such as partial, feather, or non-weight bearing on your surgical leg.

- The ward staff will help you to stand on your new joint if allowed by your surgeon.

- The nurse will assess you for pain and nausea.

- You will use a commode/raised toilet seat during the day and a bedpan/urinal at night. When you are able, you will walk to the bathroom. Some people who have spinal anesthetic find it difficult to urinate and will need a catheter (a temporary tube placed in your bladder to empty it).

- You may have blood work.

- You may have an intravenous line (IV) for medicine.

- After knee surgery, you may have a drain on your leg to collect blood from your knee.

- You are taught exercises to help reduce complications after surgery, such as:

  - breathing deeply and coughing every hour to keep your lungs clear;

  - pumping your ankles to improve circulation in your legs.

419

- You may be started on a blood thinning medicine (e.g., heparin injections) after surgery to help reduce your risk of developing a blood clot.

Length of Hospital Stay Guidelines

Your time in the hospital is short. Your health care team will work with you to make sure you are medically stable and able to manage daily tasks to go home. Before surgery, it is important to make arrangements to have someone pick you up from the hospital when going home. Discharge time is usually in the morning.

Be aware that you may go home sooner than expected. Ensure your travel arrangements are flexible.

- Total hip replacement—Three nights or less (includes resurfacing and revision surgery)

- Total knee replacement—Three nights or less (includes revision surgery)

- Partial knee replacement—Overnight

- Bilateral (both) knee replacement—Five nights or less

For example: If you have surgery on Monday and are spending three nights in the hospital, you will probably be sent home on Thursday morning.

Rehabilitation

- Physical activity is a very important part of your recovery. Not only does it help to improve the function of your joint, but it also helps clear your lungs, reduces the risk of blood clots in your legs, reduces pain, and starts your bowels moving.

- The physiotherapist (PT) will work with you throughout your stay. Your physiotherapist will teach you how to:

  - walk with a walker and/or crutches;

  - do your daily exercises;

  - use the stairs safely.

- The physiotherapist will give you exercises to do in hospital and at home. They may also refer you to a physiotherapist in your local community.

- The occupational therapist (OT) will teach you how to do daily activities, such as dressing and bathing, while following precautions and protecting your new joint.

Pain Control

Pain Control after Surgery

- Your nurse will teach you how to use the pain scale to describe your level of pain. "0" is no pain and "10" is the worst possible pain.

- It is our goal to keep your pain at "3–4" or below at all times.

- Generally, pain medicine is given as a pill taken by mouth.

- If you have had a general anesthetic, you may have a patient controlled analgesia (PCA) pump. This is when a controlled amount of pain medication is pumped into your IV tube when you push a button.

- A combination of medicines will likely be used to control your pain after surgery. This normally would include acetaminophen (e.g., Tylenol) plus possibly an anti-inflammatory (e.g., NSAID) and/or narcotic (e.g., morphine). By taking a combination of these medicines, you may be able to reduce the side effects of any one of these medicines and have improved pain control. It is important to talk to your health care team to understand how and when to take these medicines to best control your pain and symptoms.

- Some side effects of pain medicine can include: nausea, vomiting, drowsiness, itchiness, and/or constipation. Tell your nurse if you have any of these symptoms.

Pain Control at Home

Most people have less and less pain over the next 6 to 12 weeks. If pain is preventing you from caring for yourself, sleeping, and/or exercising, talk to your physiotherapist or doctor. If your pain becomes increasingly worse or if you have pain in a new part of your body, seek medical attention immediately.

Here are some ways to manage your pain:

- Take pain medicine as directed. It is normal to have some increased pain or symptoms during physical activity or physiotherapy sessions. It may be helpful to take a dose of pain medicine

1 or 2 hours before engaging in these activities in the first weeks after surgery. It is better to take medicine **before** the pain is severe.

- Ice can reduce pain and inflammation. It is particularly useful for people who have had knee replacement surgery. Place an ice pack wrapped in a towel on your joint as directed by your physiotherapist.

- Pace yourself. Do not push yourself. Regular rest is an important part of your healing process.

- Relax. Use relaxation techniques such as breathing exercises or progressive muscle relaxation (progressive muscle relaxation is when you tighten and relax each part of your body, starting with the toes and working up to your neck).

- Distract yourself. Listen to music, visit with friends, write letters, watch TV.

- Think positively. You will become more and more comfortable as you recover from your surgery.

Heparin Injections

After hip or knee replacement surgery, you are at risk for developing a blood clot. Many people are given a daily injection of a blood thinning medicine such as heparin to reduce this risk. Your doctor will decide if this medicine is right for you.

Here is some information about heparin injections:

- Low molecular weight heparin (LMWH) is also called dalteparin or Fragmin.

- Heparin is usually injected into the skin on your stomach using a very thin, short needle attached to a prefilled syringe.

- Heparin injections are usually given daily for 10–35 days after surgery.

- Your nurses will give you your heparin injections while you are in hospital. They will teach you how to give yourself the injection before you are discharged home.

- If you don't feel comfortable giving yourself the injection, have a family member or friend come to the hospital to learn how to give the injection at the same time each day.

- The main pharmacies near city hospitals carry this form of heparin. Pick up your prescription before you go home. If you are planning on using your local pharmacy, be aware that they may need 48 hours to get your heparin injections in stock.

Going Home

Most people will be discharged home, not to a rehab facility. Before leaving the hospital, plan appointments with the following people:

- The person (e.g., family doctor or physiotherapist) who will remove your staples, 7–14 days after surgery
- Your surgeon, usually around 6 weeks after surgery
- Your physiotherapist, usually within 1 week of discharge (if recommended by your surgeon)
- Your family doctor, once you are back on your feet, to review your general condition

Recovery at Home

Physiotherapy after Hospital

The hospital physiotherapist will help you to arrange a physiotherapy appointment for when you get home from the hospital. Depending on your needs, where you live, and local services, your appointment may be at a physiotherapy clinic, outpatient hospital center, rehab facility, or home health program.

Your physiotherapist will give you exercises to stretch and strengthen your legs and improve your walking and balance. As you recover, the exercises will get harder. Doing the exercises assigned by your physiotherapist will help you move your new joint and enjoy greater independence. It is important to continue with the exercises for at least 1 year after your surgery.

Talk to your physiotherapist if you have questions about your exercises or concerns about your progress.

Transportation

There are many different ways to get around after surgery. Here are some options:

- Friends/family

- Taxis

- Temporary disabled parking pass

- Transit service for those who cannot use the regular bus service. This service will pick you up and drop you off at appointments such as medical visits.

Talk to your health care providers about completing the necessary forms for these services **before** surgery.

Air travel: You may have some extra challenges traveling by plane after surgery. Be sure to give yourself extra time when flying. Your new joint may set off metal detectors at the airport. If you are flying within 3 months of having hip surgery, bring your high-density foam cushion to raise the height of your seat. While on the plane, do foot pumping exercises every hour to help reduce the risk of clots. If flying home from hospital, check with your air carrier if medical documentation is needed.

Driving: Driving is restricted after knee or hip surgery. There are a number of factors that can impact your ability to safely return to driving. These include using mobility aids and taking prescription pain medicines. Talk to your surgeon and physiotherapist before driving. Most people start to drive within 12 weeks after surgery.

Car transfer: It can be challenging to protect your joint getting into some cars, particularly following hip surgery. Talk to your occupational therapist if you have questions about car travel. Please practice these instructions before you come to the hospital.

- Park away from the sidewalk or curb so you are not stepping down from the curb to the car. If you have a high truck or sport-utility vehicle, you may need to park near the curb so that you do not have to climb up to the seat.

- Move the seat as far back as possible.

- Recline the seat.

- Place your high-density foam cushion on the seat. If it is a wedge cushion, position the thick end at the back of the seat.

- Back up to the seat until you feel the back of the seat on your legs.

- Extend your operated leg.

- Hold onto the back of the seat and the car to stabilize yourself.

- Lower yourself to the seat.

- Slide back and lift your legs into the car. (If you have had hip surgery, do **not** bend more than 90 degrees).

- A piece of plastic or a large garbage bag over the cushion may help you to slide in more easily.

- You can also try a device called a "Handybar" that can assist you to get in and out of a regular car. This can be purchased at medical supply stores.

Everyday Activities Guidelines

Walking

You can expect to use walking aids, such as a walker, crutches, or cane, for up to 3 months or longer after surgery. By 4 to 6 weeks after your surgery, you should be walking with more confidence, have more strength, and be able to walk longer distances. Regular physiotherapy after your surgery will help you get the most out of your new joint. Physical activity will help you have a faster recovery and will get your blood moving. This will also reduce your risk of developing a blood clot.

Stairs

It is a good idea to practice the stairs with the hospital physiotherapist so that you are able to manage stairs safely and independently. If you have had both knees replaced (bilateral), your physiotherapist will practice a technique with you that allows you to alternate your surgical legs when going up and down the stairs.

Going up the stairs:

- Use a handrail and/or crutches/cane.

- Step up with your good (non-operated) leg first.

- Follow with your operated leg and crutch, one stair at a time.

Going down the stairs:

- Use the handrail or your crutches.

- Place your crutch on the step below.

- Step down with your operated leg first.

- Follow with your good (nonoperated) leg, one stair at a time.

Getting into Bed

- Sit at the side of the bed. It may be easier to get into bed on your stronger side.

- Slide back across the bed using your arms for support.

- If necessary, a half bed rail can allow you to get in and out of bed more easily. A half bed rail consists of a handle with 2 long metal rods that are placed between the mattress and the box spring. A half bed rail can be obtained through the Red Cross or medical supply stores.

- Lift your operated leg into bed or use a "leg lifter" (this may be the belt from your housecoat or a crutch turned upside down, hooked over your foot so you can help lift the leg using your arms) if needed.

Getting out of Bed

- Slide your body to the edge of the bed.

- Use your arms to push yourself to a sitting position. (If you have had hip surgery, do not push yourself up past 90 degrees. Remember your hip precautions.)

- Slide your operated leg off the bed.

- Bring your body to a sitting position at the bedside.

Sitting Down

- Use a firm chair with arm rests.

- If you have had hip surgery, measure the chair height against your leg before you sit. The chair should be 2 inches above your standing knee height. Use a high density foam cushion or bed blocks to increase the chair height.

- Back up to the chair until you feel the edge behind your knees.

- Move your operated leg forward and reach back for the arm rests.

- Slowly lower yourself into the chair.

Getting Dressed

- Sit on a raised chair or bed.

- Dress your operated leg first and undress it last.

- Use adaptive aids like a long-handled reacher, sock aid, and shoehorn to reach the foot of your operated leg and put on socks, pants, shoes, etc. while protecting your new joint.

- While you are in the hospital, your occupational therapist will show you how to use these aids and give you tips on how to dress while maintaining joint precautions.

Bathroom Safety

Falls can happen anywhere but are most likely in the bathroom. Here are ways to reduce the risk:

- Do not rush. Plan to use the toilet often. Have a bedside commode if needed.

- When bathing, use a bench or chair, non-slip bath mats, grab bars, and/or a removable tub clamp.

- Make sure the route from your bedroom to the bathroom is well-lit.

- Wear sensible, non-slip shoes or slippers.

- If you feel dizzy or unsteady, talk to your family doctor.

Using the Toilet

- Use a raised toilet seat for the first 3 months after your surgery.

- Make sure that the toilet seat has secure armrests or that you can use the counter to push yourself up. You can also install grab bars to help you stand or sit. Do not use towel racks or toilet paper holders to help you stand or sit down.

- Toilet seat should be 2 inches above standing knee height.

- Sit down as you would in a chair.

Bathtub Transfer

- Use a tub transfer bench with a handheld shower (in a bathtub) or shower chair (in a shower stall) for the first 3 months after surgery. Do not try to sit on the bottom of the tub.

- Remove glass shower doors on your tub and replace with a shower curtain.

427

- Place a non-slip bath mat inside and outside the tub.

- Your transfer bench or shower chair should be 2 inches above your standing knee height. If you are tall, you may need bench leg extensions.

- Sit down as you would in a chair. Slide back as far as you can on the seat. Then lift your legs over the edge of the tub. Do not bend your hip past 90 degrees if you have had hip surgery.

- Use long-handled aids to clean your feet and other hard-to-reach places.

- A handheld shower hose will allow you to bathe more easily. If you have had a hip replacement, you will not be able to reach forward for the taps due to hip precautions.

- Some surgeons will want you to do sponge baths until your staples are removed in order to avoid getting the new incision wet.

Wound Care

You will have a cut (incision) at the site of your surgery. Your nurse will teach you how to care for your incision at home. While it is normal to have some redness and clear drainage from your wound, watch for signs of infection. You do not need a bandage unless there is drainage.

The edges of your skin may be held together with sutures, staples, or Steri-Strips. Staples are metal clips that hold the edges of your skin together while your skin heals. Your staples will be removed 7 to 14 days after surgery. If you have Steri-Strips, leave them alone. They will fall off on their own.

It is important to keep your incision dry until it is fully healed. You may find it useful to tape a plastic bag or waterproof dressing over your incision while showering unless otherwise instructed by your surgeon.

Sexual Activity after Hip Replacement

- You may return to sexual activity when you feel ready and comfortable; this is often around 4 to 6 weeks after surgery.

- You must maintain hip precautions for 3 months during all daily activities, including sexual activity.

- Think about how you will maintain your hip precautions of not twisting and not bending more than 90 degrees.

- You may need to consider trying some new positions. Talk to your partner.

- If you have questions or concerns about how to protect your new hip during sexual activity, talk to your occupational therapist, physiotherapist, or surgeon.

- Visit the website www.aboutjoints.com for illustrations of sexual positions that maintain hip precautions.

Returning to Work

Allow yourself time to recover from surgery and focus on your rehabilitation before returning to work. Some people return to some form of work quickly after surgery but others need a longer time to heal and recover. This depends on factors such as health status and the type of work you do. Talk to a health care professional, such as an occupational therapist, about what is right for you.

Work Environment Adaptations

Chair: Choose a standard chair for sitting. Avoid chairs with wheels; they can roll away from you when you are getting up. Use your high-density foam cushion to increase the seat height if necessary.

Desk: Position your phone, paperwork, and computer close to you. If you have had a hip replacement, you should not bend forward to reach these items. This will break your hip precautions.

Keyboard tray: If you have raised your chair and your desk is too low, use a height-adjustable keyboard tray so that you can sit comfortably while typing.

Schedule: Plan lots of stretch breaks. Get up and move around frequently. Avoid sitting in the same position for more than 45 minutes at a time.

Bathroom: Check the height of the toilets at the office and the location of grab bars.

Review your workstation before surgery so that you can make the necessary adjustments before you return to work.

Complications

After surgery, a few people have complications and need more medical treatment. Here are some possible complications:

- Constipation/bladder function
- Blood clots
- Swelling
- Infection
- Anemia (low blood count)
- Joint loosening
- Hip joint dislocation

Constipation/Bladder Function

Constipation can be a problem after surgery. A change in your diet, less activity, and pain medicine may make your constipation worse.

Here are some ways to stay regular at the hospital and at home:

- Drink at least eight glasses of water or low-calorie fluid a day.
- Eat fiber, such as prunes, bran, beans, lentils, fruits, and vegetables.
- Move around as much as you can—do your exercises.

Your nurse may give you laxatives and/or stool softeners. You may need to keep taking these medicines at home. If you have constipation at home, talk to your family doctor or pharmacist. Constipation can be serious so do not ignore your symptoms.

Some patients have difficulty urinating after their joint surgery. Please talk to your nurse right away if you are having problems. You may need a catheter.

Blood Clots

A small number of people may get blood clots after surgery. Blood clots usually develop in the deep veins in the legs. People who have problems with their circulation and/or are inactive are more likely to develop a blood clot.

To reduce the risk of blood clots:

- Give yourself your daily heparin blood thinner injections (if prescribed by your doctor).

430

- Walk short distances at least once an hour (except when you are sleeping).
- When you are sitting or in bed, pump your ankles and flex your leg muscles.

Tell your family doctor or surgeon immediately if you have:

- pain, aching, heat, or redness in your calf area;
- increasing severe swelling in your surgical leg.

Call 911 immediately if you have:

- shortness of breath;
- sudden chest pain.

Swelling

It is normal to have some swelling in your leg after surgery and during your recovery. Swelling may increase as you become more active. To help reduce swelling:

- Point and flex your feet hourly when awake.
- Lie down flat and raise your legs (maintain hip or knee precautions) by placing pillows under the length of your leg.
- Do short periods of activity. Walk a few steps. Rest. Repeat.
- Place an ice pack wrapped in a towel on your joint. For some people, a "Cryocuff" may be used after knee replacement surgery. This is a type of ice pack/compression device for the lower leg. For more information, talk to your physiotherapist about using ice at home.

Infection

Less than 1% of people have an infection around their new joint. An infection in the body can reach the new joint through the bloodstream.

People who develop joint infections need antibiotics and, on rare occasions, further surgery. To prevent infection or incision problems, it is important to keep the incision and dressings dry. Do not touch or pick at the incision and maintain good cleanliness of the surrounding skin.

Tell your doctor or surgeon if you have any of these signs of infection.

Incision infection:

- The area around your incision is becoming more red and the red is spreading.
- New drainage (green, yellow, or foul smelling pus) from the wound site. It is common for new surgical wounds to have some drainage for the first few (3–5) days after surgery but this will slowly stop and the wound should stay dry.
- There is increased pain or swelling of wound site and surrounding area.
- Fever above 38 degrees Celsius or 101 degrees Fahrenheit
- Call your surgeon if you think you have a possible wound infection.

Urinary tract infection:

- Pain when you urinate
- Frequent or urgent need to urinate
- Foul smelling urine
- Fever above 38 degrees Celsius or 101 degrees Fahrenheit

Sore throat/chest infection:

- Swollen neck glands; pain when you swallow
- Frequent cough, coughing up yellow or green mucus, shortness of breath
- Fever above 38 degrees Celsius or 101 degrees Fahrenheit

Anemia (Low Blood Count)

If you have signs of anemia, see your family doctor. You may need an iron supplement. The signs of anemia are:

- feeling dizzy or faint;
- feeling very tired;
- shortness of breath;
- rapid pulse.

Joint Loosening

Over many years, the bond between the joint replacement and your bone may loosen. This can cause pain and make it difficult for you to

432

move your artificial joint. To reduce the risk of this complication, avoid high-impact physical activities. If you notice increased pain in your artificial joint, talk to your doctor as soon as possible.

Hip Joint Dislocation

Call 911 if your surgical leg is suddenly extremely painful, shortens, and the hip cannot be moved.

Dental Work and Medical Procedures

It is important to tell your health care professional that you have had joint replacement surgery before having dental work or medical procedures (including procedures with the bladder, prostate, lung, or colon). You may be put on antibiotics to prevent infection from moving through your bloodstream to your new joint. Talk to your dentist or doctor about what is right for you.

Part Four

Arthritis Self-Management: Strategies to Reduce Pain and Inflammation

Chapter 38

Questions and Answers about Arthritis Pain

Over 80% of older adults experience osteoarthritis (OA), which is the most common cause of arthritis with older age. Rheumatoid arthritis (RA) is different and the second most common type of arthritis. These two arthritis conditions cause pain and can make it difficult for older people to take care of themselves. Obtaining a careful evaluation and developing a plan for treatment with your primary care provider is key to improving quality of life.

What is the difference between OA and RA?

OA is a degenerative disease caused by continued wearing down of the structure and/or tissue in the joints (e.g., cartilage and connective tissues). OA usually affects the large joints that bear the weight of the body and may not affect the same joints on opposite sides of the body. OA pain is usually located in the knees, hips, feet, ankles, joints of the hands and neck, and lower spine. RA is caused by inflammation that generally affects the same joints on opposite sides of the body (such as both hands). RA may also affect internal organs such as the heart, lungs, and eyes. Both OA and RA can result in loss of physical function and can cause people to become disabled. OA causes stiffness on rising and discomfort while using the affected joints. RA is usually felt as pain, swelling, warmth, and tenderness in various joints, with discomfort and fatigue that may last throughout the day.

Can my arthritis be cured?

There are no treatments that cure arthritis. However, a treatment plan that includes drug and non-drug treatments (such as occupational therapy, physical therapy, psychological treatments, and education) can improve pain, function, and overall quality of life.

Do I just have to learn to live with my arthritis pain?

Although many people believe that arthritis pain is a result of aging and must be tolerated, living with the pain is not good for you. Untreated pain can have serious effects such as poor healing, weakness, breathing complications, depression, anger, as well as making overall quality of life worse. There are many treatment choices that can and should be explored to help relieve pain and its impact.

Is there a difference in treatment between OA and RA?

Yes, treatments can differ depending on the type of arthritis. Pain medicines and medicines to fight inflammation are most often used for OA, and are also useful in patients with RA. However, patients with RA are also treated with drugs that change the immune system.

What can I do to help my arthritis?

One of the most important things you can do is to learn as much as possible about your disease, its treatment and ways to adjust your life to the disease. The older person who takes charge of their disease (in a self-management program) can lower pain, improve their function and overall quality of life. Many different strategies that improve health are often included in self-management programs and focus on nutrition, exercise, physical therapies, coping skills, use of canes and walkers, pacing activity, scheduling activity, and stress management. When your self-management program, including over-the counter medication, is not relieving the pain, a visit to your primary care provider is warranted.

Are the nutrition therapies advertised in magazines, television, and internet useful to manage arthritis pain?

There are many advertised alternative nutrition therapies that have no scientific evidence to show they are effective. You should be cautious about these. However, there are several treatments that have been proven helpful for patients with arthritis. Glucosamine sulfate is an example. There is no specific arthritis diet that has been shown to improve symptoms. However, keeping your body weight at a normal level, and following a balanced diet with the right amount of protein, fat, vitamins, and minerals is important. Caffeine, nicotine, and alcohol can interfere with sleep and also can impact your overall health and management of your disease.

It seems that exercise would only make joints that already have arthritis worse and cause pain. Should I limit my activity?

Actually, keeping up physical activity is important for everyone. Although it may seem that exercise would hurt joints that are already painful, exercise is an important part of an arthritis treatment program. Motion and lubricating fluid in the joint improve with mild to moderate exercise. Low activity can add to the pain and stiffness, as well as loss of function that can result from arthritis. A carefully balanced program of activity is important.

I had a small peptic ulcer years ago. Are there certain medications that are better choices for me?

Acetaminophen (such as Tylenol) is the first choice in pain medicines if your pain is mild, because acetaminophen does not have a risk of causing bleeding from the stomach. Discuss your options with your primary care provider.

Are joint injections a good treatment option for my joint pain?

Injection of steroids into joints with arthritis should be considered in patients with OA or RA who have worse or severe inflammation in one or a few joints. Injection of hyaluronic acid supplements into the knee may be an option for people whose OA pain is not getting better with other pain medications. These injections replace or supplement the body's natural lubrication in the joint.

My doctor has tried numerous drug and non-drug treatments to control my arthritis pain, but I still have severe pain that prevents me from doing any of the activities that are important to me. Are there any other options?

Strong pain medicines, such as morphine, tramadol, oxycodone, and hydrocodone, might be used if other drug and nondrug treatments have not provided enough pain relief and your overall quality of life is made worse by the pain. Some find that using stronger pain medicine is needed to treat flares of pain that only last a day or a week to supplement other medicines. Surgical options, including joint replacement, are other alternatives to consider when drug and nondrug treatments are ineffective at maintaining function and quality of life. Consult your health care provider to discuss your options.

Reference

American Pain Society. (2002). *Guideline for the Management of Pain in Osteoarthritis, Rheumatoid Arthritis, and Juvenile Onset Arthritis. Clinical Practice Guideline No. 2.* Glenview, IL: American Pain Society.

Additional Resources

The Foundation for Health in Aging—*Eldercare at Home,* Chapter 11 "Pain" www.healthinaging.org/eldercare/chap11.html.

American Chronic Pain Association
P.O. Box 850
Rocklin, CA 95677
Phone: 916-632-0922
Website: www.theacpa.org

American Pain Society
4700 West Lake Avenue
Glenview, IL 60025
Phone: 847-375-4715
Fax: 866-574-2654
Website: www.ampainsoc.org
E-mail: info@ampainsoc.org

Arthritis Foundation
P.O. Box 7669
Atlanta, GA 30357-0669
Toll-Free: 800-283-7800
Website: www.arthritis.org
E-mail: arthritisfoundation
@arthritis.org

Chapter 39

Tips on Dealing with Your Pain

Chapter Contents

Section 39.1

Pain Management Tips

Pain has been in the news lately, and not always in the ways that we would hope. On the one hand, *Time Magazine* featured the issue of treating chronic pain on its cover in February [2005], and the *Today* show featured a five-part, educational series on chronic pain in March [2005]. On the other hand, the DEA's [Drug Enforcement Agency's] withdrawal of the Frequently Asked Questions document has increased confusion about prescribing proven medications for the treatment of pain, further stigmatizing pain patients. And now, the withdrawal of two COX-2 non-steroidal anti-inflammatory (NSAID) medications and the more stringent, FDA [Food and Drug Administration]-mandated warnings on all NSAIDs have created fear and confusion about what's safe and effective for treating pain.

You may be feeling overwhelmed and confused. You may ask yourself, "What's safe? What medications can I take? Who can I trust to provide accurate and complete information about my condition and my treatment options? What can I do now that I can no longer take this medication? What can I do if my doctor is no longer willing to prescribe to me? What things can I do to improve my quality of life?"

The important thing to remember is that you are not alone. Millions of Americans suffer from chronic pain, and there are many organizations working to address this serious, life-altering, and profoundly difficult problem. Overcoming suffering and pain is difficult—sometimes it even seems impossible, but there are things you can do to help yourself. You must be your own "best" advocate.

Now, more than ever, is the time to educate yourself about your treatment options and empower yourself by doing what you can to care for yourself physically, emotionally, and spiritually.

Unfortunately, there is no magic pill or cure to relieve chronic pain or its underlying conditions. Medication alone often is not enough, especially for people who have chronic pain. As some of your medical options may be disappearing, it may be time to reevaluate what's working for you and what you can do differently to help yourself. Relieving pain requires work both on the part of the physician and on the part of the patient. People with chronic pain must be active participants in their care.

How to Feel More in Control of Your Pain Condition

Find an Understanding and Knowledgeable Pain Specialist

If you are looking for a pain specialist, you have some different options for your search. First, you can ask for a referral from your primary care physician. This is often the first step that should be taken. You can also ask others to recommend a doctor.

Many professional physician organization web sites have listings of their members available to the public. These directories oftentimes can help you locate an appropriate pain medicine physician in your area. You can print the directory and share it with your primary care physician to identify the best physician for your particular needs.

Once you have identified a physician, you should ask specific questions to help you determine whether the physician will best meet your needs. Some of the questions below can help you make an informed decision.

- How many cases of my type of pain condition have you treated?
- What are your special qualifications to treat my pain condition?
- Have you participated in any special training about pain management techniques?
- What is your philosophy of management of my pain condition in terms of medications and alternative therapies?
- What types of medications do you usually prescribe?
- What types of non-medication therapies do you use?
- Where do you refer patients who need additional treatment?
- Is your clinic listed with any professional societies?
- Are you, or is someone in the clinic, available 24 hours a day if I need help?

Finding an understanding and qualified pain specialist is one of the first steps in fighting to regain your life.

Take Care of the Things You Can Control

Part of being an active participant in your care is caring for your body. No one but you can care for your body. Getting adequate rest, eating a healthy diet, and engaging in physical activity are vitally important to maintaining function and health. It may seem like a catch-22—you're in pain, so you don't want to move or you're finally feeling a little better, but you're afraid to move because your pain might come back. Avoiding exercise can be detrimental to your health—you lose muscle tone and strength, your heart and lungs work less efficiently, and your pain can increase.[1] On the other hand, the benefits of incorporating activity into your lifestyle are immeasurable and include increased muscle strength and flexibility, improved sleep, and stress relief.[2]

Following are some suggestions for increasing your activity level:

- Choose exercises that can be incorporated into your daily routine and that you enjoy.

- Set a schedule.

- Ask your doctor about appropriate exercises and activities for your situation.

- Set appropriate goals.[3] No goal is too small—visiting friends or walking around the block may be appropriate goals, depending on your pain and physical condition.

Ask your physician which exercises are safe for you. In addition to a healthy diet and exercise, relaxation techniques such as meditation, visualization, hypnosis, and biofeedback may help you feel better. Your health care provider can help you decide which techniques may be beneficial for you.

Caring for Your Emotional Health

The effect emotions and psychosocial well-being have on pain cannot be ignored as emotions have a direct effect on your health.[4] Pain so often is accompanied by loss—loss of function, loss of employment, loss of money, loss of friends and relationships to name just a few—it's no wonder that people in chronic pain have an increased incidence of depression, anxiety, and sleep disturbances.[5] Research has shown that people in chronic pain suffering from depression have poorer outcomes than those who are not depressed.[6] It is natural for people in

444

pain to grieve for what they've lost, and it is important to remember that your family members and friends grieve too. Your emotions may range from fear, anger, denial, disappointment, guilt, and loneliness to hope and optimism. Every person feels different emotions at different times, which can make relationships and pain control difficult.

Taking care of the emotional aspects of chronic pain is necessary to treat your overall pain condition. Your physician may want to prescribe medication for depression, anxiety, and sleep disturbances and, in addition, may suggest cognitive behavioral therapy (e.g., relaxation techniques, coping strategies, psychological therapy).[7] Your doctor does not think you're crazy—he or she is treating you as a "whole"—not just the part in pain. Following are some suggestions to help you deal with the emotional aspects of pain:

- Keep a journal of your emotions. A journal can help you release some of the emotions you feel.

- Share your thoughts and feelings with loved ones and allow them to share their feelings with you. People cannot read your mind—just as pain is an invisible disease, emotions can be difficult to discern.

- Avoid isolation and loneliness by joining a support group. There are local support groups that you can attend with people who know what you are experiencing and there are online communities that offer support and understanding. The National Pain Foundation's Community section is a good way to share your story and connect with others online. The American Chronic Pain Association has support groups throughout the country. Contact the ACPA at www.theacpa.org or 800-533-3231 to find a group near you.

- Be active—exercise can help relieve the stress and emotional pain you feel.

Evaluate Your Treatment Options

Medications such as NSAIDs and selective NSAIDs (COX-2 inhibitors) are important tools in the management of chronic pain, but they are not the only tools available to help you. NSAIDs work by decreasing inflammation and pain.

Traditional NSAIDs, such as ibuprofen and naproxen, tend to irritate the stomach and can lead to ulcers and bleeding. The COX-2

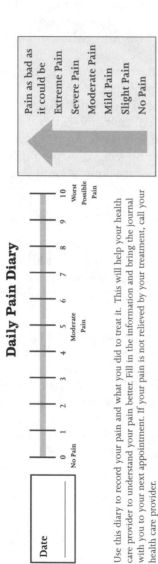

Daily Pain Diary

Date _____

No Pain 0 1 2 3 4 5 6 7 8 9 10

Moderate Pain (5)

Worst Possible Pain (10)

Pain as bad as it could be — Extreme Pain
Severe Pain
Moderate Pain
Mild Pain
Slight Pain
No Pain

Use this diary to record your pain and what you did to treat it. This will help your health care provider to understand your pain better. Fill in the information and bring the journal with you to your next appointment. If your pain is not relieved by your treatment, call your health care provider.

Time	Where is the pain? Rate the pain (0–10), or list the word from the scale that describes your pain.	What were you doing when the pain started or increased?	Did you take medicine? What did you take? How much?	What other treatments did you use?	After an hour, what is your pain rating?	Other problems or side effects? Comments.

Time	Where is the pain? Rate the pain (0-10), or list the word from the scale that describes your pain.	What were you doing when the pain started or increased?	Did you take medicine? What did you take? How much?	What other treatments did you use?	After an hour, what is your pain rating?	Other problems or side effects? Comments.

Figure 39.1. A daily pain diary can help you keep track of pain. (*Source: From "Daily Pain Diary," © 2002. Reprinted with permission from the American Geriatrics Society Foundation (www.americangeriatrics.org). For more information visit the AGS online at www.americangeriatrics.org. Reviewed by David A. Cooke, MD, FACP, July 27, 2009.*)

NSAIDs have become popular because they are less likely to cause ulcers and bleeding. News that another NSAID has been withdrawn from the market and the fact that all NSAIDs will now have additional warnings on their labels can be frightening and disheartening for patients dealing with chronic pain. The first step in determining if NSAIDs and COX-2 NSAIDs are still an option for you is to speak with your doctor. All medications have benefits and all medications have side effects and risks. Different people react differently to medications, and choosing to take a medication becomes a very personal decision that must take into account the risks and benefits, your level of functioning without a particular medication, and your overall health. You and your doctor are the only people who can determine whether a specific medication is the right choice for you.

If you are taking any NSAIDs for pain, be sure your doctor knows your medical history, including any history of heart problems, high blood pressure, ulcers, and medication allergies. Be sure your doctor knows about all the medications you currently take, including medications prescribed by other doctors, over-the-counter medications, and supplements. This information will help you and your doctor weigh the overall risk-benefit of a medication.

It is up to you to educate yourself about your health and your treatment options. There are many options for your pain, including:

- prescription and over-the-counter NSAIDs;
- other prescription medications such as opioids, anxiolytics/ hypnotics, anticonvulsants, antidepressants, muscle relaxants and more, depending on your pain condition;
- complementary and alternative therapies, such as biofeedback, meditation, relaxation techniques, yoga, acupuncture, and more;
- physical therapy;
- interventional treatments (e.g., for arthritis, injections at the pain site containing a pain reliever and corticosteroid, or for back and neck pain, spinal cord stimulators and intrathecal drug pumps).

Talk with your doctor. Developing an open and trusting relationship with your pain specialist is important to helping you determine which treatment options are best for you.

To help you locate a health care provider, visit the National Pain Foundation's Pain Care Provider Directory [http://www.nationalpain foundation.org/providers .php].

448

References

1. "Chronic pain: Exercise can bring relief," Mayo Clinic (April 23, 2001). M Nicholas et al, *Manage Your Pain: Practical and Positive Ways of Adapting to Chronic Pain* (Sydney: ABC Books, 2002) 84–89, 98–127.

2. "Chronic pain," WebMD (March 2001).

3. "Chronic pain: Exercise can bring relief," Mayo Clinic (April 23, 2001); Nicholas et al, *Manage Your Pain: Practical and Positive Ways of Adapting to Chronic Pain*, 84–89, 98–127.

4. M McCaffery, C Pasero, *Pain Clinical Manual,* second ed (St. Louis: Mosby, 1999) 499–505.

5. Ibid.

6. Ibid.

7. Ibid.

Section 39.2

Joint Protection:
What Is It and Why Is It Important?

"Joint Protection: Prevent Joint Damage and Reduce Risk of Osteoporosis," © 2005 Missouri Arthritis Rehabilitation Research and Training Center (MARRTC). Reprinted with permission. For additional information, visit http://marrtc.missouri.edu.

What Is Joint Protection?

Joint protection means using your joints in ways that avoid excess stress. That might involve changing your surroundings or how you do activities.

Why Is Joint Protection Important?

Joint protection is important to make sure that you do not cause harm to your joints. Accidents, injuries (traumatic or repetitive), or overuse of a particular joint can cause joint injuries. These injuries can cause pain and increase the odds that you may develop osteoarthritis in the future. Important parts of joint protection include muscle strength, good posture, moving around, and proper body mechanics.

Muscle Strength

Maintain muscle strength. Muscles help support joints. Keeping muscles strong may reduce the risk of wear and tear on joints and help prevent injury.

Good Posture

When standing, imagine a line separating the front half of your body from the back. For good posture, your ear lobe, tip of your shoulder, side of your hip, knee and ankle should be in line with one another.

When sitting, your elbows, hips, knees, and ankles should rest comfortably at 90-degree angles.

When working in a seated position, make sure the lower part of your spine is supported.

When resting, lie on your back with one pillow under your head and keep your arms and legs out straight.

Move Around

One way to prevent joint damage is not stay in one position too long. Here are some tips:

- Use a stool for periodic rest breaks when standing.
- During periods of sitting, change the position of your legs.
- Every so often move the ankle joints by first pulling the toes toward the head, then pointing them down.

Warning Signs of Arthritis

- Joint pain
- Swelling (sometimes)
- Stiffness in or around your joint
- Difficulty moving a joint

If you have any of these signs in or around a joint for more than two weeks, please visit your doctor.

Proper Body Mechanics

Proper body mechanics are very important when lifting objects. Here are tips on how to lift safely:

- Lift with a straight back and knees bent.
- Stay close to the object that is to be lifted.
- Keep your feet shoulder width apart for good base support.
- Avoid twisting at the waist.

Chapter 40

Lifestyle Changes to Manage Pain

Many people with arthritis find that small changes in the way they do things and in the techniques they use for pain management yield positive results. Managing moderate arthritis pain does not have to be complicated.

Exercise

Arthritis experts emphasize that a well-designed exercise program can decrease the pain and stiffness you feel—while increasing your range of motion. Talk to your doctor about the kinds of exercise that best suits your particular needs.

While high impact activities such as running and floor aerobics can increase joint pain, regular gentle exercise (such as swimming, water aerobics, and biking) has been shown to reduce or prevent joint pain. Exercise benefits your cartilage too as the action of the joints increases blood flow, which in turn brings nutrients to the joint and removes waste products. Building strong muscles around your joints can help to support them and reduce your chances of injury.

"Arthritis Exercises and Pain Management Techniques," reprinted with permission from www.allaboutarthritis.com, an informational website from DePuy Orthopaedics, Inc., a Johnson & Johnson company. © 2002 DePuy Orthopaedics, Inc. All rights reserved. Reviewed by David A. Cooke, MD, FACP, June 29, 2009.

Strengthening and Range of Motion Exercises

Try to put each of your joints through its full range of motion every day. Remember that normal daily activities such as housework, climbing stairs, lifting, and bending do not put your joints through their full range of motion.

In order to better protect your joints, the muscles surrounding a joint should be strengthened. Exercise is a good way to do this. Two basic types of exercise can help with pain relief.

Stretching or range-of-motion exercises help you stay flexible while preventing stiffness and joint deformities.

Strengthening exercises make the muscles, ligaments, and tendons that support your joints stronger, thereby making movement less painful.

Tips for beginners:

- Do these exercises slowly, without bouncing or jerking.
- Start with no more than 5 repetitions of each exercise, and take at least 2 weeks to increase to 10 repetitions.
- Do the exercises in an order that does not require you to get up and down a lot.
- Always do the same number of exercises for both sides of your body.

Exercises for Your Back

To stretch:

- Lie on the floor with your knees bent, and your feet flat on the floor.
- Bring one knee toward your chest, lifting your foot up off the floor. If you need to, tuck your hands under your thigh to help lift the leg.
- Hold for 10 seconds, then lower the leg slowly.

To strengthen:

- Lie on the floor with your knees bent and your feet flat on the floor.
- Tighten your stomach muscles and your buttocks to push the

small of your back against the floor. This is known as the pelvic tilt.

- Hold for 10 seconds and relax.

Exercises for Your Knees

To stretch some muscle groups and to strengthen others:

- Lie on your back with your legs straight.
- Straighten your knee completely to tighten the muscle just above your knee. If you are doing this correctly, your heel should come up off the floor.
- Hold for a count of 5 and relax.
- Sit in a chair and cross your legs above the ankles. Your legs can be either straight or bent.
- Push forward with the back leg and backward with the front leg, pressing evenly so that your legs do not move.
- Hold for 10 seconds and release.

Exercises for Your Hips

To stretch:

- Stand straight and hold onto a sturdy table or counter.
- Move the outside leg as far out to the side as it will go.
- Keep your foot in place, roll your knee in then out, leading with your heel.

To strengthen:

- Stand straight, face and hold onto a sturdy table or counter.
- Move one leg backward and up behind you, keeping the knee straight. Do not arch your back or lean forward.
- Hold for a count of 10, then slowly release.

Exercises for Your Ankles

- Bend and point your toes while watching TV or talking on the phone.

Exercises for Your Shoulders

- Grasping a stick or mop handle at each end, raise it as high over your head as possible. You can do this exercise sitting, standing, or lying down.

Joint Protection

- Listen to your body and stop any activity that causes ongoing pain. Alternate heavy or repeated tasks with easy tasks or breaks in your daily schedule. Change tasks often.

- Pay attention to joint positioning. Use larger, stronger joints to carry loads. For example, carry a purse on your shoulder instead of with your fingers. Don't remain in the same position for a long time; get up and walk around periodically.

- Use helpful devices. Take advantage of the many items that can help you cope with the tasks of daily life, such as items with longer or thicker handles.

- Use a chair with a straight back, high seat, and arms, so you can push on the arms when getting up.

- Use a cane, crutches, or a walker, if your doctor recommends them, to reduce stress on weight-bearing joints.

- Use carts, such as luggage carts, so you can push or pull instead of carrying heavy items.

Weight Control

By reducing stress on your joints, controlling your weight helps prevent osteoarthritis of the knees and other weight-bearing joints. And it lessens pain in those who have it. To keep weight off, lose it gradually—no more than two to five pounds per month. Eat fewer calories and exercise more to lose weight.

If you need to lose a lot of weight, work with your doctor or a registered dietitian to find the best weight loss program for you.

Heat and Cold

Applying heat or cold to sore joints can temporarily relieve the pain and stiffness of osteoarthritis. Heat helps to relax aching muscles. Cold can numb the area to reduce pain. Ask your doctor or therapist which method is best for you. And follow these tips:

- Time your use of heat or cold to give the best relief from pain or stiffness—for example, after you get out of bed in the morning or before exercise.

- Don't use heat or cold for more than 15 to 20 minutes each time. Let your skin return to normal temperature before using it again.

- Don't use heat combined with rubs or creams.

- Always put a towel or cloth between your skin and heat or cold packs.

Heat methods include: electric blankets and mitts, heating pads, hot baths or showers, hot packs, hot towels, hot tubs, heated pools, and paraffin wax.

Cold methods include: bags of frozen vegetables, cold compresses, an ice cube or cubes wrapped in a towel, ice bags, and cold packs.

Chapter 41

Arthritis and Sleep Deprivation

Arthritis sufferers often don't relate sleep deprivation effects to their disease. Awareness of the connection between arthritis and sleep deprivation and talking with your doctor may be the key to getting better sleep.

Insomnia creates a vicious cycle for arthritis patients.

- When you don't get enough sleep, the result is fatigue.
- You may not feel like exercising. Lack of physical activity may contribute to sleeplessness.
- Your aches and pain become magnified.
- Lack of sleep, over time, may contribute to weight gain by altering the body's metabolism. Weight gain may increase your arthritis pain.
- Fatigue can be caused by rheumatoid arthritis and other rheumatic conditions.

According to one study, sleep deprivation is the No. 1 reason arthritis patients see a doctor, even more than pain or other problems related to their disease "Study shows sleep disruption to be arthritis sufferers' chief complaint," University of North Carolina at Chapel Hill, February 2000).

"We believe this unexpected finding is important because it's not well recognized by either patients or physicians," said Joanne Jordan, MD, in the February 2000 press release. "As a rheumatologist, I know that you can give patients all the anti-inflammatory drugs in the world to try to control their arthritis, but if you don't take care of their sleep disruption, they may not get any better. Oftentimes, patients don't tell doctors about it because they think nothing can be done to treat problems with sleeping."

Controlling Nighttime Pain

Arthritis sufferers may tolerate their achy joints all day, but seem to notice more discomfort at night. A key to restful sleep begins with pain management. Talk with your physician about your sleep problem. It's possible a change in your evening dose of pain medication may help you sleep better. Some pain medications that cause drowsiness in certain patients may actually stimulate others. Pay close attention to your reaction to pain medications. Discuss them with your doctor and he or she may adjust your medications to help you sleep better.

Another problem sometimes associated with arthritis is "restless leg syndrome." This condition causes discomfort when the legs are at rest, creating an urge to move the legs. This interferes with sleep. If you think you have restless leg syndrome, discuss your symptoms with your doctor. This is a treatable condition for many patients.

The Mind-Body Connection

In addition to physical pain interfering with sleep, anxiety from severe arthritis may contribute to the problem. Arthritis can lead to a sense of loss resulting in anxiety or depression that may affect healthy sleep habits. Talking with a counselor may help you cope. Ask your physician for a recommendation.

Here are some additional tips:

- Talk about your problems with your doctor even if they are not arthritis specific.

- Choose a comfortable mattress and pillow. Some arthritis sufferers prefer firmer mattresses. Others prefer a softer surface. Also, there are a variety of specialized contoured pillows. Experiment, and choose what works best for you.

- Try bed linens and pajamas with silky materials. Smooth bedding helps you move under the covers and change positions comfortably.

- Avoid caffeine, nicotine and alcohol too close to bedtime.

- Don't try to force yourself to sleep. If you can't get to sleep after 15 to 20 minutes, get up and do something relaxing, such as reading or knitting.

- Avoid reading, eating, or watching TV in bed.

- Get enough exercise during the day, but not late in the evening.

- Exercising too close to bedtime can make it harder to relax your body and fall asleep.

- Avoid naps during the day until you get into a healthful nighttime sleep pattern. Also, get up at the same time every morning.

- There are many other ways to address sleep deprivation effects, depending on the combination of causes. Talking with your doctor is an important first step to improving your quality of sleep.

Chapter 42

Weight Management and Arthritis

Arthritis Basics—Frequently Asked Questions

What is recommended for people with arthritis?

Early diagnosis and appropriate management of arthritis, including self-management activities, can help people with arthritis decrease pain, improve function, stay productive, and lower health care costs. Key self-management activities include the following:

- **Learn arthritis management strategies:** Learning techniques to reduce pain and limitations can be beneficial to people with arthritis. Self-management education, such as the Arthritis Foundation Self Help Program (AFSHP), or the Chronic Disease Self Management Program (CDSMP) help you learn the strategies and develop the confidence to manage your arthritis on a day to day basis. For example, AFSHP has been shown to reduce pain even 4 years after participating in the program.

- **Be active:** Research has shown that physical activity decreases pain, improves function, and delays disability. Make sure you

This chapter contains text excerpted from "Arthritis Basics—Frequently Asked Questions," by the Centers for Disease Control and Prevention (CDC, www.cdc.gov), 2008, and excerpted from "Choosing a Safe and Successful Weight-Loss Program," by the Weight-control Information Network (win.niddk.nih.gov), part of the National Institutes of Health, April 2008.

get at least 30 minutes of moderate physical activity 3 days a week. You can get activity in 10-minute intervals.

- **Watch your weight:** The prevalence of arthritis increases with increasing weight. Research suggests that maintaining a healthy weight reduces the risk of developing arthritis and may decrease disease progression. A loss of just 11 pounds can decrease the occurrence (incidence) of new knee osteoarthritis.

- **See your doctor:** Although there is no cure for most types of arthritis, early diagnosis and appropriate management are important, especially for inflammatory types of arthritis. For example, early use of disease-modifying drugs can affect the course of rheumatoid arthritis. If you have symptoms of arthritis, see your doctor and begin appropriate management of your condition.

- **Protect your joints:** Joint injury can lead to osteoarthritis. People who experience sports or occupational injuries or have jobs with repetitive motions like repeated knee bending have more osteoarthritis. Avoid joint injury to reduce your risk of developing osteoarthritis.

Is exercise recommended for people who have arthritis?

Recent studies have shown that moderate physical activity three or more days a week can help to relieve arthritis pain and stiffness and give you more energy. Regular physical activity can also lift your mood and make you feel more positive.

An activity that produces a slight increase in heart rate or breathing is considered moderate physical activity. Low-impact activities performed at a moderate pace work best for people with arthritis. These include walking, swimming, and riding a bicycle. Everyday activities such as dancing, gardening, and washing the car can be good if done at a moderate pace that produces slight breathing and heart rate changes.

If you are having an acute flare-up of your inflammatory arthritis, it may be better to restrict your exercise to simple range of motion (carefully moving the joint as far as it can go) during the flare-up.

How does body weight influence arthritis?

Weight control is essential; research suggests that maintaining a healthy weight reduces the risk of developing osteoarthritis and may decrease disease progression. A loss of just 11 pounds can decrease the occurrence (incidence) of new knee osteoarthritis.

Choosing a Safe and Successful Weight-Loss Program

Choosing a weight-loss program may be a difficult task. You may not know what to look for in a weight-loss program or what questions to ask. This text can help you talk to your health care professional about weight loss and get the best information before choosing a program.

Should I talk with a health care professional?

If your health care provider tells you that you should lose weight and you want to find a weight-loss program to help you, look for one that is based on regular physical activity and an eating plan that is balanced, healthy, and easy to follow. You may want to talk with your doctor or other health care professional about controlling your weight before you decide on a weight-loss program. Doctors do not always address issues such as healthy eating, physical activity, and weight management during general office visits. It is important for you to start the discussion in order to get the information you need. Even if you feel uncomfortable talking about your weight with your doctor, remember that he or she is there to help you improve your health. Here are some tips:

- Tell your health care professional that you would like to talk about your weight. Share your concerns about any medical conditions you have or medicines you are taking.

- Write down your questions in advance.

- Bring pen and paper to take notes.

- Bring a friend or family member along for support if this will make you feel more comfortable.

- Make sure you understand what your health care provider is saying. Do not be afraid to ask questions if there is something you do not understand.

- Ask for other sources of information like brochures or websites.

- If you want more support, ask for a referral to a registered dietitian, a support group, or a commercial weight-loss program.

- Call your health care professional after your visit if you have more questions or need help.

What questions should I ask?

Find out as much as you can about your health needs before joining a weight-loss program. Here are some questions you might want to ask your health care professional:

Ask these questions about your weight:

- Do I need to lose weight? Or should I just avoid gaining more?
- Is my weight affecting my health?
- Could my extra weight be caused by a health problem such as hypothyroidism or by a medicine I am taking? (Hypothyroidism is when your thyroid gland does not produce enough thyroid hormone, a condition that can slow your metabolism—how your body creates and uses energy.)

Ask these questions about weight loss:

- What should my weight-loss goal be?
- How will losing weight help me?

Ask these questions about nutrition and physical activity:

- How should I change my eating habits?
- What kinds of physical activity can I do?
- How much physical activity do I need?

Ask these questions about treatment:

- Should I take weight-loss drugs?
- What about weight-loss surgery?
- What are the risks of weight-loss drugs or surgery?
- Could a weight-loss program help me?

What is a responsible and safe weight-loss program?

If your health care provider tells you that you should lose weight and you want to find a weight-loss program to help you, look for one that is based on regular physical activity and an eating plan that is balanced, healthy, and easy to follow. Weight-loss programs should encourage healthy behaviors that help you lose weight and that you can stick with every day. Safe and effective weight-loss programs should include the following:

- Healthy eating plans that reduce calories but do not forbid specific foods or food groups
- Tips to increase moderate-intensity physical activity
- Tips on healthy habits that also keep your cultural needs in mind, such as lower-fat versions of your favorite foods
- Slow and steady weight loss (Depending on your starting weight, experts recommend losing weight at a rate of 1/2 to 2 pounds per week. Weight loss may be faster at the start of a program.)
- Medical care if you are planning to lose weight by following a special formula diet, such as a very low-calorie diet (a program that requires careful monitoring from a doctor)
- A plan to keep the weight off after you have lost it

How can I get familiar with the program?

Gather as much information as you can before deciding to join a program. Professionals working for weight-loss programs should be able to answer the following questions.

- What does the weight-loss program consist of?
- Does the program offer one-on-one counseling or group classes?
- Do you have to follow a specific meal plan or keep food records?
- Do you have to purchase special food, drugs, or supplements?
- If the program requires special foods, can you make changes based on your likes and dislikes and food allergies?
- Does the program help you be more physically active, follow a specific physical activity plan, or provide exercise instruction?
- Does the program teach you to make positive and healthy behavior changes?
- Is the program sensitive to your lifestyle and cultural needs?
- Does the program provide ways to keep the weight off? Will the program provide ways to deal with such issues as what to eat at social or holiday gatherings, changes to work schedules, lack of motivation, and injury or illness?

- What are the staff qualifications?

- Who supervises the program?

- What type of weight management training, experience, education, and certifications does the staff have?

- Does the product or program carry any risks?

- Could the program hurt you?

- Could the recommended drugs or supplements harm your health?

- Do participants talk with a doctor?

- Does a doctor run the program?

- Will the program's doctors work with your personal doctor if you have a medical condition such as high blood pressure or are taking prescribed drugs?

- Is there ongoing input and follow-up from a health care professional to ensure your safety while you participate in the program?

- How much does the program cost?

- What is the total cost of the program?

- Are there other costs, such as weekly attendance fees, food and supplement purchases, etc.?

- Are there fees for a follow-up program after you lose weight?

- Are there other fees for medical tests?

- What results do participants typically have?

- How much weight does an average participant lose and how long does he or she keep the weight off?

- Does the program offer publications or materials that describe what results participants typically have?

If you are interested in finding a weight-loss program near you, ask your health care provider for a referral or contact your local hospital.

Chapter 43

Exercise and Arthritis

Chapter Contents

Section 43.1

Questions and Answers about Arthritis and Exercise

Excerpted from "Questions and Answers About Arthritis and Exercise," by the Federal Citizen Information Center (FCIC, www.pueblo.gsa.gov), and the National Institute of Arthritis and Musculoskeletal and Skin Diseases. The date of this document is unknown. Reviewed by David A. Cooke, MD, FACP, July 26, 2009.

This text answers general questions about arthritis and exercise. The amount and form of exercise recommended for each individual will vary depending on which joints are involved, the amount of inflammation, how stable the joints are, and whether a joint replacement procedure has been done. A skilled physician who is knowledgeable about the medical and rehabilitation needs of people with arthritis, working with a physical therapist also familiar with the needs of people with arthritis, can design an exercise plan for each patient.

Should people with arthritis exercise?

Yes. Studies have shown that exercise helps people with arthritis in many ways. Exercise reduces joint pain and stiffness and increases flexibility, muscle strength, and endurance. It also helps with weight reduction and contributes to an improved sense of well-being.

How does exercise fit into a treatment plan for people with arthritis?

Exercise is one part of a comprehensive arthritis treatment plan. Treatment plans also may include rest and relaxation, proper diet, medication, and instruction about proper use of joints and ways to conserve energy (that is, not waste motion) as well as the use of pain relief methods.

What types of exercise are most suitable for someone with arthritis?

Three types of exercise are best for people with arthritis:

- Range-of-motion exercises help maintain normal joint movement and relieve stiffness. This type of exercise helps maintain or increase flexibility.

- Strengthening exercises help keep or increase muscle strength. Strong muscles help support and protect joints affected by arthritis.

- Aerobic or endurance exercises improve cardiovascular fitness, help control weight, and improve overall function. Weight control can be important to people who have arthritis because extra weight puts extra pressure on many joints. Some studies show that aerobic exercise can reduce inflammation in some joints.

How does a person with arthritis start an exercise program?

People with arthritis should discuss exercise options with their doctors. Most doctors recommend exercise for their patients. Many people with arthritis begin with easy, range-of-motion exercises and low-impact aerobics. People with arthritis can participate in a variety of, but not all, sports and exercise programs. The doctor will know which, if any, sports are off-limits.

The doctor may have suggestions about how to get started or may refer the patient to a physical therapist. It is best to find a physical therapist who has experience working with people who have arthritis. The therapist will design an appropriate home exercise program and teach clients about pain-relief methods, proper body mechanics (placement of the body for a given task, such as lifting a heavy box), joint protection, and conserving energy.

How does a person with arthritis get started?

- Discuss exercise plans with your doctor.

- Start with supervision from a physical therapist or qualified athletic trainer.

- Apply heat to sore joints (optional; many people with arthritis start their exercise program this way).

- Stretch and warm up with range-of-motion exercises.

- Start strengthening exercises slowly with small weights (a 1- or 2-pound weight can make a big difference).

- Progress slowly.

- Use cold packs after exercising (optional; many people with arthritis complete their exercise routine this way).

- Add aerobic exercise.

- Consider appropriate recreational exercise (after doing range-of-motion, strengthening, and aerobic exercise). Fewer injuries to arthritic joints occur during recreational exercise if it is preceded by range-of-motion, strengthening, and aerobic exercise that gets your body in the best condition possible.

- Ease off if joints become painful, inflamed, or red and work with your doctor to find the cause and eliminate it.

- Choose the exercise program you enjoy most and make it a habit.

What are some pain relief methods?

There are known methods to stop pain for short periods of time. This temporary relief can make it easier for people who have arthritis to exercise. The doctor or physical therapist can suggest a method that is best for each patient. The following methods have worked for many people.

Moist heat supplied by warm towels, hot packs, a bath, or a shower can be used at home for 15 to 20 minutes three times a day to relieve symptoms. A health professional can use short waves, microwaves, and ultrasound to deliver deep heat to noninflamed joint areas. Deep heat is not recommended for patients with acutely inflamed joints. Deep heat is often used around the shoulder to relax tight tendons prior to stretching exercises.

Cold supplied by a bag of ice or frozen vegetables wrapped in a towel helps to stop pain and reduce swelling when used for 10 to 15 minutes at a time. It is often used for acutely inflamed joints. People who have Raynaud phenomenon should not use this method.

Hydrotherapy (water therapy) can decrease pain and stiffness. Exercising in a large pool may be easier because water takes some weight off painful joints. Community centers, YMCAs, and YWCAs have water exercise classes developed for people with arthritis. Some patients also find relief from the heat and movement provided by a whirlpool.

Mobilization therapies include traction (gentle, steady pulling), massage, and manipulation (using the hands to restore normal movement to stiff joints). When done by a trained professional, these methods can help control pain and increase joint motion and muscle and tendon flexibility.

TENS (transcutaneous electrical nerve stimulation) and biofeedback are two additional methods that may provide some pain relief, but many patients find that they cost too much money and take too much time. TENS machines cost between $80 and $800. The inexpensive units are fine. Patients can wear them during the day and turn them off and on as needed for pain control.

Relaxation therapy also helps reduce pain. Patients can learn to release the tension in their muscles to relieve pain. Physical therapists may be able to teach relaxation techniques. The Arthritis Foundation has a self-help course that includes relaxation therapy and also sells relaxation tapes. Health spas and vacation resorts sometimes have special relaxation courses.

Acupuncture is a traditional Chinese method of pain relief. A medically qualified acupuncturist places needles in certain sites. Researchers believe that the needles stimulate deep sensory nerves that tell the brain to release natural painkillers (endorphins). Acupressure is similar to acupuncture, but pressure is applied to the acupuncture sites instead of using needles.

How often should people with arthritis exercise?

- Range-of-motion exercises can be done daily and should be done at least every other day.

- Strengthening exercises also can be done daily and should be done at least every other day unless you have severe pain or swelling in your joints.

- Endurance exercises should be done for 20 to 30 minutes three times a week unless you have severe pain or swelling in your joints.

What type of strengthening program is best?

This varies depending on personal preference, the type of arthritis involved, and how active the inflammation is. Strengthening one's muscles can help take the burden off painful joints. Strength training can be done with small free weights, exercise machines, isometrics, elastic bands, and resistive water exercises. Correct positioning is critical, because if done incorrectly, strengthening exercises can cause muscle tears, more pain, and more joint swelling.

Are there different exercises for people with different types of arthritis?

There are many types of arthritis. Experienced doctors, physical therapists, and occupational therapists can recommend exercises that are particularly helpful for a specific type of arthritis. Doctors and therapists also know specific exercises for particularly painful joints. There may be exercises that are off-limits for people with a particular type of arthritis or when joints are swollen and inflamed. People with arthritis should discuss their exercise plans with a doctor. Doctors who treat people with arthritis include rheumatologists, general practitioners, family doctors, internists, and rehabilitation specialists (physiatrists).

How much exercise is too much?

Most experts agree that if exercise causes pain that lasts for more than 1 hour, it is too much. People with arthritis should work with their physical therapist or doctor to adjust their exercise program when they notice any of the following signs of too much exercise:

- Unusual or persistent fatigue
- Increased weakness
- Decreased range of motion
- Increased joint swelling
- Continuing pain (pain that lasts more than 1 hour after exercising)

Should someone with rheumatoid arthritis continue to exercise during a general flare? How about during a local joint flare?

It is appropriate to put joints gently through their full range of motion once a day, with periods of rest, during acute systemic flares or local joint flares. Patients can talk to their doctor about how much rest is best during general or joint flares.

Section 43.2

Yoga Promotes Physical Fitness and Joint Health

Excerpted from "Yoga for Health: An Introduction," by the National Center for Complementary and Alternative Medicine (NCCAM, www.nccam .nih.gov), part of the National Institutes of Health, May 2008.

Yoga is a mind-body practice in complementary and alternative medicine (CAM) with origins in ancient Indian philosophy. The various styles of yoga that people use for health purposes typically combine physical postures, breathing techniques, and meditation or relaxation.

Overview

Yoga in its full form combines physical postures, breathing exercises, meditation, and a distinct philosophy. Yoga is intended to increase relaxation and balance the mind, body, and the spirit.

Early written descriptions of yoga are in Sanskrit, the classical language of India. The word "yoga" comes from the Sanskrit word yuj, which means "yoke or union." It is believed that this describes the union between the mind and the body. The first known text, *The Yoga Sutras,* was written more than 2,000 years ago, although yoga may have been practiced as early as 5,000 years ago. Yoga was originally developed as a method of discipline and attitudes to help people reach spiritual enlightenment. The *Sutras* outline eight limbs or foundations of yoga practice that serve as spiritual guidelines:

1. Yama (moral behavior)

2. Niyama (healthy habits)

3. Asana (physical postures)

4. Pranayama (breathing exercises)

5. Pratyahara (sense withdrawal)

6. Dharana (concentration)

7. Dhyana (contemplation)

8. Samadhi (higher consciousness)

The numerous schools of yoga incorporate these eight limbs in varying proportions. Hatha yoga, the most commonly practiced in the United States and Europe, emphasizes two of the eight limbs: postures (asanas) and breathing exercises (pranayama). Some of the major styles of hatha yoga include Ananda, Anusara, Ashtanga, Bikram, Iyengar, Kripalu, Kundalini, and Viniyoga.

Use of Yoga for Health in the United States

According to the 2007 National Health Interview Survey (NHIS), which included a comprehensive survey of CAM use by Americans, yoga is one of the top 10 CAM modalities used. More than 13 million adults had used yoga in the previous year, and between the 2002 and 2007 NHIS, use of yoga among adults increased by 1 percent (or approximately 3 million people). The 2007 survey also found that more than 1.5 million children used yoga in the previous year.

People use yoga for a variety of health conditions including anxiety disorders or stress, asthma, high blood pressure, and depression. People also use yoga as part of a general health regimen—to achieve physical fitness and to relax.

The Status of Yoga Research

Research suggests that yoga might provide benefits in the following ways:

- Improve mood and sense of well-being
- Counteract stress
- Reduce heart rate and blood pressure
- Increase lung capacity
- Improve muscle relaxation and body composition
- Help with conditions such as anxiety, depression, and insomnia
- Improve overall physical fitness, strength, and flexibility
- Positively affect levels of certain brain or blood chemicals

More well-designed studies are needed before definitive conclusions can be drawn about yoga's use for specific health conditions.

Side Effects and Risks

Yoga is generally considered to be safe in healthy people when practiced appropriately. Studies have found it to be well tolerated, with few side effects.

People with certain medical conditions should not use some yoga practices. For example, people with disk disease of the spine, extremely high or low blood pressure, glaucoma, retinal detachment, fragile or atherosclerotic arteries, a risk of blood clots, ear problems, severe osteoporosis, or cervical spondylitis should avoid some inverted poses.

Although yoga during pregnancy is safe if practiced under expert guidance, pregnant women should avoid certain poses that may be problematic.

If You Are Thinking about Yoga

- Do not use yoga as a replacement for conventional care or to postpone seeing a doctor about a medical problem.

- If you have a medical condition, consult with your health care provider before starting yoga.

- Ask about the physical demands of the type of yoga in which you are interested, as well as the training and experience of the yoga teacher you are considering.

- Look for published research studies on yoga for the health condition you are interested in.

- Tell your health care providers about any complementary and alternative practices you use. Give them a full picture of what you do to manage your health. This will help ensure coordinated and safe care.

Section 43.3

Water Aerobics Can Benefit People with Arthritis

Water isn't just for drinking anymore. It's also a great place for working out. If you have arthritis, exercising in a well-heated pool has particular advantages over a health club floor. For one thing, the buoyancy of the water supports your body and reduces the stress on your weight-bearing joints.

"In fact, when you're standing in shoulder-high water, only about 10% of your body weight is acting on your joints, so exercise doesn't hurt as much," says Doreen Stiskal, MS, PT, a physical therapist at Seton Hall University who recently helped revise the Arthritis Foundation's popular water exercise program.

Since water supports your joints, it makes it easier to move freely, improving your range of motion. At the same time, water offers at least 12 times more resistance than air, strengthening your muscles. The pressure water exerts on your legs also can aid circulation, something like wearing support hose. In addition, the soothing sensation of warm water is a great stress reliever. You may be able to do things in the water you can't on land.

"I had one couple who hadn't danced in years, but they were able to dance in the water," says Donna Adler, a water exercise instructor and trainer for the Arthritis Foundation in Phoenix.

Water Workouts

Aerobic exercise refers to any activity that raises your heart rate and breathing and keeps them elevated for an extended period of time. To get this effect, you need to use the large muscles of your arms and legs in rhythmic, continuous motions. One way to do this is with water aerobics. Unlike dry-land aerobics, exercises in water are easier on your joints. And unlike lap swimming, you don't have to be able to swim a stroke to do water aerobics.

In shallow-water aerobics, you stand in waist to chest-deep water. Typical moves include many that are familiar to dry-land exercisers, such as marching, stretching, circling your arms, bending your knees, and swinging your legs. A deep-water workout, on the other hand, is done in water over your head. A flotation device is worn to keep your head above water and your body upright. Jumping jacks and moving your legs as if you were jogging, cycling, or cross-country skiing are common with deep water exercises. These can be more difficult than shallow-water ones, since they put more demands on both your cardiovascular system and your balance.

Hydro Power

Water exercise programs have been making a splash around the country. Here are some things to keep in mind when choosing a water aerobics class:

- **Water temperature:** Warm water relaxes the muscles and eases joint stiffness. For an arthritis-oriented class, "a water temperature of 84 degrees Fahrenheit to 88 degrees Fahrenheit is recommended, with an absolute minimum of 83 degrees Fahrenheit," says Adler.

- **Intensity:** Exercising in the water is so much easier, you may be tempted to overdo. "Start off slowly," says Stiskal. "If you're new to a class, don't try to compete with the veterans. Respect your limitations."

- **Instructor:** Look for a qualified instructor who is knowledgeable about arthritis. The Arthritis Foundation Aquatic Program, taught at YMCAs and community pools around the country, is a good place to start.

- **Classmates:** One of the best things about water aerobics is you can socialize as you exercise. Take a friend, or make new ones in your class. You may have so much fun, working out will start to seem like playing.

Chapter 44

Nutrition and Arthritis

Chapter Contents

Section 44.1

Eating Right with Arthritis

"Eating Right with Arthritis: Arthritis Nutrition FAQs," © 2009 Hospital for Special Surgery (www.hss.edu). Reprinted with permission. Editor's Note: Questions are answered by Laura Allman, RD, Nutritionist, Food and Nutrition Services Department, Hospital for Special Surgery.

How can a proper diet be helpful for my arthritis?

Researchers continue to look at the role diet plays in arthritis. While evidence is accumulating, anyone with arthritis can benefit from a diet that provides adequate macronutrients and micronutrients to prevent deficiencies. Some examples of these nutrients include vitamins, minerals, proteins, and carbohydrates. Doctors recommend a balanced diet with variety and moderation.

Is weight management important in helping with my arthritis?

Yes, weight management can help lower cholesterol and blood pressure. Having a healthy weight can also improve mobility, and contribute to overall well-being and health.

What are corticosteroids and how might they affect my diet?

Corticosteroids are medications used to control inflammation and pain associated with arthritis. Corticosteroids are some of the oldest, most effective and fastest-working drugs for many forms of arthritis. When used properly and sparingly, corticosteroids have the power to spare joints, eyes, and internal organs from damaging inflammation.

Unfortunately, they also have the potential to do great harm by causing increased risk of diabetes and osteoporosis. You may experience sodium retention, loss of potassium, and weight gain. Corticosteroids also can increase your appetite. If you are taking corticosteroids, it is reasonable to avoid adding extra salt to your food. Also, watch your calorie intake carefully to avoid weight gain. It's especially important for women on corticosteroids to take calcium and vitamin D supplements.

One should consume the recommended 5–7 servings of fruits and vegetables daily to help counteract the symptoms (sodium retention/ potassium loss), and to provide essential potassium and help balance any sodium retention. If a patient cannot manage their own weight gain, they can see a nutritionist for a consult and personalized meal plan.

Are sugar substitutes safe to use?

Yes.

Which one is best to use?

I like using Splenda® because it measures exactly like sugar when baking.

Are eggs okay to eat?

Eggs are a great source of protein, but also contain cholesterol and saturated fat in the yolk.

What is an appropriate amount to eat each week?

If you are watching the cholesterol in your diet, you should have fewer than four whole eggs a week.

What about egg substitutes?

Egg whites and egg substitutes do not have the yolk, so they are fat and cholesterol free.

Do nightshade vegetables contribute to arthritis?

There has been no recent data or research to show that nightshade vegetables contribute to arthritis. However, if eliminating these foods from your diet improves your symptoms, then you can choose to do so. Nightshade vegetables include white potatoes, peppers, tomatoes, and eggplant.

Does chocolate influence arthritis?

I have not seen research that shows a correlation between chocolate and arthritis. But if you find that it worsens your symptoms, try eliminating it and see if your body responds.

What is the difference between an omega-3 fatty acid and an omega-6 fatty acid?

Omega-3 and Omega-6 belong to a family of fats called essential fatty acids (EFAs). These EFAs are found in polyunsaturated fats. Two of the Omega-3 fatty acids are called eicosapentaenoic acid (EPA) and docosahexanoic (DHA). EPA and DHA are found primarily in oily cold-water fish such as tuna, salmon, and mackerel. The third omega-3 fatty acid is called alpha-linolenic acid (ALA), which is found in dark leafy vegetables, flaxseed oils, and certain vegetable oils.

Studies have shown that having omega-3 acids in your diet may reduce the severity of inflammation. Omega-6 fatty acids convert in the body producing gamma linoleic acid (GLA). Omega-6 fatty acids are found in meats, poultry, and eggs, which may contribute to inflammation.

How much fish is okay to eat without having to worry about consuming too much mercury?

Mercury is not found in all fish, and it is safe to consume fish low in mercury on a daily basis. If you eat a high mercury fish, you will not feel sick immediately. However, eating fish with high amounts of mercury regularly causes it [mercury] to build up in your blood over time.

Which kinds of fish are high in mercury?

The source for this data is the National Resources Defense Council, which compiles their information from the Food and Drug Administration and the Environmental Protection Agency:

Highest mercury (avoid when possible):

- King mackerel
- Orange roughy
- Shark
- Swordfish
- Tilefish
- Tuna (bigeye, ahi)

High mercury (limit to three or fewer servings per month):

- Bluefish
- Grouper
- Spanish mackerel
- Sea bass (Chilean)
- Tuna (canned albacore)
- Tuna (yellowfin)

Moderate mercury (limit to six servings per month):

- Bass (striped, black)
- Carp
- Cod (Alaskan)
- Croaker (White Pacific)
- Halibut (Atlantic and Pacific)
- Jacksmelt
- Lobster
- Mahi mahi
- Monkfish
- Perch
- Sablefish
- Skate
- Snapper
- Tuna (chunk light canned)
- Tuna (skipjack)
- Weakfish (sea trout)

Least mercury (enjoy these fish):

- Anchovies
- Butterfish
- Catfish
- Clam
- Crab
- Crayfish
- Crawfish
- Flounder
- Haddock
- Hake
- Herring
- Mackerel (North Atlantic)
- Mullet
- Oyster
- Pollack
- Salmon (fresh and canned)
- Sardine
- Scallop
- Sole
- Tilapia
- Squid
- Trout (freshwater)
- Whitefish
- Whiting

Section 44.2

Psoriasis, Psoriatic Arthritis, and Gluten Intolerance: Is There a Connection?

"A Connection between Psoriasis and Celiac Disease Suspected for Some," © 2004 National Psoriasis Foundation (www.psoriasis.org). Reprinted with permission. The text that follows this document under the heading "*Health Reference Series* Medical Advisor's Notes and Updates" was provided to Omnigraphics, Inc. by David A. Cooke, MD, FACP, July 5, 2009. Dr. Cooke is not affiliated with the National Psoriasis Foundation.

Have you ever wondered if something in your diet might be making your psoriasis worse? Many people have. There have been nearly as many theories about diet and psoriasis over the years as there have been people with psoriasis. But scientists have never convincingly demonstrated the effect of any particular diet on the disease. Now however, a growing body of research is beginning to establish that for a very small percentage of people with psoriasis, there may be an important connection between what goes in their mouth and what happens on their skin.

That connection could have everything to do with last night's heaping bowl of pasta and this morning's cereal, the post-breakfast donut at the office and your lunchtime sandwich. All of these meals contain gluten, which is the insoluble component of grains such as wheat, barley, and rye.

Some researchers believe that a very small subgroup of people with psoriasis may also have gluten-sensitive enteropathy, also known as gluten intolerance or celiac disease. People who have celiac disease may have mild to severe damage to the lining of the small intestine, damage that can cause chronic diarrhea, food absorption problems, and nutritional and vitamin deficiencies. According to the most recent studies, celiac disease may affect as many as 2 million Americans. Individuals with celiac disease may experience abdominal cramping and pain, bone and joint pain, bloating, flatulence, and fatigue, among other symptoms.

No More Pasta?

Researchers who have studied psoriasis and gluten intolerance believe that people with both diseases might significantly improve their psoriasis by using the only available treatment for celiac disease—a strict, limiting diet called the Gluten-Free Diet (GFD). This diet requires long-term, complete avoidance of gluten, which requires a radical change in the eating habits of most Americans.

Avoiding gluten while on the GFD means giving up common foods such as barley, beer, cereals, anything made with wheat flour, and pasta. Such a diet is definitely a complete lifestyle change, and results may appear only after weeks or months of strict adherence to the diet. Gerald Krueger, MD, professor of dermatology at the University of Utah, says no one should be misled about the GFD. "It is a very harsh diet. People with severe celiac disease will tell you it is very difficult."

Psoriasis and Gluten Research

A 1993 study by Swedish scientists led by Gerd Michaelsson, MD, PhD, professor emeritus at Uppsala University in Uppsala, Sweden (see text that follows for interview with Dr. Michaelsson), found that 16 percent of patients with psoriasis had increased antibodies to gliadin (the proteins in gluten to which some people have a reaction). Increased levels of these antibodies, called AGA, are one marker of celiac disease.

The same researchers performed another study, published in the *British Journal of Dermatology* in 2000, which evaluated the effect of a gluten-free diet in 33 people with psoriasis who were AGA-positive compared to six people with psoriasis who were AGA-negative. Participants followed the GFD for three months, followed by three months on their ordinary diet. Thirty of the 33 AGA-positive patients improved on the GFD, while none of the six AGA-negative patients improved on the diet. When the AGA-positive patients went back to their ordinary eating habits, psoriasis got worse for 18 of the 30 who had originally improved.

According to Dr. Krueger, it is encouraging to note from these small trials that many of the psoriasis patients who had tested positive for AGA did improve on the GFD. "It does look like there is an increased frequency of celiac disease among people with psoriasis," says Dr. Krueger. "I do think there could be something there, given that both psoriasis and celiac disease appear to be Th-1 type immune-mediated diseases." Both psoriasis and celiac disease are believed to be diseases driven by hyperactive, or inappropriately activated, T cells—in the skin for psoriasis, and in the gut for people with celiac disease. This is the intriguing connection that has scientists looking at the two diseases for other links in both cause and treatment.

Connection Still in Doubt

However, simple math dictates that it would be surprising if there weren't some people with both diseases. "Indeed," Dr. Krueger says, "there is a certain small percentage of people in the general population with celiac disease, and a certain small percentage of people in the general population with psoriasis, so one should not be surprised to find a significant number of people who have both. The challenge is to determine if the connection is real. The difficulty in determining a final truth is one of numbers—numbers of patients and numbers of dollars. It can be very difficult for researchers to gather enough patients to study a rare subgroup of patients in a disease that only affects about 2 percent of the population in the first place. And it is very, very expensive."

Meanwhile, it is very important to discuss celiac disease and the GFD with your doctor before changing your diet or your treatments. Symptoms may or may not be present for people with both diseases. Dr. Michaelsson believes that in fact many people with psoriasis who are AGA-positive and who could potentially be helped by the GFD may have no celiac symptoms, but instead may have what she calls "silent celiac disease."

"If you believe that gluten intolerance may be an issue for you, particularly if you have uncontrolled moderate to severe psoriasis or palmoplantar pustulosis, Dr. Krueger recommends that you discuss the situation thoroughly with your doctor. Talk about whether a screening for the markers of celiac disease (including anti-gliadin, anti-endomysial antibodies, and anti-tissue transglutaminase) might be recommended. These markers are present in the blood of a person with celiac disease who has been exposed to gluten, but the markers disappear when gluten is removed from the diet.

It is important to consult with a doctor and get the appropriate tests before starting a GFD, because following the GFD before having the proper blood tests can jeopardize the tests' accuracy. Many doctors will want to follow positive blood tests with a biopsy of the intestine to confirm celiac disease. For psoriasis patients who have been diagnosed with celiac disease, Dr. Krueger agrees with Dr. Michaelsson's recommendation that it would be worthwhile to try a GFD.

Three organizations that may also be able to provide information are:

- Celiac Sprue Association/USA, Inc.: www.csaceliacs.org;
- Gluten Intolerance Group of North America: www.gluten.net;

- University of Maryland Center for Celiac Research: www.celiaccenter.org.

Psoriasis and Gluten Intolerance: An Interview with Dr. Gerd Michaelsson

What are the key pieces of evidence that link celiac disease (or gluten intolerance) and psoriasis?

First—most patients with psoriasis are not gluten intolerant. However, there is a subgroup with silent celiac disease/gluten intolerance and it is important to identify these patients, as there is a chance to considerably improve the skin lesions on the gluten-free diet (GFD). In some patients there may be a total or nearly total clearance on the diet. When gluten is reintroduced there is a flare up of the psoriasis. The effect of the diet also seems to be very good in the type of psoriasis called palmoplantar pustulosis (PPP)—again with recurrence when gluten is reintroduced. Otherwise, in PPP the main focus is on the role of smoking, as 95% of PPP patients are smokers at the onset of their PPP. In looking at patients with psoriatic arthritis and with evidence of gluten intolerance, there is an improvement both of the skin lesions and the arthritis. But the effect on the arthritis is less impressive than that on the skin, which may indicate that there may be additional causative factors involved in the arthritis.

In your opinion, what percentage of people with psoriasis and/or psoriatic arthritis are affected by the link?

About 16% of patients with psoriasis vulgaris have serum antibodies against gliadin, which is a fraction of gluten. It is interesting that we have found no patients with psoriasis vulgaris, without arthritis, who have a previously diagnosed celiac disease (but also see following text concerning psoriatic arthritis). Probably patients with celiac disease adhering to a strict GFD do not develop psoriasis or the psoriasis clears on the diet and these patients do not need to see a dermatologist. Not all psoriasis patients with antibodies to gliadin have classical celiac disease, which is characterized by a damage of the villi in the intestinal mucosa and pronounced inflammation. Many of the patients have only mild changes in the intestine with very discrete inflammation. Still, they can improve on GFD. However, the most dramatic improvement of the psoriasis takes place in those with the most pronounced changes in the intestinal mucosa. Some of these patients also have serum antibodies against the enzyme tissue trans-glutaminase. Among patients with arthritis the percentage with antibodies to gliadin is the same as in those with psoriasis vulgaris but in addition we found that 4% had previously diagnosed celiac disease which again indicates that the arthritis does not respond in the same way to GFD as the skin. The highest percentage of serum antibodies to gliadin (20%) is found in patients with PPP. Our preliminary data indicate a very good response to the GFD in these patients.

What do you think is the most likely explanation for the connection between the two diseases? Is it likely to be genetic, or caused by other factors (i.e., immune-mediated, T-cell activation, etc.)?

Psoriasis patients with gluten intolerance may belong to a genetic subgroup with increased risk for psoriasis, celiac disease/gluten intolerance, and thyroid disease—the latter association is particularly common in women with PPP. Possibly there may be one or several autoantigens which are relevant for the inflammation in psoriasis. One of these possible autoantigens may be the enzyme tissue transglutaminase which is expressed in proliferating small blood vessels but also involved in the processing of gluten. The expression of this enzyme is increased in the blood vessels of psoriatic lesions and this expression is decreased when the patients are on GFD. At the same time there is a decrease in the number of proliferating cells in the skin lesions. Further studies are needed to clarify this issue.

Would you recommend patients with psoriasis or psoriatic arthritis look for any particular symptoms, or take any particular actions?

In our patients with previously unrecognized gluten intolerance, we found that none of them had an increased history of gastrointestinal complaints versus those who were not gluten intolerant. We recommend that patients with moderate to severe psoriasis or palmoplantar pustulosis be screened for the presence of serum antibodies against gliadin and tissue transglutaminase and for the level of serum IgA [immunoglobulin A] (if serum IgA is low the antibody screening may give false negative results). It should also be observed that in 10% of patients found to have celiac disease there are no antibodies in the serum. Other markers which may indicate the presence of celiac disease are low levels of iron, zinc, and folic acid, but in patients with only mild intestinal changes these parameters are usually normal. The costs of the screening are low and the results may be very rewarding. Thus, our first observed patients with psoriasis and silent celiac disease has been free from psoriasis for 25 years.

Health Reference Series *Medical Advisor's Notes and Updates*

The debate about whether there actually is a relationship between psoriasis and celiac disease continues unabated. While some studies such as those cited above found improvements in some psoriasis on gluten-free diets, other trials have failed to identify a relationship between psoriasis and celiac disease. For example, a 2007 study performed at the University of Michigan found no difference in the rates of positive antibody markers for celiac disease among patients with psoriasis, psoriatic arthritis, and healthy individuals. This study also found relatively high rates of these antibodies among apparently healthy individuals, so the significance of antibody results in psoriasis patients remains uncertain. Further studies are needed.

Chapter 45

Herbs, Dietary Supplements, and Arthritis

Chapter Contents

Section 45.1

Glucosamine and Chondroitin Fare No Better Than Placebo in Slowing Arthritis Damage

Excerpted from "Dietary Supplements Glucosamine and/or Chondroitin Fare No Better than Placebo in Slowing Structural Damage of Knee Osteoarthritis," by the National Institutes of Health, September 29, 2008.

The dietary supplements glucosamine and chondroitin sulfate, together or alone, appeared to fare no better than placebo in slowing loss of cartilage in osteoarthritis of the knee, researchers from the Glucosamine/chondroitin Arthritis Intervention Trial (GAIT) team report in the October 2008 issue of *Arthritis & Rheumatism*.[1] Interpreting the study results is complicated, however, because participants taking placebo had a smaller loss of cartilage, or joint space width, than predicted. Loss of cartilage, the slippery material that cushions the joints, is a hallmark of osteoarthritis and its loss is typically measured as a reduction in joint space width—the distance between the ends of bones in a joint as seen on an x-ray.

"While these results are of interest, we cannot draw definitive conclusions about the utility of glucosamine or chondroitin in reducing joint space width loss, in part because the placebo group fared better than anticipated based on prior research results," said Josephine P. Briggs, MD, director of the National Center for Complementary and Alternative Medicine, at the National Institutes of Health (NIH), one of the study's funders. "The results of the study provide interesting insights for future research."

The NIH-supported study was led by University of Utah School of Medicine's Allen D. Sawitzke, MD, and Daniel O. Clegg, MD. This study was an ancillary, or additional, trial conducted by the GAIT team with a subset of participants from the original GAIT study. The original GAIT study sought to determine whether these dietary supplements could treat the pain of knee osteoarthritis and found that overall the combination of glucosamine plus chondroitin sulfate did not provide significant relief from osteoarthritis pain among all participants. However, a smaller subgroup of study participants with moderate-to-severe pain showed significant relief with the combined supplements. These results were reported in 2006.[2]

To study whether the dietary supplements could diminish the structural damage of osteoarthritis, interested GAIT patients were offered the opportunity to continue their original study treatment in the ancillary trial for an additional 18 months, for a total of two years. The randomly assigned study treatments were 500 milligrams glucosamine hydrochloride three times daily, sodium chondroitin sulfate 400 milligrams three times daily, the combination of glucosamine plus chondroitin sulfate, placebo, or celecoxib 200 milligrams daily. The research team enrolled 572 GAIT participants for the ancillary study. Participants entering the ancillary study had x-ray evidence of moderate (grade 2) or severe (grade 3) knee osteoarthritis in one or both knees using a scale that measures osteoarthritis severity called the Kellgren-Lawrence scale. At the end of the ancillary study, the team had gathered data on 581 knees.

"At two years, no treatment showed what we determined to be a clinically important reduction in joint space width loss," said Dr. Sawitzke, associate professor of medicine and lead investigator for the ancillary study. "While we found a trend toward improvement among those with milder, Kellgren-Lawrence grade 2 osteoarthritis of the knee in those taking glucosamine alone, we were not able to draw any definitive conclusions."

The joint space width in the knee, or knees, of the patients was measured with a specific x-ray protocol on entering the ancillary study and at one and two years to determine any loss in joint width. The x-ray technique required images of the knees be taken in a standardized, weight-bearing position.

The GAIT researchers expected patients in the placebo group to have a joint space width loss of approximately 0.4 millimeters over two years, based on results of previously published large studies. The study team hypothesized that a loss of 0.2 millimeters or less would show a slowed rate of cartilage loss. The final results, adjusted for baseline joint space width, gender, and other factors, showed the following:

- Glucosamine alone group had the least average joint space width loss of 0.013 millimeters.

- Chondroitin alone group had an average loss of 0.107 millimeters.

- Glucosamine plus chondroitin group had an average loss of 0.194 millimeters.

- Celecoxib group had an average loss of 0.111 millimeters.
- Placebo group had an average loss of 0.166 millimeters.

In addition to measuring average loss of joint space width, the study also measured the percentage of participants with progression (worsening) of their osteoarthritis—defined as a joint space width loss of more than 0.48 millimeters over the two years. Overall, those with grade 2 (moderate) knee osteoarthritis were least likely to have progression of osteoarthritis compared to those with more severe disease. Approximately 24 percent of participants taking the combination of glucosamine plus chondroitin sulfate showed disease progression, which was similar to placebo, but greater than either glucosamine or chondroitin sulfate alone. The researchers theorize that this may reflect interference in absorption of the two supplements when taken together.

"Research continues to reveal that osteoarthritis, the most common form of arthritis, appears to be the result of an array of factors including age, gender, genetics, obesity, and joint injuries," said Stephen I. Katz, M.D., director of the National Institute of Arthritis and Musculoskeletal and Skin Diseases, co-funder of the study. "Because osteoarthritis affects an estimated 27 million Americans, we are seeking ways to not only treat pain, but also address the structural effects of the condition."

The researchers note that the study has limitations, such as a greater-than-expected variability in measurement of joint space width loss and a less-than-expected loss of joint space width in the placebo group. However, the team also notes that not only was the study designed to investigate whether glucosamine and chondroitin sulfate, either together or alone, may have an effect on structural damage, it was also designed to test the method of measuring joint space width loss and learning more about the natural progression of osteoarthritis.

"Despite the ancillary study's limitations, it has provided us with new insights on osteoarthritis progression, the techniques to use to more reliably measure loss of joint space width, the possible effects of these dietary supplements, and the characteristics of osteoarthritis patients that may best respond, all of which will assist investigators in future studies," said Dr. Clegg, professor of medicine and chief of rheumatology and principal investigator for GAIT.

References

1. Sawitzke AD, Shi H, Finco MF, et al. The Effect of Glucosamine and/or Chondroitin Sulfate on the Progression of

Knee Osteoarthritis: A Report from the Glucosamine/Chondroitin Arthritis Intervention Trial. *Arthritis & Rheumatism*, 2008; 58(10):3183–3191.

2. Clegg D, Reda DJ, Harris CL, et al. Glucosamine, Chondroitin Sulfate, and the Two in Combination for Painful Knee Osteoarthritis. *New England Journal of Medicine*, 2006;354:795–808.

Note: On September 30, 2008, at the request of the institute, the text in the last sentence in the ninth paragraph was changed to "an estimated 27 million" as it appears above, from "nearly 21," as originally posted.

Section 45.2

Effectiveness of Glucosamine and Chondroitin Depends on Level of Arthritis Pain

From "Efficacy of Glucosamine and Chondroitin Sulfate May Depend on Level of Osteoarthritis Pain," by the National Center for Complementary and Alternative Medicine (NCCAM, www.nccam.nih.gov), February 22, 2006.

In a study published in the *New England Journal of Medicine*, the popular dietary supplement combination of glucosamine plus chondroitin sulfate did not provide significant relief from osteoarthritis pain among all participants.

However, a smaller subgroup of study participants with moderate-to-severe pain showed significant relief with the combined supplements. This research was funded by the National Center for Complementary and Alternative Medicine (NCCAM) and the National Institute of Arthritis and Musculoskeletal and Skin Diseases (NIAMS), components of the National Institutes of Health (NIH). Researchers led by rheumatologist Daniel O. Clegg, MD, of the University of Utah, School of Medicine, Salt Lake City, conducted the 4-year study known as the Glucosamine/chondroitin Arthritis Intervention Trial (GAIT) at 16 sites across the United States.

"GAIT is another example of NIH's commitment to exploring the potential of complementary and alternative medicine to prevent and treat disease in a manner that is fair, unbiased, and scientifically rigorous," said Elias A. Zerhouni, MD, NIH Director.

GAIT enrolled nearly 1,600 participants with documented osteoarthritis of the knee. Participants were randomly assigned to receive one of five treatments daily for 24 weeks: glucosamine alone (1500 mg), chondroitin sulfate alone (1200 mg), glucosamine and chondroitin sulfate combined (same doses), a placebo, or celecoxib (200 mg). Celecoxib is an FDA-approved drug for the management of osteoarthritis pain and served as a positive control for the study. (A positive control is a treatment that investigators expect participants to respond to in a predictable way; it helps validate study results.) A positive response to treatment was defined as a 20 percent or greater reduction in pain at week 24 compared to the start of the study.

The researchers found that participants taking celecoxib experienced statistically significant pain relief, as expected, versus placebo— about 70 percent of those taking celecoxib versus 60 percent taking placebo had a 20 percent or greater pain reduction. For all participants, there were no significant differences between the other treatments tested and placebo.

However, for participants in the moderate-to-severe pain subgroup, glucosamine combined with chondroitin sulfate provided statistically significant pain relief compared to placebo—about 79 percent in this group had a 20 percent or greater pain reduction compared to 54 percent for placebo. In the subgroup of participants with mild pain, glucosamine and chondroitin sulfate together or alone did not provide statistically significant relief compared to placebo.

"This rigorous, large-scale study showed that the combination of glucosamine and chondroitin sulfate appeared to help people with moderate-to-severe pain from knee osteoarthritis, but not those with mild pain," said Stephen E. Straus, MD, NCCAM Director. "It is important to study dietary supplements with well-designed research in order to find out what works and what does not."

"Because of the small size of the moderate-to-severe pain subgroup, the findings in this group for glucosamine plus chondroitin sulfate should be considered preliminary and need to be confirmed in a study designed for this purpose," said Dr. Clegg, Professor of Medicine and Chief of Rheumatology at the University of Utah, School of Medicine.

On entering the study, a participant's level of pain was assessed as either mild or moderate to severe using standard pain assessment tools and scales, such as the Western Ontario and McMaster Universities

Osteoarthritis Index (WOMAC). Of the 1,583 study participants, 78 percent were in the mild pain subgroup and the other 22 percent were in the moderate-to-severe pain subgroup. Level of pain was evaluated at weeks 4, 8, 16, and 24 using the WOMAC scale and other tools. In addition to taking their daily study treatment, participants could take up to 4000 mg of acetaminophen daily for pain, except for the 24 hours before they were assessed by study staff. The use of acetaminophen, however, was low, overall averaging fewer than two 500 mg tablets per day. Participants could not take other non-steroidal anti-inflammatory medicines or narcotic (opioid-based) pain relievers during the study.

"More than 20 million Americans have osteoarthritis, making it a frequent cause of physical disability among adults," said Stephen I. Katz, M.D., Ph.D., NIAMS Director. "We are excited to support studies looking at new treatment options that could improve the symptoms and quality of life of people with osteoarthritis."

GAIT was conducted under an Investigational New Drug application filed with the U.S. Food and Drug Administration. Thus, all of the products used in the study were subject to the FDA's pharmaceutical regulations and evaluated and manufactured by an FDA-licensed clinical research pharmacy center. The glucosamine and chondroitin sulfate used were tested for purity, potency, quality, and consistency among batches. Products were retested for stability throughout the study. The dosages selected were based on the prevailing doses in the scientific literature. Few side effects from any of the treatments were reported. Those reported were generally mild, such as upset stomach, and distributed evenly across the treatment groups.

"The GAIT team's goal was to assess whether glucosamine and chondroitin sulfate, which we saw our osteoarthritis patients using, provided pain relief," said Dr. Clegg. "I urge people with osteoarthritis to follow a comprehensive plan for managing their arthritis pain—eat right, exercise, lose excess weight, and talk to your physician about appropriate treatment options."

Source: Clegg D, et al. Glucosamine, Chondroitin Sulfate, and the Two in Combination for Painful Knee Osteoarthritis. *New England Journal of Medicine,* 2006;354:795–808.

Section 45.3

Flaxseed and Flaxseed Oil

Excerpted from "Flaxseed and Flaxseed Oil," by the National Center for Complementary and Alternative Medicine (NCCAM, www.nccam.nih.gov), part of the National Institutes of Health, April 2008.

Flaxseed is the seed of the flax plant, which is believed to have originated in Egypt. It grows throughout Canada and the northwestern United States. Flaxseed oil comes from flaxseeds.

What It Is Used For

- Flaxseed is most commonly used as a laxative.

- Flaxseed is also used for hot flashes and breast pain.

- Flaxseed oil is used for different conditions than flaxseed, including arthritis.

- Both flaxseed and flaxseed oil have been used for high cholesterol levels and in an effort to prevent cancer.

How It Is Used

Whole or crushed flaxseed can be mixed with water or juice and taken by mouth. Flaxseed is also available in powder form. Flaxseed oil is available in liquid and capsule form. Flaxseed contains lignans (phytoestrogens, or plant estrogens), while flaxseed oil preparations lack lignans.

What the Science Says

- Flaxseed contains soluble fiber, like that found in oat bran, and is an effective laxative.

- Studies of flaxseed preparations to lower cholesterol levels report mixed results.

- Some studies suggest that alpha-linolenic acid (a substance found in flaxseed and flaxseed oil) may benefit people with heart disease. But not enough reliable data are available to determine whether flaxseed is effective for heart conditions.

- Study results are mixed on whether flaxseed decreases hot flashes.

- Recent studies have looked at the effects of flaxseed on high cholesterol levels, as well as its possible role in preventing conditions such as heart disease and osteoporosis.

Side Effects and Cautions

- Flaxseed and flaxseed oil supplements seem to be well tolerated. Few side effects have been reported.

- Flaxseed, like any supplemental fiber source, should be taken with plenty of water; otherwise, it could worsen constipation or, in rare cases, even cause intestinal blockage.

- The fiber in flaxseed may lower the body's ability to absorb medications that are taken by mouth. Flaxseed should not be taken at the same time as any conventional oral medications or other dietary supplements.

- Tell your health care providers about any complementary and alternative practices you use. Give them a full picture of what you do to manage your health. This will help ensure coordinated and safe care.

Section 45.4

Omega-3 Fatty Acids

Excerpted from "Effects of Omega-3 Fatty Acids on Lipids and Glycemic Control in Type II Diabetes and the Metabolic Syndrome and on Inflammatory Bowel Disease, Rheumatoid Arthritis, Renal Disease, Systemic Lupus Erythematosus, and Osteoporosis." MacLean CH, Mojica WA, Morton SC, et al. Summary, Evidence Report/Technology Assessment: Number 89. AHRQ Publication Number 04-E012-1, March 2004. Agency for Healthcare Research and Quality, Rockville, MD, www.ahrq.gov. Reviewed by David A. Cooke, MD, FACP, July 26, 2009.

Over the past 40 years, an increasing number of physiological functions have been attributed to omega-3 fatty acids, including movement of calcium and other substances into and out of cells, relaxation and contraction of muscles, inhibition and promotion of clotting, regulation of secretion of substances that include digestive enzymes and hormones, control of fertility, cell division, and growth. In addition, omega-3 fatty acids may play an important role in brain development and function. Some evidence has suggested that omega-3 fatty acids in the diet may protect against heart attack and stroke, as well as certain inflammatory diseases like arthritis, lupus, and asthma. The major dietary sources of omega-3 fatty acids in the U.S. population are fish, fish oil, vegetable oils (principally canola and soybean), walnuts, wheat germ, and some dietary supplements.

Rheumatoid Arthritis

Among nine studies reporting outcomes in patients with rheumatoid arthritis, omega-3 fatty acids had no effect on patient report of pain, swollen joint count, erythrocyte sedimentation rate (ESR), and patient's global assessment by meta-analysis. A previously performed meta-analysis reached the same conclusions for swollen joint count, ESR, and patient's global assessment. That meta-analysis found a statistically significant improvement in tender joint count compared to placebo. The one study that assessed the effect on joint damage found no effect. In a qualitative analysis of seven studies that assessed the effect of omega-3 fatty acids on anti-inflammatory drug or corticosteroid requirement, six demonstrated reduced requirement for these drugs. No studies assessed the effect on requirements for disease modifying anti-rheumatic drugs. None of the studies used a composite score that incorporates both subjective and objective measures of disease activity, such as the American College of Rheumatology response criteria.

Systemic Lupus Erythematosus

Among three studies that assessed the effects of omega-3 fatty acids in SLE, variable effects on clinical activity were reported. No studies were identified that assessed effect on damage or patient perception of disease. Omega-3 fatty acids had no effect on corticosteroid requirements in one study. No studies were identified that assessed the effects of omega-3 fatty acids on requirements for other immunosuppressive drugs for SLE. None of the studies used a measure of disease activity that incorporates both subjective and objective measures of disease activity.

Section 45.5

Thunder God Vine

Excerpted from "Thunder God Vine," by the National Institute of Complementary and Alternative Medicine (NCCAM, www.nccam.nih.gov), part of the National Institutes of Health, June 2008.

Introduction

Thunder god vine is a perennial vine native to China, Japan, and Korea. It has been used in China for health purposes for more than 400 years. Common names include thunder god vine and lei gong teng; Latin names include *Tripterygium wilfordii.*

What It Is Used For

Thunder god vine has been used in traditional Chinese medicine for conditions involving inflammation or overactivity of the immune system.

Orally, thunder god vine is taken for excessive menstrual periods or autoimmune diseases, including rheumatoid arthritis, multiple sclerosis, and lupus.

Thunder god vine preparations are also applied to the skin for rheumatoid arthritis.

How It Is Used

Extracts are prepared from the skinned root of thunder god vine.

What the Science Says

Laboratory findings suggest that thunder god vine may fight inflammation, suppress the immune system, and have anti-cancer effects.

Although early evidence is promising, there have been few high-quality studies of thunder god vine in people. Results from a small study funded by the National Institute of Arthritis and Musculoskeletal and Skin Diseases (NIAMS) suggest that an oral extract of the herb may improve rheumatoid arthritis symptoms in some patients. A larger NIAMS-funded study is comparing thunder god vine with a conventional medicine for rheumatoid arthritis.

A small study on thunder god vine applied to the skin also found benefits for rheumatoid arthritis symptoms.

There is not enough scientific evidence to assess thunder god vine's use for any other health conditions.

Side Effects and Cautions

Thunder god vine can cause severe side effects and can be poisonous if it is not carefully extracted from the skinned root. Other parts of the plant—including the leaves, flowers, and skin of the root—are highly poisonous and can cause death.

The extract of thunder god vine used in the NIAMS study was well tolerated. However, thunder god vine can cause diarrhea, upset stomach, hair loss, headache, menstrual changes, and skin rash.

Thunder god vine has been found to decrease bone mineral density in women who take the herb for 5 years or longer. This side effect may be of particular concern to women who have osteoporosis or are at risk for the condition.

Thunder god vine decreases sperm count and so may be associated with male infertility.

Tell your health care providers about any complementary and alternative practices you use. Give them a full picture of what you do to manage your health. This will help ensure coordinated and safe care.

Section 45.6

S-adenosylmethionine and Methyl Sulfonyl Methane

Many nutritional supplements are marketed as alternative therapies for arthritis sufferers. S-adenosylmethionine or SAM-e (pronounced "sammy") and methyl sulfonyl methane, or MSM, are two of the most popular nutritional supplements marketed to lessen arthritic pain. These pills are sold in supermarkets, health stores, and pharmacies.

About SAM-e

SAM-e, found naturally in the human body, helps produce hormones and cell membranes. For years, SAM-e has been sold as a prescription medication in Europe for the treatment of arthritis symptoms. In 1999, it became available in the United States as an over-the-counter nutritional supplement. Some studies indicate that SAM-e may relieve osteoarthritic pain just as well as nonsteroidal anti-inflammatory drugs (NSAIDs), such as ibuprofen, but with fewer side effects ("Alternative Arthritis Treatments", Mayo Clinic, [November 2002]). Some SAM-e manufacturers claim the nutritional supplement helps regenerate cartilage and improve joint disease. No scientific evidence supports this claim.

Some potential downsides to taking SAM-e include:

- No long-term studies to show what effects might occur in people who take it daily for years.

- SAM-e is not a cure. You have to keep taking it to get the effects.

- It can be expensive and is not covered by insurance.

About MSM

MSM is sold as a treatment for pain and inflammation from rheumatoid arthritis, osteoarthritis, fibromyalgia, and gout.

There is little scientific data on MSM's safety or benefits. A few animal studies suggest that MSM may have an anti-inflammatory effect, but there are no published trials demonstrating its effectiveness or safety in human beings ("Is MSM as good as it sounds?" *Harvard Health Online*, [August 2002]).

In a statement to the Arthritis Foundation, Stanley Jacob, MD, one of the developers of MSM, says MSM's major benefit for those with osteoarthritis (OA) and rheumatoid arthritis (RA) is pain relief. It hasn't been shown to preserve cartilage or to stop disease progression or joint destruction. Common side effects of taking MSM are diarrhea, stomach upsets, or mild cramps.

Summary

If you are considering the use of SAM-e or MSM, be sure to consult your doctor first. Both nutritional supplements should be used only with your doctor's advice, along with other treatments he or she may prescribe.

Chapter 46

Complementary and Alternative Medicine for Arthritis

Chapter Contents

Section 46.1

Arthritis Patients Skeptical of Conventional Medical Practices Likely to Use Alternative Medicine

From "Skeptical patients with arthritis and fibromyalgia are likely to use alternative medicine," by the Agency for Healthcare Research and Quality (AHRQ, www.ahrq.gov), June 2008.

Medical skeptics are individuals who doubt conventional medicine's ability to significantly improve their health status. Their skepticism can often lead them to seek additional care from massage therapists, church leaders, chiropractors, herbalists, and acupuncturists.

In a recent study, researchers at the University of North Carolina at Chapel Hill surveyed 1,759 patients with arthritis and fibromyalgia to determine the strength of their medical skepticism and their subsequent use of complementary and alternative medicine (CAM). Of the 721 individuals who returned the survey, 106 (15 percent) used CAM providers. When church leaders were excluded, the number fell to 75 (10 percent). Of the 106, 54 percent had rheumatoid arthritis, 23 percent had osteoarthritis, and 23 percent had fibromyalgia. Most were female (78 percent) and white (86 percent) and had spent some time in college.

Researchers measured medical skepticism using the Medical Skepticism Scale. This consists of four questions to which respondents answer using a five-point Likert scale (disagree strongly to agree strongly). In this study, medical skepticism was associated with CAM provider use. In fact, a one-point increase in the skepticism scale increased the probability of using a CAM provider by 70 percent.

The authors note that providers who treat medical skeptics can better assist these patients by thoroughly communicating what conventional medicine offers as well as which alternative therapies may be useful in treating their conditions. This study was funded in part by the Agency for Healthcare Research and Quality.

Source: "Medical skepticism and the use of complementary and alternative health care providers by patients followed by rheumatologists," by

Leigh F. Callahan, PhD, Janet K. Freburger, PT, PhD, Thelma J. Mielenz, PT, PhD, OCS, and Elizabeth K. Wiley-Exley, MPH, in the June 2008 *Journal of Clinical Rheumatology* 14(3), pp. 143–147.

Section 46.2

Acupuncture Relieves Arthritis Pain and Improves Function

From "Acupuncture Relieves Pain and Improves Function in Knee Osteoarthritis," by the National Center for Complementary and Alternative Medicine (NCCAM, nccam.nih.gov), part of the National Institutes of Health, December 20, 2004.

Acupuncture provides pain relief and improves function for people with osteoarthritis of the knee and serves as an effective complement to standard care. This landmark study was funded by the National Center for Complementary and Alternative Medicine (NCCAM) and the National Institute of Arthritis and Musculoskeletal and Skin Diseases (NIAMS), both components of the National Institutes of Health. The findings of the study—the longest and largest randomized, controlled phase III clinical trial of acupuncture ever conducted—were published in the December 21, 2004, issue of the Annals of Internal Medicine.[1]

The multi-site study team, including rheumatologists and licensed acupuncturists, enrolled 570 patients, aged 50 or older with osteoarthritis of the knee. Participants had significant pain in their knee the month before joining the study, but had never experienced acupuncture, had not had knee surgery in the previous 6 months, and had not used steroid or similar injections. Participants were randomly assigned to receive one of three treatments: acupuncture, sham acupuncture, or participation in a control group that followed the Arthritis Foundation's self-help course for managing their condition. Patients continued to receive standard medical care from their primary physicians, including anti-inflammatory medications, such as COX-2 [cyclooxygenase-II] selective inhibitors, non-steroidal anti-inflammatory drugs, and opioid pain relievers.

"For the first time, a clinical trial with sufficient rigor, size, and duration has shown that acupuncture reduces the pain and functional impairment of osteoarthritis of the knee," said Stephen E. Straus, MD, NCCAM Director.

"These results also indicate that acupuncture can serve as an effective addition to a standard regimen of care and improve quality of life for knee osteoarthritis sufferers. NCCAM has been building a portfolio of basic and clinical research that is now revealing the power and promise of applying stringent research methods to ancient practices like acupuncture."

"More than 20 million Americans have osteoarthritis. This disease is one of the most frequent causes of physical disability among adults," said Stephen I. Katz, MD, PhD, NIAMS Director. "Thus, seeking an effective means of decreasing osteoarthritis pain and increasing function is of critical importance."

During the course of the study, led by Brian M. Berman, MD, Director of the Center for Integrative Medicine and Professor of Family Medicine at the University of Maryland School of Medicine, Baltimore, Maryland, 190 patients received true acupuncture and 191 patients received sham acupuncture for 24 treatment sessions over 26 weeks. Sham acupuncture is a procedure designed to prevent patients from being able to detect if needles are actually inserted at treatment points. In both the sham and true acupuncture procedures, a screen prevented patients from seeing the knee treatment area and learning which treatment they received. In the education control group, 189 participants attended six, 2-hour group sessions over 12 weeks based on the Arthritis Foundation's Arthritis Self-Help Course, a proven, effective model.

On joining the study, patients' pain and knee function were assessed using standard arthritis research survey instruments and measurement tools, such as the Western Ontario McMasters Osteoarthritis Index (WOMAC). Patients' progress was assessed at 4, 8, 14, and 26 weeks. By week 8, participants receiving acupuncture were showing a significant increase in function and by week 14 a significant decrease in pain, compared with the sham and control groups. These results, shown by declining scores on the WOMAC index, held through week 26.

Overall, those who received acupuncture had a 40 percent decrease in pain and a nearly 40 percent improvement in function compared to baseline assessments.

"This trial, which builds upon our previous NCCAM-funded research, establishes that acupuncture is an effective complement to conventional arthritis treatment and can be successfully employed as part of a multidisciplinary approach to treating the symptoms of osteoarthritis," said Dr. Berman.

Acupuncture—the practice of inserting thin needles into specific body points to improve health and well-being—originated in China more than 2,000 years ago. In 2002, acupuncture was used by an estimated 2.1 million U.S. adults, according to the Centers for Disease Control and Prevention's 2002 National Health Interview Survey.[2] The acupuncture technique that has been most studied scientifically involves penetrating the skin with thin, solid, metallic needles that are manipulated by the hands or by electrical stimulation. In recent years, scientific inquiry has begun to shed more light on acupuncture's possible mechanisms and potential benefits, especially in treating painful conditions such as arthritis.

References

1. Berman BM, Lao L, Langenberg P, Lee WL, Gilpin AMK, Hochberg MC. Effectiveness of Acupuncture as Adjunctive Therapy in Osteoarthritis of the Knee: A Randomized, Controlled Trial. *Annals of Internal Medicine.* 2004; 141(12):901–910.

2. Barnes P, Powell-Griner E, McFann K, Nahin R. CDC Advance Data Report #343. Complementary and Alternative Medicine Use Among Adults: United States, 2002. May 27, 2004.

Section 46.3

Chiropractic Care Aids Patients with Chronic, Pain-Related Conditions

Excerpted from "Chiropractic: An Introduction," by the National Center for Complementary and Alternative Medicine (NCCAM, www.nccam.nih .gov), part of the National Institutes of Health, November 2007.

Chiropractic is a health care approach that focuses on the relationship between the body's structure—mainly the spine—and its functioning. Although practitioners may use a variety of treatment approaches, they primarily perform adjustments to the spine or other parts of the body with the goal of correcting alignment problems and supporting the body's natural ability to heal itself.

Overview and History

The term "chiropractic" combines the Greek words cheir (hand) and praxis (action) to describe a treatment done by hand. Hands-on therapy—especially adjustment of the spine—is central to chiropractic care. Chiropractic, which in the United States is considered part of complementary and alternative medicine, is based on these key concepts:

- The body has a powerful self-healing ability.

- The body's structure (primarily that of the spine) and its function are closely related, and this relationship affects health.

- Therapy aims to normalize this relationship between structure and function and assist the body as it heals.

While some procedures associated with chiropractic care can be traced back to ancient times, the modern profession of chiropractic was founded by Daniel David Palmer in 1895 in Davenport, Iowa. Palmer, a self-taught healer, believed that the body has a natural healing ability. Misalignments of the spine can interfere with the flow of energy needed to support health, Palmer theorized, and the key to health is to normalize the function of the nervous system, especially the spinal cord.

Patterns of Use

According to the 2007 National Health Interview Survey, which included a comprehensive survey of CAM use by Americans, about 8 percent of American adults and nearly 3 percent of children had received chiropractic or osteopathic manipulation in the past 12 months. Adjusted to nationally representative numbers, these percentages mean that more than 18 million adults and 2 million children received chiropractic or osteopathic manipulation in the previous year.

Many people who seek chiropractic care have chronic, pain-related health conditions. Low-back pain, neck pain, and headache are common conditions for which people seek chiropractic treatment.

What to Expect from Chiropractic Visits

During the initial visit, chiropractors typically take a health history and perform a physical examination, with a special emphasis on the spine. Other examinations or tests such as x-rays may also be performed. If chiropractic treatment is considered appropriate, a treatment plan will be developed.

During follow-up visits, practitioners may perform one or more of the many different types of adjustments used in chiropractic care. Given mainly to the spine, a chiropractic adjustment (sometimes referred to as a manipulation) involves using the hands or a device to apply a controlled, sudden force to a joint, moving it beyond its passive range of motion. The goal is to increase the range and quality of motion in the area being treated and to aid in restoring health. Other hands-on therapies such as mobilization (movement of a joint within its usual range of motion) also may be used.

Chiropractors may combine the use of spinal adjustments with several other treatments and approaches:

- Heat and ice
- Electrical stimulation
- Rest
- Rehabilitative exercise
- Counseling about diet, weight loss, and other lifestyle factors
- Dietary supplements

Side Effects and Risks

Side effects and risks depend on the specific type of chiropractic treatment used. For example, side effects from chiropractic adjustments can include temporary headaches, tiredness, or discomfort in parts of the body that were treated. The likelihood of serious complications, such as stroke, appears to be extremely low and related to the type of adjustment performed and the part of the body treated.

If dietary supplements are a part of the chiropractic treatment plan, they may interact with medicines and cause side effects. It is important that people inform their chiropractors of all medicines (whether prescription or over-the-counter) and supplements they are taking.

Other Points to Consider

Research to expand the scientific understanding of chiropractic treatment is ongoing.

If you decide to seek chiropractic care, talk to your chiropractor about the following topics:

- His education, training, and licensing
- Whether he has experience treating the health conditions for which you are seeking care
- Any special medical concerns you have and any medicines or dietary supplements you are taking

Tell all of your health care providers about any complementary and alternative practices you use. Give them a full picture of what you do to manage your health. This will help ensure coordinated and safe care.

Section 46.4

Massage Therapy for Managing Arthritis Pain

More than 2,000 years ago, the ancient Greek physician Hippocrates wrote that doctors should be experienced in "rubbing that can bind a joint that is loose and loosen a joint that is too hard." Today, massage is still a popular way to manage arthritis pain. Proponents claim that massage therapy, done correctly, can help improve joint movement, relax tense muscles, and stimulate the flow of blood and nutrients to the skin and underlying tissues. What's more, it just feels good, and the relaxation it brings can help break the cycle of pain and stress that often goes along with arthritis.

Pressing the Flesh

Technically speaking, massage involves the manipulation of soft tissues with the hands through rubbing, stroking, pressure, and so on. Trained practitioners use massage therapy techniques to improve the well-being of clients. Today, there are more than a quarter million massage therapists in the United States, and nearly one-fifth of American adults go get a professional massage each year. The American Massage Therapy Association (AMTA), the field's leading professional organization, lists arthritis as one of the conditions for which massage can help. But how well does it work? A recent journal article (*Medical Clinics of North America*, 2002) reviewed the medical literature on the use of massage to manage arthritis pain. The authors concluded that few people would dispute the short-term benefits for arthritis pain relief. However, studies of the long-term effects of the technique are still lacking.

Hands-On Approaches

Massage therapy can take a wide variety of forms. These are some of the most common ones:

- **Swedish massage:** This is what most people think of when they hear the word "massage." It's a full-body treatment that combines stroking, kneading, and friction on the top layer of muscles with gentle movement of the joints.

- **Deep tissue massage:** This technique uses slow strokes and strong pressure on the deeper layers of muscle tissue. The goal is to release tension there. However, the deep pressure can cause some soreness, so it's not for everyone.

- **Myofascial release:** This approach uses long, stretching strokes to release tension in the fascia, the connective tissue around the muscles.

- **Trigger point therapy:** This method uses concentrated finger pressure on knots of tension or pain that can trigger pain elsewhere in the body.

- **Acupuncture and shiatsu:** These Asian techniques use finger pressure on specific points on the body—the same points that are stimulated in acupuncture. The pressure is supposed to unblock the flow of life energy, called qi ("chee").

- **Reflexology:** This method involves rubbing certain points on the feet, hands, or ears that are believed to correspond to various parts of the body.

Much-Kneaded Advice

A typical massage therapy session lasts about 60 to 90 minutes. To see real improvement, though, you may need four to six sessions about a week apart. The cost runs $30 to $125 or more per hour, but insurance sometimes covers the treatment if a doctor prescribes it. The first session usually begins with the massage therapist asking questions about your current physical condition, medical history, and goals for the treatment. Next, you'll be asked to remove some or all of your clothing and lie on a padded table. A sheet or towel should be provided, and the therapist should uncover only the part of your body being massaged. This not only protects your modesty, but also helps you stay warm. Often, the therapist will use oil or lotion, so if you know you have skin allergies, be sure to mention them up front. During the massage, don't hesitate to speak up if anything feels inappropriate or causes pain. While massage therapy may provide shorter-term pain relief, massage therapy that is too rough may aggravate arthritis pain and symptoms.

Hand-y Self-Help

In addition to giving you a massage, a good therapist can show you techniques to use on yourself at home. Giving yourself a massage isn't as relaxing as having someone else do it, but it can still help ease pain and tension. Not only will the part being rubbed feel better, but so may your hands, since they're getting a workout in the process. Self-massage works best for localized trouble spots that are easily accessible. For hard-to-reach places, you might ask a partner to lend a hand or buy an electric massager. But don't try massage on an inflamed joint or when you have an infection, since it could make these problems worse.

Here are some simple techniques to try:

- **Kneading:** Grasp the muscle between your palm (or thumb) and finger. Then lift slightly and squeeze, as if you were kneading dough. Don't just pinch the skin. Work into the muscle itself with a slow, regular squeeze-and-release motion. Be careful not to overdo it. Fifteen to 20 seconds on the same spot is enough.

- **Stroking:** Cup your hand over the muscle you want to massage. Then firmly glide your hand over the length of the muscle in a slow, repeated movement. A little oil or lotion may help. Try using different amounts of pressure until you find out what works best for you.

One key to a good experience is finding the right massage therapist. Always ask about credentials and education. The main credential to watch for is Nationally Certified in Therapeutic Massage and Bodywork (NCTMB). Also, look for a graduate of a training program that has been accredited by the Commission on Massage Therapy Accreditation (COMTA). In addition, ask about which techniques the therapist uses and whether he or she has experience working with other people who have arthritis. To find a qualified therapist in your area, contact the AMTA (www.amtamassage.org, 888-843-2682).

Part Five

Living with Arthritis

Chapter 47

Depression and Arthritis

Chapter Contents

Section 47.1

Depression May Be Underdiagnosed in People with Arthritis

Dealing with a chronic disease can be emotionally draining, but when does the normal stress of being ill become clinical depression? While the exact number of people with chronic conditions who suffer from clinical depression is hard to estimate, doctors agree that people with chronic conditions should be screened more aggressively for psychological disorders.

Autoimmune diseases, such as rheumatoid arthritis, scleroderma, and lupus, may put people at an increased risk for depression. A French study, presented recently at the annual convention of the American College of Rheumatology, found that although depression is a common disorder among people with scleroderma, it remains largely unrecognized and untreated.

"Depression is underdiagnosed in the general population, so I wouldn't be surprised if it is underdiagnosed in the rheumatology clinic," says Celso Velazquez, MD, assistant professor of rheumatology at the University of Missouri-Columbia School of Medicine. The link between chronic disease and depression is not causal. Depression occurs in physically healthy people, as well as in people with chronic conditions, and is not always related to the severity of the disease. On the other hand, many people with chronic illness manage just fine.

Steroids, used in conditions such as lupus, can cause depression, and doctors should carefully monitor patients who take steroids and adjust the dosage if necessary.

In fact, many of the symptoms associated with autoimmune conditions are also signs of depression, including lack of energy, fatigue, anxiety, lethargy, sleep disturbances, mood swings, changes in appetite, and others.

Fibromyalgia is another disorder where depression screening is crucial since some of the symptoms of fibromyalgia can mimic symptoms of depression and vice versa, Velazquez says.

However, what differentiates true depression from transient blues is the persistence of symptoms—usually six weeks or more. In addition, true depression impedes a person's ability to perform normal daily activities.

"I would say we, as doctors, need to be more aware of it, and we should find ways to screen for it more often," Velazquez says. Routine screening using a standard questionnaire is relatively cheap and easy to do, but it could put an extra load on doctors' already-cramped schedules.

Symptoms of depression include:

- sadness throughout the day;
- feelings of emptiness or hopelessness;
- loss of interest in previously enjoyed activities;
- feeling stressed and overwhelmed;
- trouble concentrating;
- feelings of worthlessness or self-hatred;
- irritability or restlessness;
- thoughts of death or suicide;
- fatigue or lack of energy;
- sleeping too much or too little;
- change in appetite or weight;
- vague aches and pains;
- headache;
- back pain;
- digestive problems or change in bowel movements.

Section 47.2

Symptoms of Depression in People with Arthritis

It's perfectly normal to feel a little down and blue at times. For some people, though, the stress of arthritis pain can add up to full-blown depression. It may work something like this: You get into the habit of thinking negatively about all the changes in your life because of arthritis pain, which eventually makes you depressed. The more depressed you are, the more arthritis pain and fatigue you feel. As these symptoms get worse, your stress levels start to rise even higher. The more stress you experience, the more depressed you become. And so on. It's easy to see how you could easily get caught in this destructive cycle.

Living through the Depression

Research has shown just how closely depression and pain are linked. A medical journal article (*Rheumatic Diseases Clinics of North America*, 1999) that reviewed the scientific evidence on this subject concluded that depression is more common in people with rheumatoid arthritis than in the general population. In addition, higher levels of pain among people with arthritis seem to be tied to a greater risk of depression.

A Depressed Mood, in Turn, Can Make It Harder to Cope with Pain

"People who experience significant depression in addition to pain have a harder time overcoming their feelings of helplessness and powerlessness," says Margaret Caudill-Slosberg, MD, PhD, a pain specialist at Dartmouth Medical School.

There is good news. Depression is one of the most treatable of all mental health problems, thanks to modern advances in counseling and medications. Treating depression won't make arthritis pain magically disappear, of course. But it can make the experience of dealing with that pain much less overwhelming.

Watching for Warning Signs

These are the signs that you may need professional treatment for depression, according to the American Psychiatric Association.

A person with depression has at least one of these symptoms:

- A low mood lasting most of the day, nearly every day
- A loss of interest or pleasure in almost all activities

In addition, a person with depression has at least three or four of these symptoms:

- Weight loss or gain, or decreased or increased appetite
- Trouble falling or staying asleep, or sleeping too much
- Restless movements or movements that look slowed down
- Tiredness or loss of energy
- Feelings of worthlessness or inappropriate guilt
- Trouble thinking clearly, concentrating, or making decisions
- Frequent thoughts of death or suicide

If these symptoms last for at least two weeks, and if they start to interfere with your personal life or work, it may be time to seek help. Talk to your family doctor or a mental health professional, or call your local hospital, mental health center, or suicide prevention hotline.

Helping Yourself to Hope

Full-fledged depression needs professional treatment. However, there are things you can do on your own to help improve your mood.

- Spend time with friends and family. Socializing is a great depression-buster.
- Keep up with your normal activities. Don't give in to the urge to withdraw.

- Become more physically active. Exercise is another potent mood-lifter.

- Limit your alcohol intake. Drinking too much just makes things worse.

Chapter 48

Stress and Arthritis

Chapter Contents

Section 48.1

Coping with Arthritis Stress

Stress is an all-pervasive and unavoidable part of modern life. There are many types of stress, and just as many definitions.

"My favorite one is stress is anything that threatens the homeostasis of an organism," says Kathy Donovan Hanson, senior researcher at the Missouri Arthritis Rehabilitation Research and Training Center (MARRTC), a federally funded project at the University of Missouri-Columbia dealing with arthritis, related conditions, and disability.

Despite its mainly negative connotation, stress can be beneficial. In fact, stress is an essential coping mechanism that ensures survival. But when stress becomes a constant companion of our daily lives, it can take a toll on our bodies.

People who have a chronic disease are particularly vulnerable because their bodies are perpetually dealing with the physiological stressors caused by their conditions.

Diseases stress the body on several levels—physiological, cognitive, and emotional. For example, people with rheumatoid arthritis (RA) have to deal with purely physical stressors such as pain, stiffness, and inflammation, which in turn may affect their mood and ability to focus and think clearly.

"It's cyclical, a spiral," Donovan Hanson says. In certain situations, stress can be a lifesaver. For example, if you see a car approaching you at 100 mph, your body produces a chain of physical reactions and releases hormones that prepare you to run for your life, Donovan Hanson explains. In a situation like this adrenaline levels go up, blood pressure goes up, breathing becomes rapid and shallow, and the body is ready to physically deal with the stress. However, constant stress, as is the stress in people with chronic diseases, can cause high blood pressure, recurrent headaches, or even gastrointestinal disturbances.

If occasional stress is an essential survival mechanism, so is learning to deal with chronic stress.

One can deal with stress on two levels: by avoiding situations and factors that produce stress and by learning how to cope with stress when stress cannot be avoided.

"The single fastest thing to do to help control stress is deep breathing," Donovan Hanson says. "It triggers a relaxation response immediately."

Other techniques include:

- getting enough sleep;

- drinking plenty of water;

- proper nutrition;

- relaxation techniques such as progressive muscle relaxation, an exercise that alternates between tensing and relaxing of the muscles;

- exercise;

- staying focused on the "here" and "now" and not worrying about things you can't control;

- taking time to transition between the different roles in your life. Do not worry about personal stuff at work and don't take work home with you. Be one thing at a time.

- devoting time to things you enjoy.

Section 48.2

Stress Management for Caregivers

Caring for a person with a disability can be very rewarding and also very hard. A disability often occurs suddenly. Within a few seconds, your whole world can change and the speed and amount of recovery is unknown. There can be a lot of questions about the future in dealing with the changes resulting from the disability, for person with the disability and their loved ones. Finally, the disability can present many problems, which span physical, emotional, and mental areas. The person may be physically and mentally impaired, causing problems for the person providing care.

The term, "caregiving stress" is used to show that caring for a loved one with a disability is physically and emotionally hard. It can cause all types of problems for the caregiver, depending on the type of relationship you have with your family member (e.g., parent, spouse). Many questions may come to mind when you are caregiving:

- Can I really do this?
- Am I doing enough (too much)?
- Can I physically handle this?
- How will I ever learn all of the care tasks?
- Will I be able to take care of myself too?
- Am I neglecting others in my family?

This last question is a very important one because if you do not take care of yourself you will be unable to care for your family member. Meeting your needs and their needs is tricky yet important. When the scales tip and your stress gets to be too much, you might go through many negative effects.

Stresses caregivers can feel: anger, guilt, depression, loneliness, anxiety, and fatigue.

It is important to watch for these early signs in order for you to take steps to stop it from getting worse. Many times, caregivers wait too long before they will admit to their own exhaustion and then it is much harder to find ways to help it. When ignored, caregiver stress can lead to irritability that may lead to abuse and neglect of your family member.

Watch for some of these signs of caregiver stress:

- Changes in sleep or your eating patterns
- Moodiness and irritability
- Increased use of medicines or alcohol to "relax"
- Flare up of your own medical problems or a new illness
- Chronic fatigue
- Rough handling of the persons with the disability

What can you do if you find some of these signs in your daily life?

There are no easy answers, but sometimes even small things can help. Here are a few to follow:

- **Become comfortable asking for help.** Look beyond those old beliefs that asking others for a favor is a sign of weakness, or that others should know when and how to help.

- **Keep communication open and clear between you and your family member.** Remember the person with a disability is part of your family. It is important to allow them to make decisions and do things, as they are able.

- **Remember that sometimes your own needs must come first.** Even though it is your family member who has a disability, your needs are important too. Remember that you care for them only as well as you care for yourself.

- **Look for time for rest, have fun, and exercise.** Time away doing something different is important to your personal well being. This should happen regularly in small ways, like a phone call to a friend, a relaxing bath, or a walk on a nice day; and occasionally in a big way, like a night out with friends, or even a vacation where someone else takes over caregiving tasks.

- **Learn to set limits.** It is okay to give yourself permission to say "No" when it's necessary. Remember only so much can be done in a 24-hour day. Recognizing and setting limits can strengthen your spirit and inspire you to move forward. You're doing a lot. It is okay to give yourself a pat on the back.

- **Look for sources of support.** Support from others is very important whether it comes in the form of physical help with your family member, someone to help you get out for a while, or someone to just listen to you. You may find comfort from a minister, rabbi, or priest for spiritual support. Support groups for caregivers are a good place to find information and emotional help. You're not alone.

None of these tips are easy to follow. You will often feel as if you are not doing a good job of taking care of your loved one when you do something to take care of yourself. Just like caring for your family member takes work, caring for yourself takes work too.

Remember the old saying, "An ounce of prevention is worth a pound of cure." Even if you read these pages and feel you are handling things okay, self-care is very important. From the very start of your role as caregiver, you should build in ways to be a caregiver to yourself.

Note: Revised from *Stroke Caregiver Treatment Manual* authored by Robert J. Hartke, PhD, and Rosemarie B. King, PhD, RN, funded through the Stroke Rehabilitation Research and Training Center on Enhancing Quality of Life of Stroke Survivors, National Institute of Disability and Rehabilitation Research, 1993–1998, Grant No.: H133B30024.

Chapter 49

Maintaining Independence

Chapter Contents

Section 49.1

Modifying Your Home for Independence

From "There's No Place Like Home—For Growing Old," by the National Institute on Aging (NIA, www.nia.nih.gov), February 19, 2009.

"The stairs are getting so hard to climb."

"Since my wife died, I just open a can of soup for dinner."

"I've lived here 40 years. No other place will seem like home."

These are common concerns for older people. And, you may share an often-heard wish—"I want to stay in my own home!" The good news is that with the right help you might be able to do just that.

What do I do first?

Think about the kinds of help you might want in the near future. Planning ahead is hard because you never know how your needs might change. Maybe you live alone, so there is no one to help you. Maybe you don't need help right now, but you live with a husband or wife who does. Whatever your situation, start by looking at any illnesses like diabetes, heart disease, or emphysema that you have. Then talk to your doctor about how these health problems could make it hard for you to get around or take care of yourself in the future. Help getting dressed in the morning, fixing a meal, or remembering to take medicine may be all you need to stay at home.

As you read on, you will learn about the kinds of help that you might want to look for where you live. You will read about people and places to go to for more information about the resources near you— from people in your community to the federal government. If you are worried about how much this help will cost, you will see that we have tried to give you suggestions for free or low cost help, as well as some that cost more. There are also ways to find out if there are any benefits that apply to you. Share this information with others in your family, and use it as a stepping stone to begin talking about your needs—now and in the future.

How can I help my older relatives stay in their home?

Some people start having trouble doing everyday activities like shopping, cooking, and taking care of their home or themselves as they grow older. Is that happening to any of your relatives—your parents or an aunt or uncle, for example? If so, talk to them about getting help. Offer to get information for them. Think about what you and others in the family can do to help. Talk to your friends whose relatives may be facing the same kinds of problems. Ask about the solutions they found. Then sit down and tell your relatives what you have learned. Together you can decide what to do.

What kinds of help can I get?

You can get almost any type of help you want in your home—often for a cost. The following list includes some common things people need. You can get more information on many of these services from your local Area Agency on Aging, local and state offices on aging or social services, tribal organization, or nearby senior centers.

Personal care: Is bathing, washing your hair, or dressing getting harder to do? Maybe a relative or friend could help you. Or, you could hire someone trained to help you for a short time each day.

Homemaking: Do you need help with chores like housecleaning, yard work, grocery shopping, or laundry? Some grocery stores and drug stores will take your order over the phone and bring the items to your home. There are cleaning services you can hire, or maybe someone you know has a housekeeper to suggest. Some housekeepers will help with laundry. Some dry cleaners will pick up and deliver your clothes.

Meals: Tired of cooking every day or of eating alone? Maybe you could share cooking with a friend a few times a week or have a potluck dinner with a group of friends. Sometimes meals are served at a nearby senior center, church, or synagogue. Eating out may give you a chance to visit with others. Is it hard for you to get out? Ask someone you know to bring you a healthy meal a few times a week. Also, programs like Meals on Wheels bring hot meals into your home.

Money management: Are you paying bills late or not at all because it's tiring or hard to keep track of them? Are doctors' bills and health insurance claim forms confusing? Ask a trusted relative to lend a hand. If that's not possible, volunteers, financial counselors, or geriatric care managers can help. Just make sure you get the name from a trustworthy source, like your local Area Agency on Aging. Would you like to lighten the load of paying bills yourself? Talk with someone at your bank. You might also be able to have regular bills, like utilities and rent or mortgage, paid directly from your checking account.

Health care: Do you forget to take your medicine? There are devices available to remind you when it is time to take it. Have you just gotten out of the hospital and still need nursing care at home for a short time? Medicare might pay for a home health aide to come to your home.

Products to make life easier: Is it getting harder to turn a door knob, get out of a chair, or put on your socks? There are things available to make these activities and many of the other things you do during the day easier. The Department of Education provides a website, www.abledata.com. If you can't get to or use a computer, they will answer your questions at 800-227-0216. This website has information on more than 30,000 assistive technology products designed to make it easier for people with physical limitations to do things for themselves.

Getting around—at home and in town: Are you having trouble walking? Think about getting an electric chair or scooter. These are sometimes covered by Medicare. Do you need someone to go with you to the doctor or shopping? Volunteer escort services may be available. Don't drive a car any longer? Free or lower-priced public transportation and taxis may be offered in your area. Maybe a relative, friend, or neighbor would take you along when they go on errands or do yours for you.

Activities and friends: Are you bored staying at home? Try visiting your local senior center. They offer a variety of activities. You might see some old friends there and meet new people, too. Is it hard for you to leave your home? Maybe you would enjoy visits from someone on a regular basis. Volunteers are sometimes available to stop by or call once a week. They can just keep you company, or you can talk about any problems you are having.

Safety: Are you worried about crime in your neighborhood, physical abuse, or losing money as a result of a scam? Talk to your local Area Agency on Aging. Do you live alone and are afraid of becoming sick with no one around to help? You might want to get an emergency alert system. You just push a special button that you wear, and emergency medical personnel are called. A monthly fee is charged.

Care away from home: Do you need care but live with someone who can't stay with you during the day? For example, maybe they work. Adult day care outside the home is sometimes available for older people who need help getting around or caring for themselves. The day care center can even pick you up and bring you home. If your caretaker needs to get away overnight, there are places that will provide more extended temporary respite care.

Housing: Does your home need a few changes to make it easier and safer to live in? Think about things like a ramp at the front door, grab bars in the tub or shower, nonskid floors, more comfortable handles on doors or faucets, and better insulation. Sound expensive? You might be able to get help paying for these changes. Check with your local or State Area Agencies on Aging, state housing finance agency, welfare department, community development groups, or the federal government.

Where do I start?

Here are some resources where you can look for this help:

People you know: For many older people, family, friends, and neighbors are the biggest source of help. Talk with those close to you about the best way to get what you need. If you are physically able, think about trading services with a friend or neighbor. One could do the grocery shopping, and the other could cook dinner, for example.

Community and local government resources: Learn about the types of services and care found in your community. Health care providers and social workers may have suggestions. The local Area Agency on Aging, local and state offices on aging or social services, and your tribal organization have lists of services. Look in the phone book under "Government." If you belong to a religious group, check with its local offices. The group might have a senior services program.

Geriatric care managers: Specially trained people known as geriatric care managers can help make your daily life easier. They will work with you to form a long-term care plan and find the right services. They charge for this help, and it probably won't be covered by any insurance plan. Geriatric care managers can be very helpful when family members live far apart. They will check in with you from time to time to make sure your needs haven't changed.

Federal government sources: There are many resources from the federal government where you can start looking for information on help. Some are on the internet and only available with a computer. Federal government websites are reliable. If you don't have a computer, you might be able to find one at your local library or senior center. Or ask your local Area Agency on Aging. Perhaps a grandchild, niece, or nephew could search for you. Wherever possible, we have also given a phone number. The Eldercare Locator has information on many different services for older people. They can give you the number of your local Area Agency on Aging. To use this service call 800-677-1116, or go to www.eldercare.gov on the internet.

You can get suggestions to fit your own needs from the Medicare website at www.medicare.gov. Just click on "Long-Term Care" and then "Long-Term Care Planning Tool." Type in information about yourself (age, sex, and whether you are married), as well as your health problems and other needs. Very quickly it will give the type of help you should look for and general advice on how to find it and how to pay for it. You do not have to put in any personal information—not even your name or Social Security number.

The National Library of Medicine's website, www.medlineplus.gov, has a section "Home care services." This contains links to information that might be of help.

The National Institute on Aging (NIA) has its Resource Directory for Older People. It has the names, addresses, phone numbers, and website addresses for more than 260 government agencies, professional associations, and public and private groups that have information or help for older people. You can use it online at www.nia.nih.gov/HealthInformation or call 800-222-4225 for help finding the resource you need.

Once you have chosen some service providers, you might be able to get more information about them from www.medicare.gov. The Home Health Compare section there can tell you more about some of the providers in your state. You can also check on how well these services help people. No computer? Just call 800-MEDICARE (800-633-4227) for the same information.

How much will this cost?

Some types of help could cost a lot. Thinking about how you are going to pay for the help you need is an important part of planning.

Some things you want may cost a lot. Others may be free. Some things may be covered by Medicare, private "Medigap" policies or other private health insurance, Medicaid, or long-term care insurance. Some may not. Check with your insurance provider(s). There is a chance that paying for just a few services out of pocket could cost less in the long run than moving into an independent living, assisted living, or long-term care facility. And you will have your wish of still living in your own home.

Once you have thought about which services you need, you can find out about federal, state, and local government benefits at www.govbenefits.gov. If you can't get to a computer, call 800-FED-INFO (800-333-4636) for the same kind of help.

Another website to search for benefits is www.benefitscheckup.org from the National Council on Aging. By typing in general information about yourself, you can see a list of possible benefits you might qualify for. You don't have to give your name, address, or Social Security number in order to use this service.

Are you eligible for veterans' benefits from the Department of Veterans Affairs? The VA sometimes provides medical care in your home. In some areas they also offer homemaker/home health aide services, adult day health care, and hospice. You can learn more by going to www.va.gov, calling the toll-free VA Health Care Benefits number, 877-222-8387, or contacting the VA medical center nearest you.

What if I need more help?

At some point, support from family, friends, or local programs may not be enough. If you need help on a full-time basis, you might want to think about having someone live in your home. Or, you could have someone from a service come in for as many hours and days as you want for a fee. You might also decide to move to a senior living facility that provides many or all of the services you need. But, in the meantime, you will have enjoyed your home and neighbors for longer than you once thought. A little help from family, friends, and local services will have made that possible.

Section 49.2

Avoiding Falls and Fractures

Excerpted from "Falls and Fractures," by the National Institute on
Aging (NIA, www.nia.nih.gov), part of the National Institutes of Health,
February 19, 2009.

A simple thing can change your life—like tripping on a rug or slipping on a wet spot on the kitchen floor. If you fall, then you might be like the thousands of older men and women each year who break, or fracture, a bone. A broken bone might not sound awful. But, for older people, a break can be the start of more serious problems.

Many things can make you more likely to fall. Your eyesight, hearing, muscles, and reflexes might not be as sharp as when you were younger. Diabetes, heart disease, or problems with your thyroid, nerves, or blood vessels can affect your balance. Some medicines can cause dizziness.

Then there's osteoporosis—a disease that makes bones weak and more likely to break easily. Many people think osteoporosis is only a problem for women past menopause, but it can also affect older men. Weak bones can mean that even a minor fall might be dangerous.

Don't let a fear of falling keep you from being active. Doing things like getting together with friends, gardening, walking, or going to the local senior center are also important for staying healthy. The good news is that there are simple ways you can prevent most falls.

Take the Right Steps

If you take care of your overall health, you may be able to lower your chances of falling. Most of the time, falls and accidents don't just happen. Here are a few hints that will help you avoid falls and broken bones:

- Learn how strong your bones are. Ask your doctor about a special test called a bone mineral density test. If this test shows your bones are weak, your doctor can tell you how to make them stronger and less likely to break.

- Stay physically active. Plan an exercise program that is right for you. Regular exercise makes you stronger and improves muscles. It also helps keep your joints, tendons, and ligaments flexible. Mild weight-bearing activities, such as walking or climbing stairs, may slow bone loss from osteoporosis.

- Have your eyes and hearing tested often. Even small changes in sight and hearing can put you at risk for falling. When you get new eyeglasses, take time to get used to them. Always wear your glasses when you need them. If you have a hearing aid, be sure it fits well, and wear it.

- Find out about the side effects of any medicine you take. If a drug makes you sleepy or dizzy, tell your doctor or pharmacist.

- Get enough sleep. If you are sleepy, you are more likely to fall.

- Limit the amount of alcohol you drink. Even a small amount can affect your balance and reflexes.

- Stand up slowly after eating, lying down, or sitting. Getting up too quickly can cause your blood pressure to drop. That can make you feel faint.

- Use a cane, walking stick, or walker to help you feel steadier when you walk. This is very important when you're walking in areas you don't know well or in places where the walkways are uneven. And be very careful when walking on wet or icy surfaces. They can be very slippery! Try to have sand or salt spread on icy areas by your front or back door.

- Wear rubber-soled, low-heeled shoes that fully support your feet. Wearing only socks or shoes/slippers with smooth soles on stairs or floors without carpet can be unsafe.

- You might want to think about buying a home monitoring system service. Usually, you wear a button on a chain around your neck. If you fall or need emergency help, you just push the button to alert the service. You can find local medical alarm services in your yellow pages. Most medical-insurance companies and Medicare do not cover items like home monitoring systems. Be sure to ask about cost. You will probably have to pay for it yourself.

And, always tell your doctor if you have fallen since your last checkup—even if you aren't hurt when you fall.

Make Your Home Safe

You can help prevent falls by following a few safety rules and by making changes to unsafe areas in your home.

In stairways, hallways, and pathways, follow these suggestions:

- Have handrails on both sides of all stairs from top to bottom, and make sure they are tightly fastened.

- Hold the handrails when you use the stairs, going up or down. If you must carry something while you're on the stairs, hold it in one hand and use the handrail with the other. Don't let it block your view of the steps. Go down or up the stairs sitting on each step in turn if you think you have problems with your vision or balance.

- Make sure there is good lighting with light switches at the top and bottom of stairs and each end of a long hall.

- Keep areas where you walk tidy. Don't leave things on the floor—you might trip on them.

- Check that all carpets are fixed firmly to the floor so they won't slip. Put no-slip strips on tile and wooden floors. You can buy these strips at the hardware store.

In bathrooms and powder rooms, follow these suggestions:

- Mount grab bars near toilets and on both the inside and outside of your tub and shower.

- Place nonskid mats, strips, or carpet on all surfaces that may get wet.

- Keep night lights on.

In your bedroom, follow these suggestions:

- Put night lights and light switches close to your bed.

- Keep your telephone near your bed.

In other living areas, follow these suggestions:

- Keep electric cords and telephone wires near walls and away from walking paths.

- Tack down all carpets and area rugs firmly to the floor.

- Arrange your furniture (especially low coffee tables) and other objects so they are not in your way when you walk.

- Make sure your sofas and chairs are the right height for you, so that you can get in and out of them easily.

- Stay away from a freshly washed floor.

- Don't take chances. Keep the things you use regularly in the kitchen within easy reach. Don't stand on a chair or table to reach something that's too high—use a reach stick instead. Reach sticks are special grabbing tools that you can buy at many hardware or medical-supply stores. If you use a step stool, make sure it is stable and has a handrail on top. Try to have someone stand next to you.

- Don't let your home get too cold or too hot—being very cold or very hot can make you dizzy. In the summer, if your home is not air-conditioned, keep cool with an electric fan, drink lots of liquids, and limit physical activity. In the winter, don't let the nighttime temperature drop below 65 degrees Fahrenheit.

- Keep emergency numbers in large print near each telephone.

Section 49.3

Gadgets Can Make Life with Arthritis Easier

"Gadgets Can Make Life Easier," © 2004 Missouri Arthritis Rehabilitation Research and Training Center (MARRTC). Reprinted with permission. For additional information, visit http://marrtc.missouri.edu.

Putting on socks in the morning can be a hassle for the lazy, and sometimes a near impossibility for people with arthritis. But a device called the Sock Aid can help people with arthritis slip on their favorite foot-warmers—without having to bend over and pull them on.

For some people with arthritis, avoiding bending can mean the difference between a relatively normal day and a morning fraught with relentless pain.

The Sock Aid is just one example of the assistive devices available. Such tools are designed to help people with arthritis accomplish their everyday tasks while taking the stress off their joints. And many of these items are available locally at discount and department stores.

Assistive devices may allow people with arthritis and disabilities to retain their independence longer, said Dovie Weston, an occupational therapist. Weston, M.Ed., is a clinical instructor at the University of Missouri Health Care. She's also a member of the team working on a research project devoted to vocational issues and arthritis at the Missouri Arthritis Rehabilitation and Training Center.

Fortunately, there is an almost inexhaustible list of these contraptions.

Big buttoned telephones, designed for people with shaky hands; bottle grippers, which make opening medicine bottles possible for people with trouble gripping; and garden trowels with comfortable grips are all out there to make life easier for people with disabilities.

There are also devices to help in the workplace, including computer keyboards that curve, joint-friendly computer mice that need no rolling, and pens with large grips.

For the breadwinners out there, these devices make office work much more tolerable (though there aren't any devices that can stop the phone from ringing off the hook yet).

As an occupational therapist, Weston works to help people retain their independence through exercise and adaptive devices. That's why Weston is an expert on gadgets such as the Sock Aid. These items help occupational therapists work with people with all forms of arthritis, whether it affects their hands or their spine.

Some people with arthritis may need assistive devices for everyday activities, while others may find they only need such items during a "flare," a period of time when disease is increased, or when they experience unpredictable jolts of arthritis pain.

In some cases, these adaptive devices may even function as a type of prevention medicine, said Weston. Some items can help keep joints aligned.

"If you use adaptive devices, then the extent of deformity should be lessened," said Weston. However, the devices cannot provide a cure for the pain.

Give Them a Try

Gadgets galore are within reach for people with disabilities through Centers for Independent Living (CILs), though many people might not realize it.

These nonprofit organizations are funded by the Rehabilitation Services Administration under the U.S. Department of Education. The centers are designed to help people with arthritis and other diseases live more independently. The centers sometimes offer demonstrations of such devices, allowing people to decide for themselves what works best for them.

To find such a center, check local telephone books under disability services, medical devices, or medical technology services. Such centers generally have someone on staff who can assess a person's disability and then recommend what types of devices would be helpful.

The centers often can show visitors firsthand how the devices work, said Mary Secora, a technology specialist at the Services for Independent Living Center in Columbia, Missouri. Secora, who has arthritis herself, said some centers have a plethora of gizmos and gadgets to show off. These items can include reachers that grasp onto objects, big-grip utensils, alternate keyboards, and oversized remote controls.

When You're Ready to Buy

Some of the devices, such as a doorknob attachment that makes it easier to open doors, can be purchased at local pharmacies, supermarkets, or hardware stores, said Secora.

"We try to look for things you can buy at Wal-Mart or at the Dollar store," she said.

Assistive devices can be found and purchased through catalogs and the internet.

Centers for Independent Living, including the one in Columbia, Missouri, keep such brochures on hand for people to peruse in order to get a better idea of what types of devices are available.

"The brochures act as a point of reference, so that people have an idea of what to look for," Secora said. Acknowledging that the cost of such devices may not be covered by most health insurance coverage, she said the centers also help people find the best price available for such products.

In many cases, the brochures offer a broad selection of utensils and devices ranging from the essential to the recreational.

Rubber spoons, touch-light lamps, and prism glasses, specs that allow people to stare at the ceiling and still watch TV, are among the more common devices in brochures.

"No two people's disabilities are alike," said Secora. The task, she added, is to find an adequate device.

Section 49.4

Driving When You Have Arthritis

From "Driving when you have arthritis," a brochure by the National Highway Traffic Safety Administration (NHTSA, www.nhtsa.dot.gov), March 2004. Reviewed by David A. Cooke, MD, FACP, July 26, 2009.

For most people, driving represents freedom, control, and independence. Driving enables most people to get to the places they want or need to go. For many people, driving is important economically—some drive as part of their job or to get to and from work.

Driving is a complex skill. Our ability to drive safely can be affected by changes in our physical, emotional, and mental condition.

The goal of this text is to help you, your family, and your health care professional talk about how arthritis may affect your ability to drive safely.

How can arthritis affect my driving?

Having arthritis can make your joints swollen and stiff, which can limit how far you can bend or move your shoulders, hands, head, and neck. This can make it harder to grasp or turn the steering wheel, apply the brake and gas pedals, put on your safety belt, or look over your shoulder to check your blind spot.

As a result, arthritis can make it harder for you to drive safely. If arthritis affects your hips, knees, ankles, or feet, you also may have difficulty getting in and out of your car.

Can I still drive with arthritis?

Yes, most people can drive safely with arthritis. It depends on which joints are affected, and how well you and your doctor are able to manage your condition. Your doctor cares about your health and safety, and will work with you and your loved ones to manage your care.

If you use medicine to treat your arthritis, make sure it doesn't make you sleepy. Ask your doctor about other treatments that can help with your pain, swelling, and soreness—treatments that will not make it difficult to drive safely.

Arthritis can limit your movement and strength, so try to stay fit and active. Doing so will help you to keep driving safely. Ask your doctor about exercises to keep your joints strong and supple.

What can I do when arthritis affects my driving?

Your doctor can refer you to a rehabilitation center or a specialist who can determine if, and how, your arthritis is affecting your driving. The specialist may offer training to improve your driving skills. That training may include how to use special devices that you can have installed in your car to make it easier for you to drive safely. You will need training on the use of those devices, however, before beginning to drive with them.

Improving your driving skills could help keep you and others around you safe. To find a driver rehabilitation specialist near you, go to www.aota.org/olderdriver and look up the name of a specialist in your state. You also can call hospitals and rehabilitation facilities to find an occupational therapist who can help with the driving skills assessment, remediation, and with choosing and using the special devices to make it easier for you to drive with arthritis. Depending on where you live, you may need to travel to nearby communities to find these services.

What if I have to cut back or give up driving?

You can keep your independence even if you have to cut back or give up on your driving. It may take planning ahead on your part, but it will get you to the places you want to go and the people you want to see. Consider the following options:

- Rides with family and friends
- Taxi cabs
- Shuttle buses or vans
- Public buses, trains and subways
- Walking

Also, senior centers and religious and other local service groups often offer transportation services for older adults in your community.

Who can I call for help with transportation?

- Call the ElderCare Locator at 800-677-1116 and ask for the phone number of your local Office on Aging, or go to their website at www.eldercare.gov.

- Contact your regional transit authority to find out which bus or train to take.

- Call Easter Seals Project ACTION (Accessible Community Transportation In Our Nation) at 800-659-6428 or go to their website at www.easterseals.com/transportation.

What about my safety belt?

Always wear your safety belt when you are driving or riding in a car. If arthritis makes it difficult for you to use your safety belt, speak with a driving specialist who can often help you find devices to make buckling up much easier. Make sure that every person who is riding with you also is buckled up. Wear your safety belt even if your car has air bags.

Chapter 50

Relationships and Arthritis

Chapter Contents

Section 50.1

A Spouse Can Ease the Pain of Arthritis

From "A Spouse Can Help Ease the Pain of Osteoarthritis," by the National Institute of Arthritis and Musculoskeletal and Skin Diseases (NIAMS, www.niams.nih.gov), part of the National Institutes of Health, July 2005.

With the help of a spouse, improvement can be made in the self-management of osteoarthritis (OA) pain. According to research funded in part by the National Institute of Arthritis and Musculoskeletal and Skin Diseases (NIAMS) at Duke University Medical Center, an intervention using spouse-assisted coping skills training and exercise training can improve physical fitness, pain coping, and self-efficacy in patients with OA of the knees.

The study, undertaken by Duke University Medical Center's Francis Keefe, PhD, and his colleagues at several other institutions, tested 72 married OA patients with persistent knee pain. The patients and their spouses were randomly assigned to receive spouse-assisted pain coping skills training and exercise training either in combination or alone. Still others were randomly assigned to receive only standard care. The data suggest that a combination of both spouse-assisted pain coping skills training and exercise training leads to more improvements than could be achieved with either intervention alone.

Over the past 15 years, spouse-assisted coping skills training and exercise training were developed as two approaches toward the self-management of OA pain. This resulted from the recognition that medical treatments have limitations. In this study, spouse-assisted training, either alone or in combination with exercise training, was found to produce improvements in coping and self-esteem. Exercise training, either alone or in combination with spouse-assisted coping skills training, caused improvements in physical fitness and muscle strength. The findings emphasize the importance of self-efficacy (a sense of feeling more in control of one's health) in adjusting to living with arthritis.

Osteoarthritis is the most common type of arthritis, especially among older people. It is one of the most frequent causes of physical

disability among adults, affecting more than 20 million people nation-
wide. People with osteoarthritis usually have joint pain and limited
movement. Unlike some other forms of arthritis, osteoarthritis affects
only joints and not internal organs.

Keefe FJ, et al. Effects of spouse-assisted coping skills training and
exercise training in patients with osteoarthritic knee pain: a randomized controlled study. *Pain* 2004;110: 539–549.

Section 50.2

Sexuality and Arthritis

How to deal with the physical challenges of arthritis and enjoy a healthy sex life

Dr. Carter Multz, a rheumatologist in San Jose, California, has seen
it too many times—couples where a spouse is living with arthritis and
as a result of the pain and other physical challenges their intimacy
is suffering and their relationship is strained. "They get frustrated,
they get frightened—afraid of getting hurt or hurting their partner,"
he says. "They have to work on that."

Both experts and people living with the disease agree that you can
have a healthy sex life with an unhealthy body but you need to work
on it by communicating with your partner.

There are plenty of solutions but they all involve the same approach—talking. "Sexual energy is a warm, magnetic energy," says Dr.
Jackson Rainer, a psychologist in Valdosta, Georgia, who counsels individuals and couples with chronic disease. "If you can't generate that
out of your own sense of friskiness, then a way to really develop attraction with another is to talk intimately—each tells the truth to the
other. Those truths are related to the physical sensations, the emotional feelings, and some sense of forecast of the future—what the

individual would like to happen." This talk should occur not after something has gone wrong in bed but when the couple is fully clothed, in an informal setting and with a cup of coffee since that's much less intimidating for discussing hot topics, Rainer says.

The couple should discuss what the person with arthritis can and can't do physically and how to adjust their sex life. The communication would then move into the bedroom and involve every little detail that may create tension. And if the couple does not feel like talking in bed, signs or code words can be used to show pleasure or pain. Both pleasure and pain vary in intensity and sometimes a scale of 1–10 is more precise than just a "yes" or "no" response.

The process of teaching the body map to a partner can be pleasurable and sexual. After all, that's what every couple goes through when they first discover each other sexually and it can rekindle their curiosity and desire to experiment.

"It takes a lot of work on both sides," says Waynette Porter, 28, of Myrtle Beach, South Carolina, who was diagnosed with juvenile rheumatoid arthritis when she was 7. "There's less spontaneity. There's times that I feel bad because I can't stand to be touched and I feel bad about that and thankfully he [her husband] understands that it's not me rejecting him, it's me rejecting to get more pain." The key to a successful marriage and a healthy sex life for Porter lies in communication and creativity.

One way to circumvent the pain and joint stiffness is to change the time of the day when the couple is sexually active, says Multz. "Usually late in the day fatigue and increased pain are in the way, in the morning there's stiffness, but you can take time before dinner to cuddle," he says. "Do little things that you can do. Love in the afternoon is a solution for people who are too stiff in the morning and too painful in the evening."

Another solution may be to take a dose of painkillers an hour or so earlier. A hot shower or bath before sex will also ease the joints and it can be shared with the partner as part of the foreplay. Pillows could be used to support various parts of the body and thus ease the pressure on the joints. If arthritis medications are causing dryness for women, over-the-counter lubricants can be helpful.

If none of those ideas relief the pain or stiffness, sex can be substituted for a gentle massage with a cream, skin to skin contact, tender touches, or just sleeping naked. "We focus too much on our genitals for sex," Rainer says. "It's critical to expand our definition to what is sexual, our biggest sex organ is our skin and our most powerful sex organ is our brain."

Whatever way a couple chooses to maintain intimacy, one thing is certain—benefits from sex are both psychological and physical. "During sex and especially after orgasm, the hormones released, most importantly oxytocin, act like an endorphin, a painkiller. It's a very significant source of pain relief during delivery and it also relieves the pain of arthritis," says Multz, who recently published a book titled *How to Treat Arthritis with Sex and Alcohol*. The physical and emotional benefits from sex can last for up to one or two days, Multz says.

It's all in your head: How to deal with the emotional challenges of arthritis and enjoy a healthy sex life

For Lyn Gottschalk, 50, from Green Bay, Wisconsin, living with rheumatoid arthritis for the past 20 years has meant not only constant pain and loss of motion, but also the loss of a marriage. When Gottschalk first got married, the disease had just begun to disable her and had little effect on her daily life or sexuality. As the rheumatoid arthritis progressed, it started taking its toll on her body and her sexual experience.

"I was certainly interested in him [her husband] and wanted to please him but I couldn't do the 'acrobatics' of it," she says. "Some days I couldn't at all. Although he said it was OK with him, it wasn't." Tensions in the bedroom went unaddressed and soon transferred to other aspects of daily life until the marriage slowly disintegrated. "I know what he wanted and he wanted the me that he first met," Gottschalk says. "In retrospect we should have sat down and talked about it."

Indeed, for some experts talking is such an integral part of the sexual experience as are kissing and fondling. "My favorite four-letter word for sex is talk," says Dr. Jackson Rainer, a psychologist in Valdosta, Georgia, who counsels individuals and couples with a chronic disease. "If a couple can't do this on their own, they can talk to a specialist that can walk them through the ways to talk intimately. It's a learned skill. If a couple is willing, they learn it just like they can learn a new dance."

Talking is a healthy way to communicate the physical and psychological problems associated with arthritis, but it's often seen as a last and much dreaded resource. In his long practice as a rheumatologist, Dr. Carter Multz of San Jose, California, has seen lots of patients who are embarrassed to talk about sex. For him that resistance comes from a combination of fear, apprehension, and maybe some embarrassment. "People don't want to admit that they are having a problem with sex," he says. "There's an emotional apprehension that they are a failure or just a psychosocial reluctance."

Problems with sexuality can arise not only from the physical challenges of arthritis but also from the psychological problems it often triggers such as depression, low self-esteem, and lack of desire. "Depression is defined as a numbing effect and so when you feel numb, it's hard to have any sense of liveliness and sexuality," Rainer says. "And sexuality is based on liveliness. And many medications are going to contribute as a side effect some type of depression."

Rainer says that many physicians will not interview for depression and so it's underreported among people with a chronic illness. "If they [people with arthritis] begin to lose any appetite for pleasure, zest for life, have difficulty concentrating, or are sleeping more than is normal for them, those may be markers for depression," he says. "A family practitioner or rheumatologist can prescribe an antidepressant and often that can be an excellent get-together drug. If it completely disrupts all activities of daily living, that's the time to turn to specialized help."

A lack of desire and low self-esteem are other common side effects of arthritis, which can be attributed to both certain medications and a person's emotional and physical pressure from the disease. "Loss of sexual desire is in many ways like a thermostat that's turned to low," Rainer says. "It's not unusual when people have experienced a change in health status and perception of themselves or a sense of disability, they'll find that their sexual energy is diminished." Rainer recommends talking to the partner and explaining the situation, as well as consulting a specialist who can help with the loss, limitations from the disease, and ways to regenerate sexual energy. If a partner gets defensive or takes some of those problems personally, then they can't speak with any degree of authenticity and that's a red flag for couples to seek professional help, Rainer says.

The thing to remember is that you need to redefine what it means to be sexual with your partner, Rainer says. "There's no one sex life. Every couple has its own sex life. You need to sit down with your partner and talk about how it can happen. There's no right or wrong answer. Touch, feel, shower together, all of that is very sexual."

Chapter 51

Starting a Family:
Pregnancy and Arthritis

Introduction

Background

Rheumatoid arthritis (RA) is a systemic, chronic, autoimmune inflammatory disease that affects about 1% of the U.S. population. The disease is approximately three times more common in women than in men and often affects women during their reproductive years.

Pregnancy alters the immune state, possibly contributing to a change in the course of RA. For decades, the ameliorating effects of pregnancy on the disease activity in women with RA have been observed. In 1998, researchers reported on a large prospective study of RA in women from late pregnancy to 6 months postpartum. In retrospect, 63% of the study patients reported improvement in disease activity, but only 16% were in remission at the third trimester.

In a 2008 study, researchers monitored 84 patients with RA for disease activity before conception, if possible, at each trimester of pregnancy, and at 6, 12, and 26 weeks postpartum. Disease activity was found to decrease during pregnancy but to increase after delivery. Among patients with at least moderate disease activity in the first trimester, at least 48% had a moderate response during pregnancy, while patients with low disease activity in the first trimester reported that their disease activity remained stable during pregnancy. Thirty-nine percent of patients had at least one moderate flare postpartum.

Pathophysiology

The pathophysiology of the ameliorating effect of pregnancy on RA activity during pregnancy remains unknown, but various theories have been proposed. Nonetheless, no single mechanism satisfactorily explains the observed improvement, and multiple factors are probably responsible for the decreased disease severity.

Some of the proposed theories are as follows:

- The effect of pregnancy on cell-mediated immunity (e.g., decreased cell-mediated immunity, predominance of helper T-cell 2 [TH2] cytokine profile)

- Elevated levels of anti-inflammatory cytokines, such as interleukin-1 receptor antagonist (IL-1Ra) and soluble tumor necrosis factor-alpha receptors (sTNFRs), and down-regulation of Th1 cytokines during pregnancy

- The effect of hormonal changes during pregnancy (e.g., increased cortisol, estrogen, and progestin levels)

- The effect of pregnancy on humoral immunity (e.g., a proportional decrease in immunoglobulin G lacking terminal galactose units, an elevated serum alpha-2 pregnancy-associated globulin [PAG] level)

- Altered neutrophil function during pregnancy (e.g., decreased neutrophil respiratory burst)

- The degree of HLA disparity between the mother and the fetus (the less genetically similar the mother and fetus, the more likely the RA will remit)

Possible causes for flare-ups during the postpartum period include the following:

- A decrease in the anti-inflammatory steroid levels
- Elevated levels of prolactin (i.e., proinflammatory hormone)
- Change in the neuroendocrine axis
- Change from a TH2 to a helper T-cell 1 cytokine profile

Frequency

United States: RA is observed in 1%–2% of the general population. Women of reproductive age are commonly affected; hence, pregnancy complicated by RA is not rare.

Mortality/Morbidity

- **Effect of RA on pregnancy:** Few studies have addressed the
  effects of RA on pregnancy. A 2006 study suggests that RA during pregnancy does not affect the rate of spontaneous abortion.

- **Effect of RA on fetal outcome:** There has been some contro-
  versy regarding fetal complications in mothers with RA; however,
  a 2006 study showed an increased risk for prematurity but no increased risk for low birth weight after adjusting for gestational
  age. In contrast, another 2006 study did show an increased rate
  of intrauterine growth restriction associated with RA.

- **Effect of RA on fertility:** RA does not appear to affect the
  likelihood of fertility; however, lower birth rates among women
  with RA have been reported. This may reflect choices by women
  to limit family sizes, as a recent study found that women diagnosed with RA prior to the birth of their first child had the few-
  est pregnancies and children.

Sex

RA is two to three times more common in women than in men.

Treatment

Medical Care

Preconception counseling:

- It is important to counsel patients about the teratogenicity and
  adverse effects of the medications used to treat rheumatoid arthritis (RA) before starting therapy. Patients may need a reminder
  about the importance of using contraception during DMARD [dis-
  ease-modifying antirheumatic drug] therapy, especially methotrexate, leflunomide, and cyclophosphamide.

- Educate patients that, because of a prolonged half-life, some of
  these medications may need to be discontinued several months
  before conception is planned.

- In addition to discontinuation, some patients who take DMARDs may require treatment with other medications to enhance their clearance.

Surgical Care

Cesarean delivery does not appear to be performed more commonly in patients with RA.

Consultations

- Obstetrician and gynecologist: Work closely with the rheumatologist, especially if patients are on disease-modifying agents or steroids.

- Ophthalmologist: Patients on hydroxychloroquine may need an eye examination to assess for drug toxicity.

Diet

- A low-fat, high-carbohydrate, high-fiber diet is recommended in pregnant patients with RA. Fish oils in moderate quantities can be taken during pregnancy.

- Over-the-counter herbal remedies should probably be avoided.

- Calcium supplementation is recommended to prevent osteoporosis.

Activity

Strenuous activity is best avoided in patients who experience RA flare-ups. Physical and occupational therapy can be beneficial in patients with RA.

Medication

The goals of pharmacotherapy are to reduce morbidity and to prevent complications.

None of the medications used in the treatment of arthritis is absolutely safe during pregnancy. Hence, the decision to use medications should be made after careful assessment of the risks and benefits in consultation with the patient. Pain control through nonpharmacologic management (e.g., paraffin baths, decreased physical activity, splinting, cold packs) can be used as adjunctive care.

Nonsteroidal Anti-Inflammatory Drugs

Nonsteroidal anti-inflammatory drugs (NSAIDs) should be stopped at the beginning of a menstrual cycle when conception is planned, as NSAIDs have been shown to interfere with blastocyst implantation in animal studies. Most traditional NSAIDs are considered Category B medications but should be used with caution in pregnancy. Possible effects on the mother include prolonged gestation and labor, increased peripartum blood loss, and increased anemia. The potential adverse effects in the fetus include impaired fetal renal function with oligohydramnios and increased cutaneous and intracranial bleeding. Monitoring for oligohydramnios should be considered if the pregnant patient is on prolonged NSAID therapy.

NSAIDs are contraindicated in the third trimester, as they promote premature closure of the ductus arteriosus, leading to fetal pulmonary hypertension. Ductal constriction can occur at any gestational age; however, one study noted a dramatic increase in indomethacin-induced ductal constriction at 31 weeks' gestation. Stopping NSAID therapy prior to 31 weeks' gestational age is prudent for potentially avoiding adverse effects in the fetus. Short-acting NSAIDs (e.g., ibuprofen, indomethacin, diclofenac) are preferred over long-acting agents.

Cyclooxygenase-2 (COX-2) inhibitors are generally considered Category C medications and potentially share the same side effects as traditional NSAIDs.

Corticosteroids

Corticosteroids are potent anti-inflammatory agents. They are considered relatively safe in pregnancy when used in low doses (i.e., <20 mg) and are considered Category B medications. Nonetheless, they may increase the maternal risk of hypertension, edema, gestational diabetes, osteoporosis, premature rupture of membranes, and small-for-gestational-age babies. One meta-analysis found a three and a half-fold increase in risk of cleft palate in fetuses with first-trimester exposure to corticosteroids.

The choice of glucocorticoid depends on whether the mother or the fetus needs to be treated. Hydrocortisone and cortisone cross the placenta, but 11 beta-dehydrogenase, a placental enzyme, converts hydrocortisone to cortisone, which is biologically inactive; thus, the fetus is exposed to only approximately 10% of the maternal dose. Therefore, if steroid treatment is desired for the mother, hydrocortisone,

cortisone, or prednisone should be chosen. Dexamethasone and beta-methasone cross the placenta with similar maternal and fetal concentrations; thus, they are the treatment of choice for fetal respiratory distress.

The lowest possible steroid dose needed to control activity should be used in pregnancy. Routine oral calcium and vitamin D supplementation is recommended. Stress doses of steroids should be used during labor and delivery if the mother received steroids (even low-dose) for more than 2–3 weeks during pregnancy, and the neonate should be monitored for evidence of adrenal insufficiency and infection.

Disease-Modifying Antirheumatic Drugs

Methotrexate, a folic acid antagonist, is contraindicated in pregnancy (Category X medication) because it is an abortifacient and has teratogenic effects, including craniofacial abnormalities, limb defects, and CNS [central nervous system] defects such as anencephaly, hydrocephaly, and meningomyelopathy, especially with first-trimester exposure. Because the active metabolites have a long half-life, methotrexate must be discontinued at least 3 months prior to conception; treatment with folic acid should be continued in that period and throughout pregnancy.

Leflunomide, a pyrimidine synthesis inhibitor, is also a Category X medication, and is extremely teratogenic and absolutely contraindicated in pregnancy. Its half-life is 14–15 days, but the active metabolite undergoes extensive enterohepatic circulation; thus, the drug takes up to 2 years to be undetectable in plasma. Therefore, discontinuation of the drug before conception is insufficient. The drug needs to be eliminated with administration of cholestyramine 8 g 3 times daily for 11 days. Plasma levels of less than 0.02 mg/L should be verified with two separate tests at least 2 weeks apart. If unacceptably high levels persist, additional cholestyramine may be given.

Sulfasalazine, a dihydrofolate reductase inhibitor, is a Category B medication. Sulfasalazine does not increase fetal morbidity or mortality and is considered safe in pregnancy.

Azathioprine, although a Category D medication, can be used if the benefits outweigh the risks. Although fewer women who received azathioprine for renal transplantation completed their pregnancies, no increase in fetal anomalies was observed. Azathioprine crosses the placenta, but the fetal liver lacks the enzyme inosinate pyrophosphorylase, which converts azathioprine to its active metabolite, 6-mercaptopurine;

thus, the fetus is protected from the agent's teratogenic effects. A retrospective cohort study of 155 patients found no statistical difference in conception failures, abortion secondary to a birth defect, major congenital malformations, neoplasia, or increased infections among patients taking 6-mercaptopurine compared with controls. A study of 101 pregnancies of women with inflammatory bowel disease on azathioprine at doses of 100 mg/day revealed no association with poor pregnancy outcomes.

Hydroxychloroquine, an antimalarial agent, is considered a Category C medication. Previous reports of fetal toxicity with hydroxychloroquine were based on effects of chloroquine, which has two and a half times the amount of tissue deposition as hydroxychloroquine. No real fetal toxicity is associated with hydroxychloroquine at the dosage used for rheumatoid arthritis (RA) and connective-tissue disease (6.5 mg/kg body weight). Several studies and case series have provided further evidence that no fetal toxicity was associated with hydroxychloroquine therapy in mothers.

Biologic Agents

Biologic agents are now commonly used for the treatment of RA; however, limited data are available on their use in pregnancy.

Medications in the anti-TNF [tumor necrosis factor]-alpha class (i.e., currently, etanercept, adalimumab, and infliximab) are commonly used in the treatment of RA. They have been labeled by the FDA [U.S. Food and Drug Administration] as Class B medications, as no adequate human studies have shown risk, but animal studies have shown no harm done to the fetus. Thus far, no randomized, blinded, placebo-controlled trials have been completed to demonstrate any potential teratogenicity. Numerous case reports have shown positive outcomes with anti-TNF-alpha use in pregnancy, with an incidence of spontaneous abortion and birth defects similar to that in the general population. Compared with healthy controls, the risk of preterm delivery and poor growth of offspring in all patients with RA is increased, but this is believed to be more attributable to the underlying systemic disease rather than to use of TNF blockers.

The Organization of Teratology and Information Specialist (OTIS) Project is the largest prospective cohort study to date evaluating anti-TNF-alpha medications and other medications used to treat autoimmune disease. This study, led by the University of California at San Diego, is maintaining a database of patients taking etanercept and adalimumab during first-trimester gestation.

The results for adalimumab have been updated and analyzed to May 2008. So far in this group, 30 patients have been enrolled, with an additional retrospective case series involving 66 patients whose outcomes have been monitored. Based on preliminary data, no concerns have been raised regarding the risks of adverse outcomes with adalimumab exposure, and rates of congenital defects are in range of the general population. As of October 2006, 48 pregnant patients had been enrolled and received treatment in the OTIS etanercept prospective cohort study. Based on preliminary data from this ongoing study, no concerns have been raised or consistent abnormalities found. Because of the small sample size, no definitive conclusions about adalimumab or etanercept can be made at this time.

Rituximab (Rituxan), a monoclonal antibody that inhibits CD20 antigen on B lymphocytes, is currently a Pregnancy Category C medication. Rituximab is indicated for the treatment for moderate to severe RA. Case reports on the use of rituximab during pregnancy have been reported in the oncology literature. Case reports have also shown that rituximab therapy results in detectable levels of the drug in cord blood and results in B-cell depletion in both mother and neonate. Recovery of B-cell levels in the neonate has been reported to occur at age 3–4 months and does not appear to impair antibody formation to immunizations. The dosing of rituximab in case reports was 375 mg/m^2 in one to six cycles. Although it is unknown whether rituximab is excreted in human milk, IgG [immunoglobulin G] is present in human milk, and rituximab has been detected in the milk of monkeys.

Immunomodulators

Anakinra (Kineret), an interleukin-1 receptor antagonist, is used to treat severe RA. No studies or case reports using this medication during human pregnancy or lactation were found in the literature nor reported in data provided by the drug manufacturer. Anakinra is a Pregnancy Category B medication. No adverse effects have been reported in rats and rabbits receiving up to 100 times the recommended human dose. No data are available to indicate whether anakinra is excreted in human milk.

Abatacept (Orencia) is a selective costimulation modulator that binds to CD80 and CD86, thereby inhibiting activation of T lymphocytes and interactions with CD28. Abatacept is indicated for the treatment of moderate to severe RA. No human studies have investigated the use of this medication during pregnancy or lactation. Similarly, no case reports have described abatacept therapy in human pregnancy or lactation in the literature or in drug company records.

Abatacept, which is a Pregnancy Category C medication, has been found to cross the placenta and be excreted in rat milk. No teratogenic effects were reported in mice or rabbits treated with a dose 29 times greater than that recommended for humans. Similarly, no adverse effects in offspring were reported when rats were treated with three times the human dose throughout the lactation period. In a sample of 20 rats (10 male, 10 female) treated with 11 times the human dose of abatacept, one female offspring had an increased response of T-cell–dependent antibodies and experienced thyroid inflammation.

Chapter 52

Financial, Employment, and Legal Concerns

Chapter Contents

Section 52.1

Financial Planning Questions for People with Rheumatic Disease

"A Few Financial Planning Questions for People with Fibromyalgia,"
reprinted with permission of the National Fibromyalgia Association
(www.fmaware.org), © 2007.

Everyone struggles with financial planning—just look at all the books and magazines published on the topic. For those of us with fibromyalgia, or any chronic illness, making decisions about finances can seem overwhelming. Here are 10 questions to help you get started.

1. Is 'fibro-fog' affecting your ability to make financial decisions?

Making major decisions requires a clear head, yet we often forget that minor decisions can have a profound impact on our financial health. If you suffer from 'fibro-fog,' you may not even realize that you forgot to pay a bill or are making subtraction errors in your checkbook. Trying to analyze your health insurance options or other more complex tasks may be impossible. If you are having trouble with day-to-day financial tasks, ask a family member or friend to help out.

2. Are you compromising your health because you cannot afford to visit your doctor?

Going to the doctor is expensive, but the long-term cost of not going will be greater. You will miss symptom and medication monitoring, possible new treatment options, and an objective look at your health. Ask the office manager about payment options. Another alternative is to participate in a research study as a way of getting medical care. (You can find studies at http://www.fmaware.org in the research section and http://www.clinicaltrials.gov.)

3. Are you compromising your health because you cannot afford prescription medication?

Discuss alternatives with your doctor. Is the benefit from a newer drug worth the added cost? Are sample packs available so you can try a new drug before purchasing a month's supply? Is a generic available? Some drug manufacturers have programs to assist people who cannot afford their medications; check with your pharmacist.

4. Do you have, or can you get, affordable health insurance?

Private health insurance is prohibitively expensive; last year I was given a quote of $2,200.00 per month for minimal coverage! Affordability is the key here. Can you get insurance through your employer? Do you have a spouse or domestic partner whose employer offers health insurance for family members? Online, visit *Kiplinger Personal Finance*'s article, "Your Own Health Insurance" for advice on purchasing private insurance: http://www.kiplinger.com.

5. Are you taking good care of yourself physically and emotionally?

Planning for wellness, not just illness, has benefits far beyond the physical. Medical bills are one of the leading causes for personal bankruptcy, so doing what you can to stay healthy only makes sense. Walking, for example, is a free activity which lessens the chances that you will develop diabetes or arthritis—thus improving your health and saving you health care costs, lost days of work, and so forth.

6. Is there someone you trust to discuss financial plans with?

Certified financial planners can do this, but a trusted family member may be the first person you want to talk to. Be honest, and don't forget that fibro-fog may be affecting you.

7. Are you planning for the future?

If you are working, are you contributing to a 401(k) or other plan? Have you considered the pros and cons of long-term care insurance? The federal government has publications on these topics available online and in print form, as do other organizations such as Consumer

Action and AARP [American Association of Retired Persons]. (See http://www.consumerreports.org and http://www.consumer-action .org.)

8. Are you spending more than you can afford?

We're addicted to credit and to having things now. The movement to simplify your life stems, in part, from a desire to stop the credit merry-go-round. Can't figure out where your money goes? Get a notebook and write down every cent you spend; just writing it down will help you curb impulse spending. If you have concerns about your spending habits, the federal government has publications to assist you. (See "Taking Control of Your Finances." http://www.pueblo.gsa.gov.)

9. Is your health so compromised that you should be on disability?

The National Fibromyalgia Association provides information about disability issues. Getting disability from the Social Security Administration is not easy and takes perseverance, but can ease your financial problems if you succeed.

10. Are you expecting to make any major life changes in the near future?

Retirement, becoming a parent, getting married, moving, getting divorced, changing jobs—the list is long, and every change can have serious ramifications for your financial health. Will you have health insurance after your divorce? Does your new employer offer it? Look before you make changes. Ask questions. Plan carefully.

Section 52.2

Work and Legal Rights If You're Disabled by Arthritis

"Your Legal Rights If Disabled by Arthritis," © 2002 Hospital
for Special Surgery (www.hss.edu). Reprinted with permission.
Reviewed by David A. Cooke, MD, FACP, July 5, 2009.

If your arthritis is severe enough to interfere with your work, you may benefit from the Americans with Disabilities Act (ADA). Passed by Congress in 1990, the ADA guarantees equal opportunity for individuals with disabilities in public accommodations, transportation, state and local government services, telecommunications, and, most importantly, employment.

The ADA defines a disability as a physical or mental impairment that substantially limits one or more major life activities, such as seeing, hearing, speaking, walking, breathing, performing manual tasks, learning, caring for yourself, and working. The law requires employers with 15 or more workers to provide the same opportunities to the disabled as those available to people without disabilities. It prohibits discrimination in hiring, promotions, training, pay, social activities, and other employment benefits and privileges. And they are required to make a "reasonable accommodation" if you have a known physical or mental limitation, unless such accommodation results in undue hardship for the employer.

Employers cannot ask questions about your disability before a job offer is made. You must meet all the requirements of a position that you hold or seek. You should be able to perform the functions of that position, either with or without reasonable accommodation. An employer may select an applicant who is the most qualified—not based on a disability. However, if you have a disability, you may seek a reasonable accommodation that would enable you to perform the essential functions of the job.

Arthritis is the number one cause of disability. Symptoms such as painful or stiff joints, fatigue, and limitations in movement can make walking, lifting, and other tasks difficult. Unlike some other disabilities, people with rheumatic diseases often have disabilities that their employers can't "see"—and you may feel uncomfortable speaking up about your problems.

So what are reasonable, and unreasonable, accommodations? How can you talk about your disability and express your need for accommodation? And what can you do to ensure that your rights are protected?

Reasonable Accommodations

The ADA defines "reasonable accommodations" as changes or modifications in the workplace that allow you to perform the job's essential functions without causing undue hardship on the employer. An accommodation that causes significant expense or difficulty is considered an undue hardship under the ADA. However, keep in mind that the nature and cost of the accommodation are weighed against the financial resources of the company, the number of employees, and the size of the budget, among other factors. That means that the same accommodation could be reasonable in one workplace but create an undue hardship in another. The Job Accommodation Network, a service of the President's Committee on the Employment of People with Disabilities, suggests that most accommodations cost less than $1,000.

Reasonable accommodations by employers might include:

- part-time or modified work schedule;
- adaptive tools, supplies or equipment, such as a chair with armrests, changing the height of a desk, a computer armrest, or an electric stapler;
- restructuring a job to cut out activities you have trouble with, such as lifting, reaching, kneeling, stooping, or sitting for long periods;
- reassignment to a vacant position you are qualified for (if you are still unable to perform the original job, even with accommodations).

Unreasonable accommodations might include:

- changing the job requirements to fit your qualifications;
- creating a new position that you can do despite your disability;
- hiring an additional worker to handle the workload you can't handle because of your disability;

- providing an accommodation that is too costly or extensive for the company's resources or that disrupts business operations.

Talking to Your Employer and Confidentiality

An employer is not required to make accommodations until an employee with a disability asks for them. But it can become a "Catch-22" as you weigh the pros and cons between a need to ask for changes that help you do your job and a desire to protect your privacy. The ADA protects the confidentiality of an employee's medical information, such as on any forms you may complete. However, little can be done to control the way information may get passed around through office gossip.

Disclosure in the workplace is a very personal decision, so that's a good time to ask yourself: Why am I doing this? What are my goals? If you decide that the pros outweigh the cons, arm yourself with knowledge of the law and your rights, and schedule a meeting with your employer. In discussing your situation, describe how your arthritis may affect your work. A doctor's note can help to explain your disability. Explain that you are trying to find ways to resolve the problem that will benefit the company and yourself. You can also offer suggestions for the changes—and provide an estimate of the costs of such changes, based on your research. Be assertive about your needs without imposing or placing burdens on the company or co-workers.

Relationship with Coworkers

When coworkers see that you are getting additional assistance, or when some of the duties that you have difficulty doing are given to them, conflict may arise. Roberta Horton, who is the Program and Research Manager, Department of Patient Care and Quality Management at Hospital for Special Surgery, suggests the following:

- Decide how much of your diagnosis you want to share with co-workers.

- Discuss with your employer how best to share your information.

- Have your employer's support before speaking to coworkers.

- Understand how any accommodations made by your employer may affect your coworkers, including possible increased responsibilities for them.

571

- If feasible, offer to take on duties from coworkers in exchange for their doing tasks that you find difficult.

- Acknowledge your appreciation of accommodations made by your employer and coworkers.

The Evolving Law

More than a decade after the ADA was passed, interpretation of the fine points of the law continues to evolve. For example, in *Sutton v. United Airlines, Inc.* and in *Murphy v. United Parcel Service, Inc.*, the Supreme Court ruled that the plaintiffs were not substantially limited in any major life activity if the limiting effects of their impairment were controlled by corrective measures, such as medications or assistive aids.

Such decisions narrow the scope of the ADA and could affect the number of claims filed under the ADA. It is therefore important to keep up to date on changes that might affect you.

Protecting Your Rights under the ADA

If you have disagreements with your employer, try to settle them through negotiation, mediation, and other forms of communication. If you still feel that you have been treated unfairly, you may consider filing a complaint with the Equal Employment Opportunity Commission (EEOC). To do so, you must file within 180 days from the time the discriminatory incident occurred. (You may also hire an attorney or contact the Bar Association for help in finding attorneys specializing in labor and employment law.)

Keep copies of memos, letters, and reports regarding your case. If your complaint is upheld, you may be entitled to hiring, promotion, reinstatement, back pay, or reasonable accommodation.

Where to Get Help

New York

Arthritis Foundation
New York Chapter
122 East 42nd Street, 18th Floor
New York, NY 10168
Phone: 212-984-8700

The Association of the Bar of the City of New York
42 West 44th Street
New York, NY 10036
Phone: 212-382-6665

EEOC New York District Office
201 Varick Street, Room 1009
New York, NY 10014
Phone: 212-741-8815/
212-741-2783
TTY: 212-741-3080

Nationwide

Americans with Disabilities Act
U.S. Department of Justice
950 Pennsylvania Avenue, NW
Civil Rights Division
Disability Rights Section—NYA
Washington, DC 20530
Toll-Free: 800-514-0301
TTY: 800-514-0383
Website: www.ada.gov

Arthritis Foundation
P.O. Box 7669
Atlanta, GA 30357-0669
Toll-Free: 800-283-7800
Website: www.arthritis.org
E-mail: arthritisfoundation
@arthritis.org

U.S. Equal Employment Opportunity Commission
EEOC Headquarters
1801 L Street, NW
Washington, DC 20507
Phone: 202-663-4900
TTY: 202-663-4494
EEOC Field Offices
Toll-Free: 800-669-4000
TTY: 800-669-6820

Job Accommodation Network
P.O. Box 6080
Morgantown, WV 26506-6080
Toll-Free: 800-526-7234
TTY: 877-781-9403
Fax: 304-293-5407
Website: www.jan.wvu.edu
E-mail: jan@jan.wvu.edu

For information on the ADA, accommodations, resources, and products designed for people with disabilities.

Part Six

Additional Help
and Information

Chapter 53

Glossary of Terms Related to Arthritis and Rheumatic Diseases

acupuncture: The use of fine needles inserted at specific points on the skin. Primarily used for pain relief, acupuncture may be a helpful component of an osteoarthritis treatment plan for some people.

acute pain: Acute pain often begins suddenly—after a fall or injury, for example—and lasts no longer than 6 weeks.

analgesics: Medications designed to relieve pain. Analgesics used for pain include both prescription and over-the-counter products. Some are made to be taken orally, and others are rubbed onto the skin.

ankylosing spondylitis: A form of arthritis that affects the spine, the sacroiliac joints, and sometimes the hips and shoulders. In severe cases, the joints of the spine fuse and the spine becomes rigid.

antinuclear antibody (ANA): A type of antibody directed against the nuclei of the body's cells. Because these antibodies can be found in the blood of children with lupus and some other rheumatic disorders, testing for them can be useful in diagnosis.

arthritis: Literally means joint inflammation. It is a general term for more than 100 of the rheumatic diseases. Arthritis causes joint swelling, pain, and stiffness.

This glossary contains terms excerpted from documents produced by the National Institute of Arthritis and Musculoskeletal and Skin Diseases (NIAMS, www.niams.nih.gov).

577

arthroscopic surgery: Repairing the interior of a joint by inserting a microscope-like device and surgical tools through small cuts rather than one, large surgical cut.

autoimmune disease: A disease that results when the immune system mistakenly attacks the body's own tissues.

biologics: A class of drugs, also known as biologic response modifiers, which target the immune response.

biomarkers: Physical signs or biological substances that indicate changes in bone or cartilage. Doctors believe they may one day be able to use biomarkers for diagnosing osteoarthritis before it causes noticeable joint damage and for monitoring the progression of the disease and its responsiveness to treatment.

bone spurs: Small growths of bone that can occur on the edges of a joint affected by osteoarthritis. These growths are also known as osteophytes.

Bouchard nodes: Small, bony knobs associated with osteoarthritis of the hand that can occur on the middle joints of the fingers.

bursa: A small sac of tissue located between a bone and other moving structures such as muscles, skin, or tendons. The bursa contains a lubricating fluid that allows these structures to glide smoothly.

bursitis: Inflammation or irritation of a bursa.

cartilage: A hard but slippery coating on the end of each bone. The breakdown of joint cartilage is the primary feature of osteoarthritis.

cervical spine: The upper portion of the spine closest to the skull. The cervical spine comprises seven vertebrae.

chondrocytes: Components of cartilage. Chondrocytes are cells that produce cartilage, are found throughout cartilage, and help it stay healthy as it grows. Sometimes, however, they release certain enzymes that destroy collagen and other proteins.

chondroitin sulfate: A naturally existing substance in joint cartilage that is believed to draw fluid into the cartilage. Chondroitin is often taken in supplement form along with glucosamine as a treatment for osteoarthritis.

chronic pain: Chronic pain may begin either quickly or slowly; it generally lasts for 3 months or more.

collagen: A family of fibrous proteins that are components of cartilage. Collagens are the building blocks of skin, tendon, bone, and other connective tissues.

corticosteroids: Powerful anti-inflammatory hormones made naturally in the body or synthetically for use as medicine. Corticosteroids may be taken by mouth or intravenously, or they may be injected into the affected joints to temporarily suppress the inflammation that causes arthritis-related swelling, warmth, loss of motion, and pain.

Crohn disease: Inflammation of the small intestine or colon that causes diarrhea, cramps, and weight loss.

cyclooxygenase-2 (COX-2) inhibitors: A relatively new class of nonsteroidal anti-inflammatory drugs that are formulated to relieve pain and inflammation.

disk: A circular piece of cushioning tissue situated between each of the spine's vertebrae. Each disk has a strong outer cover and a soft jelly-like filling.

disease-modifying antirheumatic drugs: A class of medication that can slow or potentially stop the activity of rheumatic disorders, such as rheumatoid arthritis, often by suppressing the overactive immune system.

epicondylitis: A painful and sometimes disabling swelling of the tissues of the elbow.

erythrocyte sedimentation rate (ESR or sed rate): A test that measures how quickly red blood cells fall to the bottom of a test tube of unclotted blood. Rapidly descending cells (an elevated sed rate) indicate inflammation in the body.

estrogen: The major sex hormone in women. Estrogen is known to play a role in regulation of bone growth. Research suggests that estrogen may also have a protective effect on cartilage.

facet joints: The joints where the vertebrae of the spine connect to one another. Arthritis of the facet joints is believed to be an uncommon cause of back pain.

fibromyalgia: A condition of widespread muscle pain, fatigue, and tender points on the body. Fibromyalgia is one cause of low back pain.

flare: A period in the course of disease in which symptoms become worse.

glucosamine: A substance that occurs naturally in the body, providing the building blocks to make and repair cartilage.

gout: Gout is a painful condition that occurs when the bodily waste product uric acid is deposited as needle-like crystals in the joints and/or soft tissues. In the joints, these uric acid crystals cause inflammatory arthritis, which in turn leads to intermittent swelling, redness, heat, pain, and stiffness in the joints.

Heberden nodes: Small, bony knobs associated with osteoarthritis of the hand that can occur on the joints of the fingers closest to the nail.

hyaluronic acid: A substance that gives healthy joint fluid its viscous (slippery) property and that may be reduced in people with osteoarthritis. For some people with osteoarthritis of the knee, replacing hyaluronic acid with injections of agents referred to as viscosupplements is useful for increasing lubrication, reducing pain, and improving function.

immune response modifiers: A relatively new class of medications used in arthritis treatment that are based on compounds made by living cells. These compounds modify the action of the immune system by blocking chemicals that fuel inflammation and tissue destruction.

immune system: A complex network of specialized cells and organs that work together to defend the body against attacks by "foreign" invaders such as bacteria and viruses. In some rheumatic conditions, it appears that the immune system does not function properly and may even work against the body.

immunosuppressive drugs: Medicines that reduce the immune response and therefore may relieve some symptoms of arthritis and rheumatic disease.

inflammation: A reaction of tissues to injury or disease, marked by four signs: swelling, redness, heat, and pain.

joint: A junction where two bones meet. Most joints are composed of cartilage, joint space, the fibrous capsule, the synovium, and ligaments.

joint capsule: A tough membrane sac that holds the bones and other joint parts together.

juvenile idiopathic arthritis (JIA): A term for various types of chronic arthritis in children. JIA can cause swelling, pain, damage to the joints, and, in some cases, damage to other parts of the body. Juvenile idiopathic arthritis has replaced juvenile rheumatoid arthritis as the preferred term for the same condition.

juvenile rheumatoid arthritis (JRA): A term used to describe the most common types of arthritis in children. It is characterized by joint pain, swelling, tenderness, warmth, and stiffness that lasts for more than 6 weeks and cannot be explained by other causes. Previously, juvenile rheumatoid arthritis was the preferred term, but recently it has been replaced by juvenile idiopathic arthritis.

ligaments: Tough bands of connective tissue that attach bones to each other, providing stability.

lumbar spine: The lower portion of the spine. The lumbar spine comprises five vertebrae.

magnetic resonance imaging (MRI): A procedure that provides high resolution computerized images of internal body tissues. This procedure uses a strong magnet that passes a force through the body to create these images.

muscles: Bundles of specialized cells that contract and relax to produce movement when stimulated by nerves.

nonsteroidal anti-inflammatory drugs (NSAIDs): A class of medications that work to reduce pain, fever, and inflammation by blocking substances called prostaglandins. Some NSAIDs, such as ibuprofen (Motrin) and naproxen sodium (Aleve), are available over the counter, while many are available only with a doctor's prescription.

osteoarthritis: A disease in which the cartilage that cushions the ends of the bones at the joints wears away, leading to pain, stiffness, and bony overgrowths, called spurs. It is the most common form of arthritis and becomes more likely with age.

osteophytes: Small growths of bone that can appear on the edges of a joint affected by osteoarthritis. These growths are also known as bone spurs.

osteoporosis: A condition in which the bones become porous and brittle and break easily.

pericarditis: Inflammation of the pericardium, the membrane that surrounds the heart. Pericarditis is a feature of some rheumatic disorders, including systemic arthritis.

pleuritis: Inflammation of the pleura, the membrane that covers the lungs and lines the inner chest wall. Pleuritis is a feature of some rheumatic disorders, including systemic arthritis.

prolotherapy: An unregulated, unproven therapy for chronic musculoskeletal pain. Prolotherapy uses an irritant solution, which is injected into painful ligaments and adjacent joint spaces to promote inflammation and subsequent healing.

proteoglycans: Components of cartilage. Made up of proteins and sugars, strands of proteoglycans interweave with collagens and form a mesh-like tissue. This allows cartilage to flex and absorb physical shock.

pseudogout: A condition often mistaken for gout that results from the deposit of calcium phosphate crystals (not uric acid crystals as in gout) in the joints and other tissues. This condition is also called chondrocalcinosis.

psoriasis: An autoimmune disease characterized by a red scaly rash that is often located over the surfaces of the elbows, knees, and scalp, and around or in the ears, navel, genitals, or buttocks. Approximately 10 to 15 percent of people with psoriasis develop an associated arthritis referred to as psoriatic arthritis.

reactive arthritis: A form of arthritis that can develop after an intestinal or urinary tract infection. The disease causes pain and swelling around the joints and in the spine. People with the disease may also experience swelling of the eye and the reproductive and urinary tracts.

remission: A period when the symptoms of arthritis improve or disappear completely. Sometimes remission is permanent, but more often it is punctuated by flares of the disease.

rheumatic disorders: Disorders that affect the joints and soft tissues, causing pain, and sometimes inflammation, tissue damage, or disability.

rheumatoid arthritis: A form of arthritis in which the immune system attacks the tissues of the joints, leading to pain, inflammation, and eventually joint damage and malformation. It typically begins at a younger age than osteoarthritis does, causes swelling and redness in joints, and may make people feel sick, tired, and uncommonly feverish. Rheumatoid arthritis may also affect skin tissue, the lungs, the eyes, or the blood vessels.

rheumatoid factor: An antibody that is found often in the blood of adults with rheumatoid arthritis and once in a while in children with juvenile arthritis. Testing for the antibody may be useful as a diagnostic tool.

sacroiliac joints: The joints where the spine and pelvis attach. The sacroiliac joints are often affected by types of arthritis referred to as spondyloarthropathies.

spinal fusion: The surgical joining of two more vertebrae together, usually with bone grafts and hardware. The resulting fused vertebrae are stable but immobile. Spinal fusion is used as a treatment for spondylolisthesis, scoliosis, herniated disks, and spinal stenosis.

spinal stenosis: The narrowing of the spinal canal (through which the spinal cord runs), often by the overgrowth of bone caused by osteoarthritis of the spine.

spondyloarthropathy: A form of arthritis that primarily affects the spine and sacroiliac joints.

stem cells: Primitive cells, usually taken from the bone marrow, which can transform into other kinds of cells, such as muscle or bone cells. In the future, researchers hope to be able to insert stem cells into cartilage and stimulate them to replace cartilage damaged by arthritis or injury.

synovial fluid: A fluid secreted by the synovium that lubricates the joint and keeps the cartilage smooth and healthy.

synovium: A thin membrane inside the joint capsule that secretes synovial fluid.

systemic: Refers to a disease that can affect the whole body, rather than just a specific organ or joints.

tendonitis: Inflammation or irritation of a tendon.

tendons: Tough, fibrous cords that connect muscles to bones.

topical treatment: Medicine, such as a cream or rinse, which is put directly on the affected body part.

transcutaneous electrical nerve stimulation (TENS): A technique that uses a small electronic device to direct mild electric pulses to nerve endings that lie beneath the skin in a painful area. TENS may relieve some arthritis pain. It seems to work by blocking pain messages to the brain and by modifying pain perception.

uric acid: A substance that results from the breakdown of purines, which are part of all human tissue and are found in many foods.

vasculitis: Inflammation of the blood vessels. Vasculitis is a feature of a number of rheumatic disorders.

vertebrae: The individual bones that make up the spinal column.

vertebroplasty: A minimally invasive surgical procedure that involves injecting a cement-like mixture into a fractured vertebra to relieve pain and stabilize the spine.

x-ray: A procedure in which low-level radiation is passed through the body to produce a picture called a radiograph. X-rays of joints affected by osteoarthritis can show such things as cartilage loss, bone damage, and bone spurs.

Chapter 54

Directory of Organizations That Help People with Arthritis and Their Families

Government Agencies That Provide Information about Arthritis

Agency for Healthcare Research and Quality
Office of Communications and Knowledge Transfer
540 Gaither Road
Second Floor
Rockville, MD 20850
Phone: 301-427-1364
Fax: 301-427-1873
Website: www.ahrq.gov

Americans with Disabilities Act
U.S. Department of Justice
950 Pennsylvania Avenue, NW
Civil Rights Division
Disability Rights Section—NYA
Washington, DC 20530
Toll-Free: 800-514-0301
TTY: 800-514-0383
Website: www.ada.gov

Resources in this chapter were compiled from several sources deemed reliable; all contact information was verified and updated in July 2009. This chapter contains text from "Patient Assistance Programs for Rheumatology-Related Drugs," © 2009 American College of Rheumatology (www.rheumatology.org). Reprinted with permission.

Centers for Disease Control and Prevention
1600 Clifton Road
Atlanta, GA 30333
Toll-Free: 800-CDC-INFO
(232-4636)
Phone: 404-639-3311
Website: www.cdc.gov
E-mail: cdcinfo@cdc.gov

Centers for Medicare and Medicaid Services
7500 Security Boulevard
Baltimore, MD 21244-1850
Toll-Free: 800-633-4227
Website: www.medicare.gov

Healthfinder®
National Health Information Center
P.O. Box 1133
Washington, DC 20013-1133
Toll-Free: 800-336-4797
Phone: 301-565-4167
Fax: 301-984-4256
Website: www.healthfinder.gov
E-mail: healthfinder@nhic.org

National Cancer Institute
Cancer Information Service
6116 Executive Boulevard
Room 3036A
Bethesda, MD 20892-8322
Toll-Free: 800-4-CANCER
(422-6237)
TTY Toll-Free: 800-332-8615
Website: www.cancer.gov
E-mail:
cancergovstaff@mail.nih.gov

National Center for Complementary and Alternative Medicine
National Institutes of Health
9000 Rockville Pike
Bethesda, MD 20892
Toll-Free: 888-644-6226
TTY: 866-464-3615
Fax: 866-464-3616
Website: nccam.nih.gov
E-mail: info@nccam.nih.gov

National Heart, Lung and Blood Institute
P.O. Box 30105
Bethesda, MD 20824-0105
Phone: 301 592 8573
Fax: 301-592-8563
Website: www.nhlbi.nih.gov
E-mail: nhlbiinfo@nhlbi.nih.gov

National Institute of Arthritis and Musculoskeletal and Skin Diseases
National Institutes of Health
1 AMS Circle
Bethesda, MD 20892-3675
Toll Free: 877-22-NIAMS
(226-4267)
TTY: 301–565–2966
Phone: 301-495-4484
Fax: 301-718-6366
Website: www.niams.nih.gov
E-mail:
NIAMSinfo@mail.nih.gov

National Institute of Diabetes, Digestive and Kidney Diseases
Building 31, Rm. 9A06
31 Center Drive, MSC 2560
Bethesda, MD 20892-2560
Phone: 301-496-3583
Website: www.niddk.nih.gov

National Institute of Neurological Disorders and Stroke
NIH Neurological Institute
P.O. Box 5801
Bethesda, MD 20824
Toll-Free: 800-352-9424
Phone: 301-496-5751
TTY: 301-468-5981
Website: www.ninds.nih.gov
E-mail: braininfo@ninds.nih.gov

National Institutes of Health
9000 Rockville Pike
Bethesda, MD 20892
Phone: 301-496-4000
TTY: 301-402-9612
Website: www.nih.gov
E-mail: NIHinfo@od.nih.gov

National Institute on Aging
Building 31, Room 5C27
31 Center Drive, MSC 2292
Bethesda, MD 20892
Phone: 301-496-1752
TTY: 800-222-4225
Fax: 301-496-1072
Website: www.nia.nih.gov

National Women's Health Information Center
8270 Willow Oaks Corporate Dr.
Fairfax, VA 22031
Toll-Free: 800-994-9662
TDD: 888-220-5446
Website:
www.womenshealth.gov

U.S. Department of Health and Human Services
200 Independent Avenue, SW
Washington, DC 20201
Toll-Free: 877-696-6775
Website: www.hhs.gov

U.S. Food and Drug Administration
10903 New Hampshire Avenue
Silver Spring, MD 20903
Toll-Free: 888-463-6332
Website: www.fda.gov

U.S. National Library of Medicine
8600 Rockville Pike
Bethesda, MD 20894
Toll-Free: 888-346-3656
Phone: 301-594-5983
TDD: 800-735-2258
Fax: 301-402-1384
Website: www.nlm.nih.gov
E-mail: custserv@nlm.nih.gov

Private Agencies That Provide Information about Arthritis

AllAboutArthritis.com
DePuy Orthopaedics, Inc.
700 Orthopaedic Drive
Warsaw, IN 46582
Phone: 574-267-8143
Fax: 574-371-4865
Website:
www.allaboutarthritis.com

American Academy of Family Physicians
11400 Tomahawk Creek Parkway
Leawood, KS 66211-2680
Toll-Free: 800-274-2237
Fax: 913-906-6075
Website: www.aafp.org

American Academy of Orthopaedic Surgeons
6300 North River Road
Rosemont, IL 60018-4262
Phone: 847-823-7186
Fax: 847-823-8125
Website: www.aaos.org
E-mail: pemr@aaos.org

American Academy of Pain Management
13947 Mono Way #A
Sonora, CA 95370
Phone: 209-533-9744
Fax: 209-533-9750
Website:
www.aapainmanage.org
E-mail:
rosemary@aapainmanage.org

American Academy of Physical Medicine and Rehabilitation
330 North Wabash Avenue,
Suite 2500
Chicago, IL 60611-7617
Phone: 312-464-9700
Fax: 312-464-0227
Website: www.aapmr.org
E-mail: info@aapmr.org

American Behçet's Disease Foundation
P.O. Box 869
Smithtown, NY 11787-0869
Toll-Free: 800-723-4287
Phone: 631-656-0537
Fax: 480-247-5377
E-mail: webmaster@behcets.com
Website: www.behcets.com

American College of Allergy, Asthma and Immunology
85 West Algonquin Road
Suite 550
Arlington Heights, IL 60005
Website: www.acaai.org
E-mail: mail@acaai.org

American College of Foot and Ankle Surgeons
8725 West Higgins Road
Suite 555
Chicago, IL 60631
Phone: 773-693-9300
Fax: 773-693-9304
Website: www.acfas.org
E-mail: info@acfas.org

American College of Rheumatology
1800 Century Place, Suite 250
Atlanta, GA 30345-4300
Phone: 404-633-3777
Fax: 404-633-1870
Website: www.rheumatology.org

American College of Sports Medicine
401 West Michigan Street
Indianapolis, IN 46202-3233
Phone: 317-637-9200
Fax: 317-634-7817
Website: www.acsm.org

American Fibromyalgia Syndrome Association, Inc.
P.O. Box 32698
7371 E. Tanque Verde Road
Tucson, AZ 85715
Phone: 520-733-1570
Fax: 520-290-5550
E-mail: kthorson@afsafund.org
Website: www.afsafund.org

American Geriatrics Society Foundation for Health in Aging
The Empire State Building
350 Fifth Avenue, Suite 801
New York, NY 10118
Toll-Free: 800-563-4916
Phone: 212-755-6810
Fax: 212-832-8646
Website: www.healthinaging.org

American Lyme Disease Foundation
P.O. Box 466
Lyme, CT 06371
Website: www.aldf.com
E-mail: inquire@aldf.com

American Occupational Therapy Association
4720 Montgomery Lane
P.O. Box 31220
Bethesda, MD 20824-1220
Phone: 301-652-2682
TDD: 800-377-8555
Fax: 301-652-7711
Website: www.aota.org

American Orthopaedic Foot and Ankle Society
6300 North River Road, Suite 510
Rosemont, IL 60018
Toll-Free: 800-235-4855
Phone: 847-698-4654
Fax: 847-692-3315
Website: www.aofas.org
E-mail: aofasinfo@aofas.org

American Pain Society
4700 West Lake Avenue
Glenview, IL 60025
Phone: 847-375-4715
Fax: 866-574-2654
Website: www.ampainsoc.org
E-mail: info@ampainsoc.org

American Physical Therapy Association
1111 North Fairfax Street
Alexandria, VA 22314-1488
Toll-Free: 800-999-2782
Phone: 703-684-2782
TDD: 703-683-6748
Fax: 703-684-7343
Website: www.apta.org

American Podiatric Medical Association
9312 Old Georgetown Road
Bethesda, MD 20814-1621
Phone: 301-581-9200
Website: www.apma.org

American Society for Surgery of the Hand
6300 North River Road
Suite 600
Rosemont, IL 60018
Phone: 847-384-8300
Fax: 847-384-1435
Website: www.assh.org
E-mail: info@assh.org

Arthritis Foundation
P.O. Box 7669
Atlanta, GA 30357-0669
Toll-Free: 800-283-7800
Website: www.arthritis.org
E-mail: arthritisfoundation
@arthritis.org

Arthritis Research Campaign
Copeman House, St. Mary's
Court, St. Mary's Gate
Chesterfield, Derbyshire S41 7TD
United Kingdom
Phone: +44 124-655-8033
Website: www.arc.org.uk
E-mail: info@arc.org.uk

Arthritis Source
Department of Orthopedics and
Sports Medicine
University of Washington
P.O. Box 356500
1959 NE Pacific Street
Seattle, WA 98195-6500
Phone: 206-543-3690
Fax: 206-685-3139
Website:
www.orthop.washington.edu

Center for Assistive Technology and Environmental Access
Georgia Institute of Technology,
College of Architecture
490 Tenth Street, NW
Atlanta, GA 30332-0156
Phone: 404-894-4960
Fax: 404-894-9320
Website: www.catea.gatech.edu

Cleveland Clinic
9500 Euclid Avenue
Cleveland, OH 44195
Toll-Free: 866-594-2091
Phone: 216-444-2200
TTY: 216-444-0261
Website:
www.clevelandclinic.org

Crohn's and Colitis Foundation of America
386 Park Avenue South
17th Floor
New York, NY 10016
Toll-Free: 800-932-2423
Website: www.ccfa.org
E-mail: info@ccfa.org

Hip Society
6300 North River Road, Suite 727
Rosemont, IL 60018-4226
Phone: 847-698-1638
Fax: 847-823-0536
Website: www.hipsoc.org
E-mail: hip@aaos.org

Job Accommodation Network
P.O. Box 6080
Morgantown, WV 26506-6080
Toll-Free: 800-526-7234
TTY: 877-781-9403
Fax: 304-293-5407
Website: www.jan.wvu.edu
E-mail: jan@jan.wvu.edu

Johns Hopkins Arthritis Center
5200 Eastern Avenue, Suite 4100
Baltimore, MD 21224
E-mail: jhuarthritis@jhmi.edu
Website: www.hopkins-arthritis.org

Hospital for Special Surgery
535 East 70th Street
New York, NY 10021
Phone: 212-606-1000
Website: www.hss.edu

International Still's Disease Foundation
1123 South Kimbrel Avenue
Panama City, FL 32404
Phone: 850-871-6656
Fax: 850-871-6656
Website: www.stillsdisease.org

Knee Society
6300 North River Road, Suite 727
Rosemont, IL 60018-4226
Phone: 847-698-1632
Fax: 847-823-0536
Website: www.kneesociety.org
E-mail: knee@aaos.org

Lupus Foundation of America
2000 L Street NW, Suite 710
Washington, DC 20036
Toll-Free: 800-558-0121
Phone: 202-349-1155
Fax: 202-349-1156
Website: www.lupus.org

Lyme Disease Foundation
P.O. Box 332
Tolland, CT 06084-0332
Toll-Free: 800-886-5963
Phone: 860-870-0070
Fax: 860-870-0080
Website: www.lyme.org
E-mail: info@lyme.org

**Missouri Arthritis
Rehabilitation Research
and Training Center**
Missouri School of Journalism
1 Hospital DC 018.00
Columbia, MO 65212
Phone: 573-884-9073
Website: www.marrtc.org
E-mail: marrtc@missouri.edu

**National Center on
Physical Activity and
Disability**
1640 West Roosevelt Road
Chicago, IL 60608-6904
Toll-Free: 800-900-8086
Fax: 312-355-4058
Website: www.ncpad.org
E-mail: ncpad@uic.edu

**National Fibromyalgia
Association**
2121 South Towne Centre Place
Suite 300
Anaheim, CA 92806
Phone: 714-921-0150
Fax: 714-921-6920
Website: www.fmaware.org

**National Organization on
Disability**
888 Sixteenth Street NW
Suite 800
Washington, DC 20006
Phone: 202-293-5960
Fax: 202-293-7999
TTY: 202-293-5968
Website: www.nod.org
E-mail: ability@nod.org

**National Osteoporosis
Foundation**
1232 22nd Street NW
Washington, DC 20037-1202
Toll-Free: 800-231-4222
Phone: 202-223-2226
Website: www.nof.org

National Pain Foundation
300 East Hampden Avenue
Suite 100
Englewood, CO 80113
Website: www
.nationalpainfoundation.org

**National Psoriasis
Foundation**
6600 SW 92nd Avenue, Suite 300
Portland, OR 97223-7195
Toll-Free: 800-723-9166
Phone: 503-244-7404
Fax: 503-245-0626
Website: www.psoriasis.org
E-mail: getinfo@psoriasis.org

**Nemours Foundation
Center for Children's
Health Media**
1600 Rockland Road
Wilmington, DE 19803
Phone: 302-651-4000
Website: www.kidshealth.org
E-mail: info@kidshealth.org

Paget Foundation
120 Wall Street, Suite 1602
New York, NY 10005-4001
Phone: 212-509-5335
Toll-Free: 800-237-2438
Fax: 212-509-8492
Website: www.paget.org
E-mail: PagetFdn@aol.com

Road Back Foundation
P.O. Box 410184
Cambridge, MA 02141
Phone: 614-227-1556
Website: www.roadback.org
E-mail: rbfcontact@roadback.org

Scleroderma Foundation
300 Rosewood Drive, Suite 105
Danvers, MA 01923
Toll-Free: 800-722-4673
Phone: 978-463-5843
Fax: 978-463-5809
Website: www.scleroderma.org

Sjögren's Syndrome Foundation
6707 Democracy Boulevard,
Suite 325
Bethesda, MD 20817
Toll-Free: 800-475-6473
Phone: 301-530-4420
Fax: 301-530-4415
Website: www.sjogrens.org

Spondylitis Association of America
P.O. Box 5872
Sherman Oaks, CA 91413
Toll-Free: 800-777-8189
Phone: 818-981-1616
Website: www.spondylitis.org
E-mail: info@spondylitis.org

Patient Assistance Programs for Rheumatology-Related Drugs

This list is not meant to be exhaustive. The American College of Rheumatology (ACR) does not endorse any of the products or manufacturers listed below.

Adalimumab (Humira®)
Abbott Immunology
Toll-Free: 866-4-HUMIRA
(448-6472)

Alendronate (Fosamax®)
Express Scripts Specialty Distribution Services/Rx Outreach
P.O. Box 66536
St. Louis, MO 63166-6536
Toll-Free: 800-769-3880

Xubex Pharmaceutical Services
P.O. Box 1244
Winter Park, FL 32790-1244
Phone: 866-699-8239
Fax: 407-671-7960

Celecoxib (Celebrex®)
Pfizer Helpful Answers
Toll-Free: 866-706-2400
Website:
www.pfizerhelpfulanswers.com

Cyclosporine (Neoral®)
Novartis Pharmaceuticals Patient Assistance Program
P.O. Box 66556
St. Louis, MO 63166-6566
Toll-Free: 800-277-2254

Etanercept (Enbrel®)
ENcourage Foundation™
Toll-Free: 888-436-2735
Website: www.enbrel.com

Etidronate (Didronel®)
Express Scripts Specialty Distribution Services/Rx Outreach
P.O. Box 66536
St. Louis, MO 63166-6536
Toll-Free: 800-769-3880

Hydroxychloroquine (Plaquenil®)
Express Scripts Specialty Distribution Services/Rx Outreach
P.O. Box 66536
St. Louis, MO 63166-6536
Toll-Free: 800-769-3880

Xubex Pharmaceutical Services
P.O. Box 1244
Winter Park, FL 32790-1244
Phone: 866-699-8239
Fax: 407-671-7960

Infliximab (Remicade®)
Remicade® (Infliximab) Patient Assistance Program
P.O. Box 221857
Charlotte, NC 28222-1857
Toll-Free: 800-652-6227
Fax: 888-526-5168

Leflunomide (Arava®)
Sanofi Aventis Pharmaceuticals Patient Assistance Program
55 Corporate Drive
Bridgewater, NJ 08807
Toll-Free: 866-325-8233
Website: www.arava.com;
www.sanofi-aventis.us

Meloxicam (Mobic®)
Express Scripts Specialty Distribution Services/Rx Outreach
P.O. Box 66536
St. Louis, MO 63166-6536
Toll-Free: 800-769-3880

Xubex Pharmaceutical Services
P.O. Box 1244
Winter Park, FL 32790-1244
Phone: 866-699-8239
Fax: 407-671-7960

Mycophenolate Mofetil (CellCept®)
Roche Medical Needs Program
Roche Laboratories, Inc.
340 Kingsland Street
Nutley, NJ 07110
Toll-Free: 877-757-6243 (select option 1, then option 2)

Nabumetone (Relafen®)
Express Scripts Specialty Distribution Services/Rx Outreach
P.O. Box 66536
St. Louis, MO 63166-6536
Toll-Free: 800-769-3880

Naproxen (Naprosyn®)
Express Scripts Specialty Distribution Services/Rx Outreach
P.O. Box 66536
St. Louis, MO 63166-6536
Toll-Free: 800-769-3880

Xubex Pharmaceutical Services
P.O. Box 1244
Winter Park, FL 32790-1244
Phone: 866-699-8239
Fax: 407-671-7960

**Nitrofurantoin
(Macrodantin®, Macrobid®)**
Express Scripts Specialty Distribution Services/Rx Outreach
P.O. Box 66536
St. Louis, MO 63166-6536
Toll-Free: 800-769-3880

Omeprazole (Prilosec®)
Express Scripts Specialty Distribution Services/Rx Outreach
P.O. Box 66536
St. Louis, MO 63166-6536
Toll-Free: 800-769-3880

Xubex Pharmaceutical Services
P.O. Box 1244
Winter Park, FL 32790-1244
Phone: 866-699-8239
Fax: 407-671-7960

Paroxetine (Paxil®)
Xubex Pharmaceutical Services
P.O. Box 1244
Winter Park, FL 32790-1244
Phone: 866-699-8239
Fax: 407-671-7960

Raloxifene (Evista®)
Eli Lilly and Company
Toll-Free: 800-488-2133
Website: www.lilly.com

Risedronate (Actonel®)
Express Scripts Specialty Distribution Services/Rx Outreach
P.O. Box 66536
St. Louis, MO 63166-6536
Toll-Free: 800-769-3880

**Sodium Hyaluronate
(Hyalgan®)**
Sanofi Patient Assistance
Program (Hyalgan®)
55 Corporate Drive
Bridgewater, NJ 08807
Toll-Free: 800-992-9022

Teriparatide (Forteo®)
Eli Lilly and Company
Toll-Free: 877-RX-LILLY
(795-4559)
Website: www.lilly.com

**Tramadol (Ultram®,
Ultracet®)**
Express Scripts Specialty Distribution Services/Rx Outreach
P.O. Box 66536
St. Louis, MO 63166-6536
Toll-Free: 800-769-3880

Xubex Pharmaceutical Services
P.O. Box 1244
Winter Park, FL 32790-1244
Phone: 866-699-8239
Fax: 407-671-7960

Prescription Drug Assistance Programs

Medicare Part D Prescription Drug Plans
Website: www.medicare.gov

Low Income Subsidy (LIS)
Toll-Free: 800-772-1213
Website: www.socialsecurity.gov

NeedyMeds.com
Website: www.needymeds.com

Prescription Assistance (PPA)
Toll-Free: 888-477-2669
Website: www.pparx.org

National Alliance on Mental Illness (NAMI)
Toll-Free: 800-950-6264
Website: www.nami.org

Index

Index

Page numbers followed by 'n' indicate a footnote. Page numbers in *italics* indicate a table or illustration.

Health Reference Series

Complete Catalog

List price $93 per volume. School and library price $84 per volume.

Adolescent Health Sourcebook, 2nd Edition

Basic Consumer Health Information about the Physical, Mental, and Emotional Growth and Development of Adolescents, Including Medical Care, Nutritional and Physical Activity Requirements, Puberty, Sexual Activity, Acne, Tanning, Body Piercing, Common Physical Illnesses and Disorders, Eating Disorders, Attention Deficit Hyperactivity Disorder, Depression, Bullying, Hazing, and Adolescent Injuries Related to Sports, Driving, and Work

Along with Substance Abuse Information about Nicotine, Alcohol, and Drug Use, a Glossary, and Directory of Additional Resources

Edited by Joyce Brennfleck Shannon. 655 pages. 2007. 978-0-7808-0943-7.

"A particularly good resource for both parents and teens. The concise presentation of the material in brief and well-organized chapters creates an easy volume to browse."
—*School Library Journal*, Jun '07

"I don't believe there are any other books written in such easy to understand language that encompass such a breadth of topics. This is a complete revision of the book and is an excellent resource for parents and teens."
—*Doody's Review Service*, 2007

Adult Health Concerns Sourcebook

Basic Consumer Health Information about Medical and Mental Concerns of Adults, Including Facts about Choosing Healthcare Providers, Navigating Insurance Options, Maintaining Wellness, Preventing Cancer, Heart Disease, Stroke, Diabetes, and Osteoporosis, and Understanding Aging-Related Health Concerns, Including Menopause, Cognitive Changes, and Changes in the Coronary and Vascular Systems

Along with Tips on Caring for Aging Parents and Dealing with Health-Related Work and Travel Issues, a Glossary, and a Directory of Resources for Additional Help and Information

Edited by Sandra J. Judd. 648 pages. 2008. 978-0-7808-0999-4.

"Provides a thorough list of topics that are important to adult health and for caregivers."
—*CHOICE*, Nov '08

"Written in easy-to-understand language . . . the content is well-organized and is intended to aid adults in making health care-related decisions."
—*AORN Journal*, Dec '08

AIDS Sourcebook, 4th Edition

Basic Consumer Health Information about Human Immunodeficiency Virus (HIV) and Acquired Immunodeficiency Syndrome (AIDS), Featuring Updated Statistics and Facts about Risks, Prevention, Screening, Diagnosis, Treatments, Side Effects, and Complications, and Including a Section about the Impact of HIV/AIDS on the Health of Women, Children, and Adolescents

Along with Tips on Managing Life with AIDS, Reports on Current Research Initiatives and Clinical Trials, a Glossary of Related Terms, and Resource Directories for Further Help and Information

Edited by Ivy L. Alexander. 680 pages. 2008. 978-0-7808-0997-0.

SEE ALSO *Contagious Diseases Sourcebook, 2nd Edition*

Alcoholism Sourcebook, 2nd Edition

Basic Consumer Health Information about Alcohol Use, Abuse, and Dependence, Featuring Facts about the Physical, Mental, and Social Health Effects of Alcohol Addiction, Including Alcoholic Liver Disease, Pancreatic Disease, Cardiovascular Disease, Neurological Disorders, and the Effects of Drinking during Pregnancy

Along with Information about Alcohol Treatment, Medications, and Recovery Programs, in Addition to Tips for Reducing the Prevalence of Underage Drinking, Statistics about Alcohol Use, a Glossary of Related Terms, and Directories of Resources for More Help and Information

Edited by Amy L. Sutton. 625 pages. 2007. 978-0-7808-0942-0.

"A comprehensive look at the adverse effects of alcohol on people of all ages . . . It serves to whet the reader's appetite to continue learning using other resources. It is practical, easy to read, and enlightening, and is the first book a lay person should consult to learn about alcoholism."
—*Doody's Review Service, 2007*

"Should be a basic acquisition for any serious public or college-level library including health reference titles for general-interest readers."
—*California Bookwatch, Feb '07*

SEE ALSO *Drug Abuse Sourcebook, 2nd Edition*

Allergies Sourcebook, 3rd Edition

Basic Consumer Health Information about Allergic Disorders, Such as Anaphylaxis, Hives, Eczema, Rhinitis, Sinusitis, and Conjunctivitis, and Their Triggers, Including Pollen, Mold, Dust Mites, Animal Dander, Insects, Chemicals, Food, Food Additives, and Medications

Along with Advice about the Diagnosis and Treatment of Allergy Symptoms, a Glossary of Related Terms, a Directory of Resources for Help and Information, and Suggestions for Additional Reading

Edited by Amy L. Sutton. 588 pages. 2007. 978-0-7808-0950-5.

SEE ALSO *Asthma Sourcebook, 2nd Edition*

Alzheimer Disease Sourcebook, 4th Edition

Basic Consumer Health Information about Alzheimer Disease, Other Dementias, and Related Disorders, Including Multi-Infarct Dementia, Dementia with Lewy Bodies, Fronto-temporal Dementia (Pick Disease), Wernicke-Korsakoff Syndrome (Alcohol-Related Dementia), AIDS Dementia Complex, Huntington Disease, Creutzfeldt-Jacob Disease, and Delirium

Along with Information about Coping with Memory Loss and Forgetfulness, Maintaining

Skills, and Long-Term Planning for People with Dementia, and Suggestions Addressing Common Caregiver Concerns, Updated Information about Current Research Efforts, a Glossary of Related Terms, and Directories of Sources for Additional Help and Information

Edited by Karen Bellenir. 603 pages. 2008. 978-0-7808-1001-3.

"An invaluable resource for persons who have received a diagnosis, for caregivers, and for family members dealing with this insidious disease. It is recommended for public, community college, and ready-reference sections in academic libraries."
—*ARBAonline, Jul '08*

SEE ALSO *Brain Disorders Sourcebook, 2nd Edition*

Arthritis Sourcebook, 2nd Edition

Basic Consumer Health Information about Osteoarthritis, Rheumatoid Arthritis, Other Rheumatic Disorders, Infectious Forms of Arthritis, and Diseases with Symptoms Linked to Arthritis, Featuring Facts about Diagnosis, Pain Management, and Surgical Therapies

Along with Coping Strategies, Research Updates, a Glossary, and Resources for Additional Help and Information

Edited by Amy L. Sutton. 567 pages. 2004. 978-0-7808-0667-2.

"This easy-to-read volume is recommended for consumer health collections within public or academic libraries."
—*E-Streams, May '05*

"As expected, this updated edition continues the excellent reputation of this series in providing sound, usable health information. . . . Highly recommended."
—*American Reference Books Annual, 2005*

Asthma Sourcebook, 2nd Edition

Basic Consumer Health Information about the Causes, Symptoms, Diagnosis, and Treatment of Asthma in Infants, Children, Teenagers, and Adults, Including Facts about Different Types of Asthma, Common Co-Occurring Conditions, Asthma Management Plans, Triggers, Medications, and Medication Delivery Devices

Along with Asthma Statistics, Research Updates, a Glossary, a Directory of Asthma-Related Resources, and More

Edited by Karen Bellenir. 581 pages. 2006. 978-0-7808-0866-9.

Attention Deficit Disorder Sourcebook

Basic Consumer Health Information about Attention Deficit/Hyperactivity Disorder in Children and Adults, Including Facts about Causes, Symptoms, Diagnostic Criteria, and Treatment Options Such as Medications, Behavior Therapy, Coaching, and Homeopathy

Along with Reports on Current Research Initiatives, Legal Issues, and Government Regulations, and Featuring a Glossary of Related Terms, Internet Resources, and a List of Additional Reading Material

Edited by Dawn D. Matthews. 447 pages. 2002. 978-0-7808-0624-5.

"Recommended reference source."
—*Booklist, Jan '03*

SEE ALSO *Learning Disabilities Sourcebook, 3rd Edition*

Autism and Pervasive Developmental Disorders Sourcebook

Basic Consumer Health Information about Autism Spectrum and Pervasive Developmental Disorders, Such as Classical Autism, Asperger Syndrome, Rett Syndrome, and Childhood Disintegrative Disorder, Including Information about Related Genetic Disorders and Medical Problems and Facts about Causes, Screening Methods, Diagnostic Criteria, Treatments and Interventions, and Family and Education Issues

Along with a Glossary of Related Terms, Tips for Evaluating the Validity of Health Claims, and a Directory of Resources for Additional Help and Information

Edited by Sandra J. Judd. 603 pages. 2007. 978-0-7808-0953-6.

"Recommended for public libraries"
—*SciTech Book News, Mar '08*

SEE ALSO *Learning Disabilities Sourcebook, 3rd Edition*

Back and Neck Disorders Sourcebook, 2nd Edition

Basic Consumer Health Information about Spinal Pain, Spinal Cord Injuries, and Related Disorders, Such as Degenerative Disk Disease, Osteoarthritis, Scoliosis, Sciatica, Spina Bifida, and Spinal Stenosis, and Featuring Facts about Maintaining Spinal Health, Self-Care, Pain Management, Rehabilitative Care, Chiropractic Care, Spinal Surgeries, and Complementary Therapies

Along with Suggestions for Preventing Back and Neck Pain, a Glossary of Related Terms, and a Directory of Resources

Edited by Amy L. Sutton. 607 pages. 2004. 978-0-7808-0738-9.

"Recommended. ...An easy to use, comprehensive medical reference book."
—*E-Streams, Sep '05*

"For anyone who has back or neck problems, this book is ideal. Its easy-to-understand language and variety of topics makes this sourcebook a worthwhile read. The price...is reasonable for the amount of information contained in the book"
—*Occupational Therapy in Health Care, 2007*

Blood and Circulatory Disorders Sourcebook, 2nd Edition

Basic Consumer Health Information about the Blood and Circulatory System and Related Disorders, Such as Anemia and Other Hemoglobin Diseases, Cancer of the Blood and Associated Bone Marrow Disorders, Clotting and Bleeding Problems, and Conditions That Affect the Veins, Blood Vessels, and Arteries, Including Facts about the Donation and Transplantation of Bone Marrow, Stem Cells, and Blood and Tips for Keeping the Blood and Circulatory System Healthy

Along with a Glossary of Related Terms and Resources for Additional Help and Information

Edited by Amy L. Sutton. 634 pages. 2005. 978-0-7808-0746-4.

"Highly recommended pick for basic consumer health reference holdings at all levels."
—*The Bookwatch, Aug '05*

Brain Disorders Sourcebook, 2nd Edition

Basic Consumer Health Information about Acquired and Traumatic Brain Injuries, Infections of the Brain, Epilepsy and Seizure Disorders, Cerebral Palsy, and Degenerative Neurological Disorders, Including Amyotrophic Lateral Sclerosis (ALS), Dementias, Multiple Sclerosis, and More

Along with Information on the Brain's Structure and Function, Treatment and Rehabilitation Options, Reports on Current Research Initiatives, a Glossary of Terms Related to Brain Disorders and Injuries, and a Directory of Sources for Further Help and Information

Edited by Sandra J. Judd. 600 pages. 2005. 978-0-7808-0744-0.

"This easy-to-read volume provides up-to-date health information... Recommended for consumer health collections within public or academic libraries."

—*E-Streams, Feb '06*

SEE ALSO *Alzheimer Disease Sourcebook, 4th Edition*

Breast Cancer Sourcebook, 3rd Edition

Basic Consumer Health Information about Breast Health and Breast Cancer, Including Facts about Environmental, Genetic, and Other Risk Factors, Prevention Efforts, Screening and Diagnostic Methods, Surgical Treatment Options and Other Care Choices, Complementary and Alternative Therapies, and Post-Treatment Concerns

Along with Statistical Data, News about Research Advances, a Glossary of Related Terms, and Directories of Resources for Additional Information and Support

Edited by Karen Bellenir. 606 pages. 2009. 978-0-7808-1030-3.

SEE ALSO *Cancer Sourcebook for Women, 3rd Edition, Women's Health Concerns Sourcebook, 3rd Edition*

Breastfeeding Sourcebook

Basic Consumer Health Information about the Benefits of Breastmilk, Preparing to Breastfeed, Breastfeeding as a Baby Grows,

Nutrition, and More, Including Information on Special Situations and Concerns Such as Mastitis, Illness, Medications, Allergies, Multiple Births, Prematurity, Special Needs, and Adoption

Along with a Glossary and Resources for Additional Help and Information

Edited by Jenni Lynn Colson. 367 pages. 2002. 978-0-7808-0332-9.

SEE ALSO *Pregnancy and Birth Sourcebook, 2nd Edition*

Burns Sourcebook

Basic Consumer Health Information about Various Types of Burns and Scalds, Including Flame, Heat, Cold, Electrical, Chemical, and Sun Burns

Along with Information on Short-Term and Long-Term Treatments, Tissue Reconstruction, Plastic Surgery, Prevention Suggestions, and First Aid

Edited by Allan R. Cook. 604 pages. 1999. 978-0-7808-0204-9.

"This is an exceptional addition to the series and is highly recommended for all consumer health collections, hospital libraries, and academic medical centers."

—*E-Streams, Mar '00*

"This key reference guide is an invaluable addition to all health care and public libraries in confronting this ongoing health issue."

—*American Reference Books Annual, 2000*

SEE ALSO *Dermatological Disorders Sourcebook, 2nd Edition*

Cancer Sourcebook, 5th Edition

Basic Consumer Health Information about Major Forms and Stages of Cancer, Featuring Facts about Head and Neck Cancers, Lung Cancers, Gastrointestinal Cancers, Genitourinary Cancers, Lymphomas, Blood Cell Cancers, Endocrine Cancers, Skin Cancers, Bone Cancers, Metastatic Cancers, and More

Along with Facts about Cancer Treatments, Cancer Risks and Prevention, a Glossary of Related Terms, Statistical Data, and a Directory of Resources for Additional Information

Edited by Karen Bellenir. 1105 pages. 2007. 978-0-7808-0947-5.

"The 5th, updated edition of *Cancer Sourcebook* should be in every public and health lending library collection... An unparalleled discussion essential for any health collections considering an all-in-one basic general reference."

—*California Bookwatch, Aug '07*

SEE ALSO *Breast Cancer Sourcebook, 3rd Edition, Cancer Sourcebook for Women, 3rd Edition, Cancer Survivorship Sourcebook, Leukemia Sourcebook*

Cancer Sourcebook for Women, 3rd Edition

Basic Consumer Health Information about Leading Causes of Cancer in Women, Featuring Facts about Gynecologic Cancers and Related Concerns, Such as Breast Cancer, Cervical Cancer, Endometrial Cancer, Uterine Sarcoma, Vaginal Cancer, Vulvar Cancer, and Common Non-Cancerous Gynecologic Conditions, in Addition to Facts about Lung Cancer, Colorectal Cancer, and Thyroid Cancer in Women

Along with Information about Cancer Risk Factors, Screening and Prevention, Treatment Options, and Tips on Coping with Life after Cancer Treatment, a Glossary of Cancer Terms, and a Directory of Resources for Additional Help and Information

Edited by Amy L. Sutton. 687 pages. 2006. 978-0-7808-0867-6.

"This excellent book provides the general public with information compiled in a way that will help them to gain the knowledge they need. 4 Stars!"

—*Doody's Review Service, Dec '06*

"An indispensable reference for health consumers and cancer patients. Recommended for public libraries and academic libraries with a medical department."

—*E-Streams, Sep '08*

Cancer Survivorship Sourcebook

Basic Consumer Health Information about the Physical, Educational, Emotional, Social, and Financial Needs of Cancer Patients from Diagnosis, through Cancer Treatment, and Beyond, Including Facts about Researching Specific Types of Cancer and Learning about Clinical Trials and Treatment Options, and

Featuring Tips for Coping with the Side Effects of Cancer Treatments and Adjusting to Life after Cancer Treatment Concludes

Along with Suggestions for Caregivers, Friends, and Family Members of Cancer Patients, a Glossary of Cancer Care Terms, and Directories of Related Resources

Edited by Karen Bellenir. 633 pages. 2007. 978-0-7808-0985-7.

"Well organized and comprehensive in coverage, the book speaks to issues encountered both during and after cancer treatment. Recommended for consumer health and public libraries."

—*Library Journal, Aug 1 '07*

"*Cancer Survivorship Sourcebook* will be useful to anyone who has a friend or loved one with a cancer diagnosis."

—*American Reference Books Annual, 2008*

SEE ALSO *Cancer Sourcebook, 5th Edition*

Cardiovascular Diseases and Disorders Sourcebook, 3rd Edition

Basic Consumer Health Information about Heart and Vascular Diseases and Disorders, Such as Angina, Heart Attacks, Arrhythmias, Cardiomyopathy, Valve Disease, Atherosclerosis, and Aneurysms, with Information about Managing Cardiovascular Risk Factors and Maintaining Heart Health, Medications and Procedures Used to Treat Cardiovascular Disorders, and Concerns of Special Significance to Women

Along with Reports on Current Research Initiatives, a Glossary of Related Medical Terms, and a Directory of Sources for Further Help and Information

Edited by Sandra J. Judd. 687 pages. 2005. 978-0-7808-0739-6.

"This updated sourcebook is still the best first stop for comprehensive introductory information on cardiovascular diseases."

—*American Reference Books Annual, 2006*

"Recommended for public libraries and libraries supporting health care professionals."

—*E-Streams, Sep '05*

Caregiving Sourcebook

Basic Consumer Health Information for Caregivers, Including a Profile of Caregivers, Caregiving Responsibilities and Concerns, Tips for Specific Conditions, Care Environments, and the Effects of Caregiving

Along with Facts about Legal Issues, Financial Information, and Future Planning, a Glossary, and a Listing of Additional Resources

Edited by Joyce Brennfleck Shannon. 583 pages. 2001. 978-0-7808-0331-2.

"Essential for most collections."
—*Library Journal, Apr 1 '02*

"An ideal addition to the reference collection of any public library. Health sciences information professionals may also want to acquire the *Caregiving Sourcebook* for their hospital or academic library for use as a ready reference tool by health care workers interested in aging and caregiving."
—*E-Streams, Jan '02*

Child Abuse Sourcebook, 2nd Edition

Basic Consumer Health Information about the Physical, Sexual, and Emotional Abuse of Children, Neglect, Münchhausen Syndrome by Proxy (MSBP), and Shaken Baby Syndrome, and Featuring Facts about Withholding Medical Care, Corporal Punishment, Child Maltreatment in Youth Sports, and Parental Substance Abuse

Along with Information about Child Protective Services, Foster Care, Adoption, Parenting Challenges, Abuse Prevention Programs, and Intervention, Treatment, and Recovery Guidelines, a Glossary of Related Terms, and Resources for Additional Help and Information

Edited by Joyce Brennfleck Shannon. 600 pages. 2009. 978-0-7808-1037-2.

SEE ALSO *Domestic Violence Sourcebook, 3rd Edition*

Childhood Diseases and Disorders Sourcebook, 2nd Edition

Basic Consumer Health Information about the Physical, Mental, and Developmental Health of Pre-Adolescent Children, Including Facts about Infectious Diseases, Asthma, Allergies, Diabetes, and Other Acute and Chronic Conditions Affecting the Gastrointestinal Tract, Ears, Nose, Throat, Liver, Kidneys, Heart, Blood, Brain, Muscles, Bones, and Skin

Along with Reports on Recommended Childhood Vaccinations, Wellness Guidelines, a Glossary of Related Medical Terms, and a List of Resources for Parents

Edited by Sandra J. Judd. 694 pages. 2009. 978-0-7808-1031-0.

SEE ALSO *Healthy Children Sourcebook*

Colds, Flu and Other Common Ailments Sourcebook

Basic Consumer Health Information about Common Ailments and Injuries, Including Colds, Coughs, the Flu, Sinus Problems, Headaches, Fever, Nausea and Vomiting, Menstrual Cramps, Diarrhea, Constipation, Hemorrhoids, Back Pain, Dandruff, Dry and Itchy Skin, Cuts, Scrapes, Sprains, Bruises, and More

Along with Information about Prevention, Self-Care, Choosing a Doctor, Over-the-Counter Medications, Folk Remedies, and Alternative Therapies, and Including a Glossary of Important Terms and a Directory of Resources for Further Help and Information

Edited by Chad T. Kimball. 622 pages. 2001. 978-0-7808-0435-7.

"A good starting point for research on common illnesses. It will be a useful addition to public and consumer health library collections."
—*American Reference Books Annual, 2002*

"Will prove valuable to any library seeking to maintain a current, comprehensive reference collection of health resources. . . Excellent reference."
—*The Bookwatch, Aug '01*

Communication Disorders Sourcebook

Basic Information about Deafness and Hearing Loss, Speech and Language Disorders, Voice Disorders, Balance and Vestibular Disorders, and Disorders of Smell, Taste, and Touch

Edited by Linda M. Ross. 533 pages. 1996. 978-0-7808-0077-9.

"This is skillfully edited and is a welcome resource for the layperson. It should be found in every public and medical library."
—*Booklist Health Sciences Supplement,*
Oct '97

Complementary and Alternative Medicine Sourcebook, 3rd Edition

Basic Consumer Health Information about Complementary and Alternative Medical Therapies, Including Acupuncture, Ayurveda, Traditional Chinese Medicine, Herbal Medicine, Homeopathy, Naturopathy, Biofeedback, Hypnotherapy, Yoga, Art Therapy, Aromatherapy, Clinical Nutrition, Vitamin and Mineral Supplements, Chiropractic, Massage, Reflexology, Crystal Therapy, Therapeutic Touch, and More

Along with Facts about Alternative and Complementary Treatments for Specific Conditions Such as Cancer, Diabetes, Osteoarthritis, Chronic Pain, Menopause, Gastrointestinal Disorders, Headaches, and Mental Illness, a Glossary, and a Resource List for Additional Help and Information

Edited by Sandra J. Judd. 630 pages. 2006. 978-0-7808-0864-5.

"A 'must' reference for any serious healthcare collection. Public library holdings, too, will welcome it as a popular reference."
—*California Bookwatch, Oct '06*

"Both basic and informative at the same time. . . a useful resource for health care professionals as well as consumers interested in learning more information about CAM therapies."
—*AORN Journal, Jan '08*

"A quality, indexed, referenced guideline for many alternative practices that are quite popular around the world...It is neatly organized to find facts quickly, is peer-reviewed, and stays current with the most recent advances."
—*Journal of Dental Hygiene, Jul '07*

Congenital Disorders Sourcebook, 2nd Edition

Basic Consumer Health Information about Nonhereditary Birth Defects and Disorders Related to Prematurity, Gestational Injuries, Congenital Infections, and Birth Complications, Including Heart Defects, Hydrocephalus, Spina Bifida, Cleft Lip and Palate, Cerebral Palsy, and More

Along with Facts about the Prevention of Birth Defects, Fetal Surgery and Other Treatment Options, Research Initiatives, a Glossary of Related Terms, and Resources for Additional Information and Support

Edited by Sandra J. Judd. 619 pages. 2007. 978-0-7808-0945-1.

"Congenital Disorders Sourcebook provides an excellent, non-technical overview of many aspects of pregnancy with the focus on congenital disorders."
—*American Reference Books Annual, 2008*

"An excellent readable reference aimed at the lay public for difficult to understand medical problems. An excellent starting point for the interested parent or family member who may then be motivated to seek more information."
—*Doody's Review Service, 2007*

SEE ALSO Pregnancy and Birth Sourcebook, 2nd Edition

Contagious Diseases Sourcebook, 2nd Edition

Basic Consumer Health Information about Diseases Spread from Person to Person through Direct Physical Contact, Airborne Transmissions, Sexual Contact, or Contact with Blood or Other Body Fluids, Including Pneumococcal, Staphylococcal, and Streptococcal Diseases, Colds, Influenza, Lice, Measles, Mumps, Tuberculosis, and Others

Along with Facts about Self-Care and Over-the-Counter Medications, Antibiotics and Drug Resistance, Disease Prevention, Vaccines, and Bioterrorism, a Glossary, and a Directory of Resources for More Information

Edited by Joyce Brennfleck Shannon. 600 pages. 2009. 978-0-7808-1075-4.

SEE ALSO AIDS Sourcebook, 4th Edition, Hepatitis Sourcebook

Cosmetic and Reconstructive Surgery Sourcebook, 2nd Edition

Basic Consumer Information about Plastic Surgery and Non-Surgical Appearance-Enhancing Procedures, Including Facts about Botulinum Toxin, Collagen Replacement, Dermabrasion,

Chemical Peels, Eyelid Surgery, Nose Reshaping, Lip Augmentation, Liposuction, Breast Enlargement and Reduction, Tummy Tucking, and Other Skin, Hair, Facial, and Body Shaping Procedures

Along with Information about Reconstructive Procedures for Congenital Disorders, Disfiguring Diseases, Burns, and Traumatic Injuries, a Glossary of Related Terms, and a Directory of Additional Resources

Edited by Karen Bellenir. 483 pages. 2007. 978-0-7808-0951-2.

"A practical guide for health care consumers and health care workers. . . . This easy-to-read reference guide would be useful for novice and veteran health care consumers, surgical technology students, nursing students, and perioperative nurses new to plastic and reconstructive surgery. It also may be helpful for medical-surgical nurses as a guide for patient teaching in their practices."

—AORN Journal, Aug '08

SEE ALSO Surgery Sourcebook, 2nd Edition

Death and Dying Sourcebook, 2nd Edition

Basic Consumer Health Information about End-of-Life Care and Related Perspectives and Ethical Issues, Including End-of-Life Symptoms and Treatments, Pain Management, Quality-of-Life Concerns, the Use of Life Support, Patients' Rights and Privacy Issues, Advance Directives, Physician-Assisted Suicide, Caregiving, Organ and Tissue Donation, Autopsies, Funeral Arrangements, and Grief

Along with Statistical Data, Information about the Leading Causes of Death, a Glossary, and Directories of Support Groups and Other Resources

Edited by Joyce Brennfleck Shannon. 626 pages. 2006. 978-0-7808-0871-3.

Dental Care and Oral Health Sourcebook, 3rd Edition

Basic Consumer Health Information about Dental Care and Oral Health Throughout the Lifespan, Including Facts about Cavities, Bad Breath, Cold and Canker Sores, Dry Mouth,

Toothaches, Gum Disease, Malocclusion, Temporomandibular Joint and Muscle Disorders, Oral Cancers, and Dental Emergencies

Along with Information about Mouth Hygiene, Crowns, Bridges, Implants, and Fillings, Surgical, Orthodontic, and Cosmetic Dental Procedures, Pain Management, Health Conditions that Impact Oral Care, a Glossary of Related Terms, and a Directory of Additional Resources

Edited by Amy L. Sutton. 619 pages. 2008. 978-0-7808-1032-7.

Depression Sourcebook, 2nd Edition

Basic Consumer Health Information about Unipolar Depression, Bipolar Disorder, Dysthymia, Seasonal Affective Disorder, Postpartum Depression, and Other Depressive Disorders, Including Facts about Populations at Special Risk, Coexisting Medical Conditions, Symptoms, Treatment Options, and Suicide Prevention

Along with Statistical Data, a Glossary of Related Terms, and a Directory of Resources for Additional Help and Information

Edited by Sandra J. Judd. 646 pages. 2008. 978-0-7808-1003-7.

"Recommended for public libraries."
—ARBAonline, Nov '08

SEE ALSO Mental Health Disorders Sourcebook, 4th Edition

Dermatological Disorders Sourcebook, 2nd Edition

Basic Consumer Health Information about Conditions and Disorders Affecting the Skin, Hair, and Nails, Such as Acne, Rosacea, Rashes, Dermatitis, Pigmentation Disorders, Birthmarks, Skin Cancer, Skin Injuries, Psoriasis, Scleroderma, and Hair Loss, Including Facts about Medications and Treatments for Dermatological Disorders and Tips for Maintaining Healthy Skin, Hair, and Nails

Along with Information about How Aging Affects the Skin, a Glossary of Related Terms, and a Directory of Resources for Additional Help and Information

Edited by Amy L. Sutton. 617 pages. 2006. 978-0-7808-0795-2.

"Helpfully brings together. . . sources in one convenient place, saving the user hours of research time."
—*American Reference Books Annual, 2006*

SEE ALSO Burns Sourcebook

Diabetes Sourcebook, 4th Edition

Basic Consumer Health Information about Type 1 and Type 2 Diabetes Mellitus, Gestational Diabetes, Monogenic Forms of Diabetes, and Insulin Resistance, with Guidelines for Lifestyle Modifications and the Medical Management of Diabetes, Including Facts about Insulin, Insulin Delivery Devices, Oral Diabetes Medications, Self-Monitoring of Blood Glucose, Meal Planning, Physical Activity Recommendations, Foot Care, and Treatment Options for People with Kidney Failure

Along with a Section about Diabetes Complications and Co-Occurring Conditions, a Glossary of Related Terms, and Directories of Resources for Additional Help and Information

Edited by Karen Bellenir. 627 pages. 2008. 978-0-7808-1005-1.

"Completely and comprehensively covering almost everything a student or physician would need to know.... well worth the investment."
—*Internet Bookwatch, Dec '08*

SEE ALSO Endocrine and Metabolic Disorders Sourcebook, 2nd Edition

Diet and Nutrition Sourcebook, 3rd Edition

Basic Consumer Health Information about Dietary Guidelines and the Food Guidance System, Recommended Daily Nutrient Intakes, Serving Proportions, Weight Control, Vitamins and Supplements, Nutrition Issues for Different Life Stages and Lifestyles, and the Needs of People with Specific Medical Concerns, Including Cancer, Celiac Disease, Diabetes, Eating Disorders, Food Allergies, and Cardiovascular Disease

Along with Facts about Federal Nutrition Support Programs, a Glossary of Nutrition and Dietary Terms, and Directories of Additional Resources for More Information about Nutrition

Edited by Joyce Brennfleck Shannon. 605 pages. 2006. 978-0-7808-0800-3.

"A valuable resource tool for any individual."
—*Journal of Dental Hygiene, Apr '07*

"From different recommended eating habits to reduce disease and common ailments to nutrition advice for those with specific conditions, *Diet and Nutrition Sourcebook* is especially important because so much is changing in this area, and so rapidly."
—*California Bookwatch, Jun '06*

SEE ALSO Digestive Diseases and Disorders Sourcebook, Eating Disorders Sourcebook, 2nd Edition, Gastrointestinal Diseases and Disorders Sourcebook, 2nd Edition, Vegetarian Sourcebook

Digestive Diseases and Disorders Sourcebook

Basic Consumer Health Information about Diseases and Disorders that Impact the Upper and Lower Digestive System, Including Celiac Disease, Constipation, Crohn's Disease, Cyclic Vomiting Syndrome, Diarrhea, Diverticulosis and Diverticulitis, Gallstones, Heartburn, Hemorrhoids, Hernias, Indigestion (Dyspepsia), Irritable Bowel Syndrome, Lactose Intolerance, Ulcers, and More

Along with Information about Medications and Other Treatments, Tips for Maintaining a Healthy Digestive Tract, a Glossary, and Directory of Digestive Diseases Organizations

Edited by Karen Bellenir. 323 pages. 2000. 978-0-7808-0327-5.

"An excellent addition to all public or patient-research libraries."
—*American Reference Books Annual, 2001*

"Recommended reference source."
—*Booklist, May '00*

SEE ALSO Diet and Nutrition Sourcebook, 3rd Edition, Gastrointestinal Diseases and Disorders Sourcebook, 2nd Edition

Disabilities Sourcebook

Basic Consumer Health Information about Physical and Psychiatric Disabilities, Including Descriptions of Major Causes of Disability, Assistive and Adaptive Aids, Workplace Issues, and Accessibility Concerns

Along with Information about the Americans with Disabilities Act, a Glossary, and Resources for Additional Help and Information

Edited by Dawn D. Matthews. 602 pages. 2000. 978-0-7808-0389-3.

"A must for libraries with a consumer health section."
—*American Reference Books Annual, 2002*

"A much needed addition to the Omnigraphics *Health Reference Series*. A current reference work to provide people with disabilities, their families, caregivers or those who work with them, a broad range of information in one volume, has not been available until now. . . . It is recommended for all public and academic library reference collections."
—*E-Streams, May '01*

"An excellent source book in easy-to-read format covering many current topics; highly recommended for all libraries."
—*CHOICE, Jan '01*

Disease Management Sourcebook

Basic Consumer Health Information about Coping with Chronic and Serious Illnesses, Navigating the Health Care System, Communicating with Health Care Providers, Assessing Health Care Quality, and Making Informed Health Care Decisions, Including Facts about Second Opinions, Hospitalization, Surgery, and Medications

Along with a Section about Children with Chronic Conditions, Information about Legal, Financial, and Insurance Issues, a Glossary of Related Terms, and Directories of Additional Resources

Edited by Joyce Brennfleck Shannon. 621 pages. 2008. 978-0-7808-1002-0.

"Consumers need to know how to manage their health care the same way they manage anything else in their lives. The text is very readable and is written for the layperson and consumer. The cost is not prohibitive. This book should be in all collections of health care libraries and public libraries."
—*ARBAonline, Jul '08*

"The information is very current, and the selection of font and layout make the book easy to read. A hardback that will stand up to much usage, this is an excellent resource for consumers. . . . Recommended. General readers."
—*CHOICE, Nov '08*

"Intended for lay readers, this resource clarifies the many confusing and overwhelming details associated with chronic disease care. Meticulous and clearly explained, the book even includes diagrams intended to ease comprehension of over-the-counter medication labels. An essential guide to navigating the health-care rapids."
—*Library Journal, Aug '08*

Domestic Violence Sourcebook, 3rd Edition

Basic Consumer Health Information about Warning Signs, Risk Factors, and Health Consequences of Intimate Partner Violence, Sexual Violence and Rape, Stalking, Human Trafficking, Child Maltreatment, Teen Dating Violence, and Elder Abuse

Along with Facts about Victims and Perpetrators, Strategies for Violence Prevention, and Emergency Interventions, Safety Plans, and Financial and Legal Tips for Victims, a Glossary of Related Terms, and Directories of Resources for Additional Information and Support

Edited by Joyce Brennfleck Shannon. 600 pages. 2009. 978-0-7808-1038-9.

SEE ALSO *Child Abuse Sourcebook, 2nd Edition*

Drug Abuse Sourcebook, 2nd Edition

Basic Consumer Health Information about Illicit Substances of Abuse and the Misuse of Prescription and Over-the-Counter Medications, Including Depressants, Hallucinogens, Inhalants, Marijuana, Stimulants, and Anabolic Steroids

Along with Facts about Related Health Risks, Treatment Programs, Prevention Programs, a Glossary of Abuse and Addiction Terms, a Glossary of Drug-Related Street Terms, and a Directory of Resources for More Information

Edited by Catherine Ginther. 581 pages. 2004. 978-0-7808-0740-2.

"Commendable for organizing useful, normally scattered government and association-produced data into a logical sequence."
—*American Reference Books Annual, 2006*

"An excellent library reference."
—*The Bookwatch, May '05*

SEE ALSO *Alcoholism Sourcebook, 2nd Edition*

Ear, Nose, and Throat Disorders Sourcebook, 2nd Edition

Basic Consumer Health Information about Disorders of the Ears, Hearing Loss, Vestibular Disorders, Nasal and Sinus Problems, Throat and Vocal Cord Disorders, and Otolaryngologic Cancers, Including Facts about Ear Infections and Injuries, Genetic and Congenital Deafness, Sensorineural Hearing Disorders, Tinnitus, Vertigo, Ménière Disease, Rhinitis, Sinusitis, Snoring, Sore Throats, Hoarseness, and More

Along with Reports on Current Research Initiatives, a Glossary of Related Medical Terms, and a Directory of Sources for Further Help and Information

Edited by Sandra J. Judd. 631 pages. 2007. 978-0-7808-0872-0.

"A resource book for the general public that provides comprehensive coverage of basic up-to-date medical information about the causes, symptoms, diagnosis, and treatment of diseases and disorders that affect the ears, nose, sinuses, throat, and voice. . . . The majority of information is presented in question and answer format, much like questions a patient might ask of a health care provider. An extensive index facilitates the reader's ability to easily access information on any specific topic."
—*Journal of Dental Hygiene, Oct '07*

"A handy compilation of information on common and some not so common ailments of the ears, nose, and throat."
—*Doody's Review Service, 2007*

Eating Disorders Sourcebook, 2nd Edition

Basic Consumer Health Information about Anorexia Nervosa, Bulimia, Binge Eating, Compulsive Exercise, Female Athlete Triad, and Other Eating Disorders, Including Facts about Body Image and Other Cultural and Age-Related Risk Factors, Prevention Efforts, Adverse Health Effects, Treatment Options, and the Recovery Process

Along with Guidelines for Healthy Weight Control, a Glossary, and Directories of Additional Resources

Edited by Joyce Brennfleck Shannon. 557 pages. 2007. 978-0-7808-0948-2.

"Recommended for the reference collection of large public libraries."
—*American Reference Books Annual, 2008*

"A basic health reference any health or general library needs."
—*Internet Bookwatch, Jun '07*

SEE ALSO *Diet and Nutrition Sourcebook, 3rd Edition, Mental Health Disorders Sourcebook, 4th Edition*

Emergency Medical Services Sourcebook

Basic Consumer Health Information about Preventing, Preparing for, and Managing Emergency Situations, When and Who to Call for Help, What to Expect in the Emergency Room, the Emergency Medical Team, Patient Issues, and Current Topics in Emergency Medicine

Along with Statistical Data, a Glossary, and Sources of Additional Help and Information

Edited by Jenni Lynn Colson. 472 pages. 2002. 978-0-7808-0420-3.

"Handy and convenient for home, public, school, and college libraries. Recommended."
—*CHOICE, Apr '03*

"This reference can provide the consumer with answers to most questions about emergency care in the United States, or it will direct them to a resource where the answer can be found."
—*American Reference Books Annual, 2003*

SEE ALSO *Injury and Trauma Sourcebook*

Endocrine and Metabolic Disorders Sourcebook, 2nd Edition

Basic Consumer Health Information about Hormonal and Metabolic Disorders that Affect the Body's Growth, Development, and Functioning, Including Disorders of the Pancreas, Ovaries and Testes, and Pituitary, Thyroid, Parathyroid, and Adrenal Glands, with Facts about Growth Disorders, Addison Disease, Cushing Syndrome, Conn Syndrome, Diabetic Disorders, Multiple Endocrine Neoplasia, Inborn Errors of Metabolism, and More

Along with Information about Endocrine Functioning, Diagnostic and Screening Tests, a Glossary of Related Terms, and Directories of Additional Resources

Edited by Joyce Brennfleck Shannon. 597 pages. 2007. 978-0-7808-0952-9.

SEE ALSO Diabetes Sourcebook, 4th Edition

▪

Environmental Health Sourcebook, 2nd Edition

Basic Consumer Health Information about the Environment and Its Effect on Human Health, Including the Effects of Air Pollution, Water Pollution, Hazardous Chemicals, Food Hazards, Radiation Hazards, Biological Agents, Household Hazards, Such as Radon, Asbestos, Carbon Monoxide, and Mold, and Information about Associated Diseases and Disorders, Including Cancer, Allergies, Respiratory Problems, and Skin Disorders

Along with Information about Environmental Concerns for Specific Populations, a Glossary of Related Terms, and Resources for Further Help and Information

Edited by Dawn D. Matthews. 650 pages. 2003. 978-0-7808-0632-0.

"Recommended for teenage and adult students and readers, and for public and academic libraries, as well as any library focusing on consumer health."
—E-Streams, May '04

"This recently updated edition continues the level of quality and the reputation of the numerous other volumes in Omnigraphics' Health Reference Series."
—American Reference Books Annual, 2004

▪

Ethnic Diseases Sourcebook

Basic Consumer Health Information for Ethnic and Racial Minority Groups in the United States, Including General Health Indicators and Behaviors, Ethnic Diseases, Genetic Testing, the Impact of Chronic Diseases, Women's Health, Mental Health Issues, and Preventive Health Care Services

Along with a Glossary and a Listing of Additional Resources

Edited by Joyce Brennfleck Shannon. 648 pages. 2001. 978-0-7808-0336-7.

"Not many books have been written on this topic to date, and the Ethnic Diseases Sourcebook is a strong addition to the list. It will be an important introductory resource for health consumers, students, health care personnel, and social scientists. It is recommended for public, academic, and large hospital libraries."
—American Reference Books Annual, 2002

"Will prove valuable to any library seeking to maintain a current, comprehensive reference collection of health resources. . . . An excellent source of health information about genetic disorders which affect particular ethnic and racial minorities in the U.S."
—The Bookwatch, Aug '01

▪

Eye Care Sourcebook, 3rd Edition

Basic Consumer Health Information about Eye Care and Eye Disorders, Including Facts about the Diagnosis, Prevention, and Treatment of Refractive Disorders, Cataracts, Glaucoma, Macular Degeneration, and Problems Affecting the Cornea, Retina, and Lacrimal Glands

Along with Advice about Preventing Eye Injuries and Tips for Living with Low Vision or Blindness, a Glossary of Related Terms, and Directories of Resources for More Help and Information

Edited by Amy L. Sutton. 646 pages. 2008. 978-0-7808-1000-6.

▪

Family Planning Sourcebook

Basic Consumer Health Information about Planning for Pregnancy and Contraception, Including Traditional Methods, Barrier Methods, Hormonal Methods, Permanent Methods, Future Methods, Emergency Contraception, and Birth Control Choices for Women at Each Stage of Life

Along with Statistics, a Glossary, and Sources of Additional Information

Edited by Amy Marcaccio Keyzer. 503 pages. 2001. 978-0-7808-0379-4.

"Recommended for public, health, and undergraduate libraries as part of the circulating collection."
—E-Streams, Mar '02

"Will prove valuable to any library seeking to maintain a current, comprehensive reference collection of health resources. . . . Excellent reference."
— *The Bookwatch, Aug '01*

SEE ALSO Pregnancy and Birth Sourcebook, 2nd Edition

Fitness and Exercise Sourcebook, 3rd Edition

Basic Consumer Health Information about the Physical and Mental Benefits of Fitness, Including Cardiorespiratory Endurance, Muscular Strength, Muscular Endurance, and Flexibility, with Facts about Sports Nutrition and Exercise-Related Injuries and Tips about Physical Activity and Exercises for People of All Ages and for People with Health Concerns

Along with Advice on Selecting and Using Exercise Equipment, Maintaining Exercise Motivation, a Glossary of Related Terms, and a Directory of Resources for More Help and Information

Edited by Amy L. Sutton. 635 pages. 2007. 978-0-7808-0946-8.

"Updates the consumer information on the physical and mental benefits of physical activity throughout the lifespan offered in earlier editions. . . . Recommended. All readers; all levels."
— *CHOICE, Oct '07*

"An exceptionally well-rounded coverage perfect for any concerned about developing and understanding a fitness program."
— *California Bookwatch, Jun '07*

SEE ALSO Sports Injuries Sourcebook, 3rd Edition

Food Safety Sourcebook

Basic Consumer Health Information about the Safe Handling of Meat, Poultry, Seafood, Eggs, Fruit Juices, and Other Food Items, and Facts about Pesticides, Drinking Water, Food Safety Overseas, and the Onset, Duration, and Symptoms of Foodborne Illnesses, Including Types of Pathogenic Bacteria, Parasitic Protozoa, Worms, Viruses, and Natural Toxins

Along with the Role of the Consumer, the Food Handler, and the Government in Food Safety; a Glossary, and Resources for Additional Help and Information

Edited by Dawn D. Matthews. 327 pages. 1999. 978-0-7808-0326-8.

"Recommended reference source."
— *Booklist, May '00*

"This book takes the complex issues of food safety and foodborne pathogens and presents them in an easily understood manner. [It does] an excellent job of covering a large and often confusing topic."
— *American Reference Books Annual, 2000*

Forensic Medicine Sourcebook

Basic Consumer Information for the Layperson about Forensic Medicine, Including Crime Scene Investigation, Evidence Collection and Analysis, Expert Testimony, Computer-Aided Criminal Identification, Digital Imaging in the Courtroom, DNA Profiling, Accident Reconstruction, Autopsies, Ballistics, Drugs and Explosives Detection, Latent Fingerprints, Product Tampering, and Questioned Document Examination

Along with Statistical Data, a Glossary of Forensics Terminology, and Listings of Sources for Further Help and Information

Edited by Annemarie S. Muth. 574 pages. 1999. 978-0-7808-0232-2.

"Given the expected widespread interest in its content and its easy to read style, this book is recommended for most public and all college and university libraries."
— *E-Streams, Feb '01*

"A wealth of information, useful statistics, references are up-to-date and extremely complete. This wonderful collection of data will help students who are interested in a career in any type of forensic field. It is a great resource for attorneys who need information about types of expert witnesses needed in a particular case. It also offers useful information for fiction and nonfiction writers whose work involves a crime. A fascinating compilation. All levels."
— *CHOICE, Jan '00*

"There are several items that make this book attractive to consumers who are seeking certain forensic data. . . . This is a useful current

source for those seeking general forensic medical answers."
—*American Reference Books Annual, 2000*

◾

Gastrointestinal Diseases and Disorders Sourcebook, 2nd Edition

Basic Consumer Health Information about the Upper and Lower Gastrointestinal (GI) Tract, Including the Esophagus, Stomach, Intestines, Rectum, Liver, and Pancreas, with Facts about Gastroesophageal Reflux Disease, Gastritis, Hernias, Ulcers, Celiac Disease, Diverticulitis, Irritable Bowel Syndrome, Hemorrhoids, Gastrointestinal Cancers, and Other Diseases and Disorders Related to the Digestive Process

Along with Information about Commonly Used Diagnostic and Surgical Procedures, Statistics, Reports on Current Research Initiatives and Clinical Trials, a Glossary, and Resources for Additional Help and Information

Edited by Sandra J. Judd. 654 pages. 2006. 978-0-7808-0798-3.

"The text is designed for the general reader seeking information on prevention, disease warning signs, diagnostic and therapeutic questions. . . . It is an excellent resource for the general reader to conveniently locate credible, coordinated and indexed information. . . . The sourcebook will prove very helpful for patients, caregivers and should be available in every physician waiting room."
—*Doody's Review Service, 2006*

SEE ALSO *Diet and Nutrition Sourcebook, 3rd Edition, Digestive Diseases and Disorders Sourcebook*

◾

Genetic Disorders Sourcebook, 4th Edition

Basic Consumer Health Information about Hereditary Diseases and Disorders, Including Facts about the Human Genome, Genetic Inheritance Patterns, Disorders Associated with Specific Genes, Such as Sickle Cell Disease, Hemophilia, and Cystic Fibrosis, Chromosome Disorders, Such as Down Syndrome, Fragile X Syndrome, and Turner Syndrome, and Complex Diseases and Disorders Resulting from the Interaction of Environmental and Genetic Factors, Such as Allergies, Cancer, and Obesity

Along with Facts about Genetic Testing, Suggestions for Parents of Children with Special Needs, Reports on Current Research Initiatives, a Glossary of Genetic Terminology, and Resources for Additional Help and Information

Edited by Sandra J. Judd. 600 pages. 2009. 978-0-7808-1076-1.

◾

Head Trauma Sourcebook

Basic Information for the Layperson about Open-Head and Closed-Head Injuries, Treatment Advances, Recovery, and Rehabilitation

Along with Reports on Current Research Initiatives

Edited by Karen Bellenir. 414 pages. 1997. 978-0-7808-0208-7.

◾

Headache Sourcebook

Basic Consumer Health Information about Migraine, Tension, Cluster, Rebound and Other Types of Headaches, with Facts about the Cause and Prevention of Headaches, the Effects of Stress and the Environment, Headaches during Pregnancy and Menopause, and Childhood Headaches

Along with a Glossary and Other Resources for Additional Help and Information

Edited by Dawn D. Matthews. 342 pages. 2002. 978-0-7808-0337-4.

"Highly recommended for academic and medical reference collections."
—*Library Bookwatch, Sep '02*

SEE ALSO *Pain Sourcebook, 3rd Edition*

◾

Healthy Aging Sourcebook

Basic Consumer Health Information about Maintaining Health through the Aging Process, Including Advice on Nutrition, Exercise, and Sleep, Help in Making Decisions about Midlife Issues and Retirement, and Guidance Concerning Practical and Informed Choices in Health Consumerism

Along with Data Concerning the Theories of Aging, Different Experiences in Aging by Minority Groups, and Facts about Aging Now and Aging in the Future; and Featuring a Glossary, a Guide to Consumer Help, Additional Suggested Reading, and Practical Resource Directory

Edited by Jenifer Swanson. 537 pages. 1999. 978-0-7808-0390-9.

"Recommended reference source."
— *Booklist, Feb '00*

SEE ALSO Physical and Mental Issues in Aging Sourcebook

Healthy Children Sourcebook

Basic Consumer Health Information about the Physical and Mental Development of Children between the Ages of 3 and 12, Including Routine Health Care, Preventative Health Services, Safety and First Aid, Healthy Sleep, Dental Care, Nutrition, and Fitness, and Featuring Parenting Tips on Such Topics as Bedwetting, Choosing Day Care, Monitoring TV and Other Media, and Establishing a Foundation for Substance Abuse Prevention

Along with a Glossary of Commonly Used Pediatric Terms and Resources for Additional Help and Information.

Edited by Chad T. Kimball. 624 pages. 2003. 978-0-7808-0247-6.

"Should be required reading for parents and teachers."
— *E-Streams, Jun '04*

"It is hard to imagine that any other single resource exists that would provide such a comprehensive guide of timely information on health promotion and disease prevention for children aged 3 to 12."
— *American Reference Books Annual, 2004*

"This easy-to-read volume is a tremendous resource."
— *AORN Journal, May '05*

SEE ALSO Childhood Diseases and Disorders Sourcebook, 2nd Edition

Healthy Heart Sourcebook for Women

Basic Consumer Health Information about Cardiac Issues Specific to Women, Including Facts about Major Risk Factors and Prevention, Treatment and Control Strategies, and Important Dietary Issues

Along with a Special Section Regarding the Pros and Cons of Hormone Replacement Therapy and Its Impact on Heart Health, and Additional Help, Including Recipes, a Glossary, and a Directory of Resources

Edited by Dawn D. Matthews. 321 pages. 2000. 978-0-7808-0329-9.

"A good reference source and recommended for all public, academic, medical, and hospital libraries."
— *Medical Reference Services Quarterly, Summer '01*

"Contains very important information about coronary artery disease that all women should know. The information is current and presented in an easy-to-read format. The book will make a good addition to any library."
— *American Medical Writers Association Journal, Summer '00*

SEE ALSO Cardiovascular Diseases and Disorders Sourcebook, 3rd Edition, Women's Health Concerns Sourcebook, 3rd Edition

Hepatitis Sourcebook

Basic Consumer Health Information about Hepatitis A, Hepatitis B, Hepatitis C, and Other Forms of Hepatitis, Including Autoimmune Hepatitis, Alcoholic Hepatitis, Nonalcoholic Steatohepatitis, and Toxic Hepatitis, with Facts about Risk Factors, Screening Methods, Diagnostic Tests, and Treatment Options

Along with Information on Liver Health, Tips for People Living with Chronic Hepatitis, Reports on Current Research Initiatives, a Glossary of Terms Related to Hepatitis, and a Directory of Sources for Further Help and Information

Edited by Sandra J. Judd. 570 pages. 2006. 978-0-7808-0749-5.

"The breadth of information found in this one book would not be readily found in another source. Highly recommended."
— *American Reference Books Annual, 2006*

SEE ALSO Contagious Diseases Sourcebook

Household Safety Sourcebook

Basic Consumer Health Information about Household Safety, Including Information about Poisons, Chemicals, Fire, and Water Hazards in the Home

Along with Advice about the Safe Use of Home Maintenance Equipment, Choosing Toys and Nursery Furniture, Holiday and Recreation Safety, a Glossary, and Resources for Further Help and Information

Edited by Dawn D. Matthews. 587 pages. 2002. 978-0-7808-0338-1.

"As a sourcebook on household safety this book meets its mark. It is encyclopedic in scope and covers a wide range of safety issues that are commonly seen in the home."
—*E-Streams, Jul '02*

Hypertension Sourcebook

Basic Consumer Health Information about the Causes, Diagnosis, and Treatment of High Blood Pressure, with Facts about Consequences, Complications, and Co-Occurring Disorders, Such as Coronary Heart Disease, Diabetes, Stroke, Kidney Disease, and Hypertensive Retinopathy, and Issues in Blood Pressure Control, Including Dietary Choices, Stress Management, and Medications

Along with Reports on Current Research Initiatives and Clinical Trials, a Glossary, and Resources for Additional Help and Information

Edited by Dawn D. Matthews and Karen Bellenir. 588 pages. 2004. 978-0-7808-0674-0.

"Academic, public, and medical libraries will want to add the *Hypertension Sourcebook* to their collections."
—*E-Streams, Aug '05*

"The strength of this source is the wide range of information given about hypertension."
—*American Reference Books Annual, 2005*

SEE ALSO *Stroke Sourcebook, 2nd Edition*

Immune System Disorders Sourcebook, 2nd Edition

Basic Consumer Health Information about Disorders of the Immune System, Including Immune System Function and Response, Diagnosis of Immune Disorders, Information about Inherited Immune Disease, Acquired Immune Disease, and Autoimmune Diseases, Including Primary Immune Deficiency, Acquired Immunodeficiency Syndrome (AIDS), Lupus, Multiple Sclerosis, Type 1 Diabetes, Rheumatoid Arthritis, and Graves' Disease

Along with Treatments, Tips for Coping with Immune Disorders, a Glossary, and a Directory of Additional Resources

Edited by Joyce Brennfleck Shannon. 643 pages. 2005. 978-0-7808-0748-8.

"Highly recommended for academic and public libraries."
—*American Reference Books Annual, 2006*

"The updated second edition is a 'must' for any consumer health library seeking a solid resource covering the treatments, symptoms, and options for immune disorder sufferers. . . . An excellent guide."
—*MBR Bookwatch, Jan '06*

SEE ALSO *AIDS Sourcebook, 4th Edition, Arthritis Sourcebook, 2nd Edition*

Infant and Toddler Health Sourcebook

Basic Consumer Health Information about the Physical and Mental Development of Newborns, Infants, and Toddlers, Including Neonatal Concerns, Nutrition Recommendations, Immunization Schedules, Common Pediatric Disorders, Assessments and Milestones, Safety Tips, and Advice for Parents and Other Caregivers

Along with a Glossary of Terms and Resource Listings for Additional Help

Edited by Jenifer Swanson. 570 pages. 2000. 978-0-7808-0246-9.

"As a reference for the general public, this would be useful in any library."
—*E-Streams, May '01*

"Recommended reference source."
—*Booklist, Feb '01*

Infectious Diseases Sourcebook

Basic Consumer Health Information about Non-Contagious Bacterial, Viral, Prion, Fungal, and Parasitic Diseases Spread by Food and Water, Insects and Animals, or Environmental Contact, Including Botulism, E. Coli, Encephalitis, Legionnaires' Disease, Lyme Disease, Malaria, Plague, Rabies, Salmonella, Tetanus, and Others, and Facts about Newly Emerging Diseases, Such as Hantavirus, Mad Cow Disease, Monkeypox, and West Nile Virus

Along with Information about Preventing Disease Transmission, the Threat of Bioterrorism, and Current Research Initiatives, with a Glossary and Directory of Resources for More Information

Edited by Karen Bellenir. 610 pages. 2004. 978-0-7808-0675-7.

"This reference continues the excellent tradition of the *Health Reference Series* in consolidating a wealth of information on a selected topic into a format that is easy to use and accessible to the general public."
—*American Reference Books Annual, 2005*

"Recommended for public and academic libraries."
—*E-Streams, Jan '05*

Injury and Trauma Sourcebook

Basic Consumer Health Information about the Impact of Injury, the Diagnosis and Treatment of Common and Traumatic Injuries, Emergency Care, and Specific Injuries Related to Home, Community, Workplace, Transportation, and Recreation

Along with Guidelines for Injury Prevention, a Glossary, and a Directory of Additional Resources

Edited by Joyce Brennfleck Shannon. 675 pages. 2002. 978-0-7808-0421-0.

"Practitioners should be aware of guides such as this in order to facilitate their use by patients and their families."
—*Doody's Health Sciences Book Review Journal, Sep-Oct '02*

"Recommended reference source."
—*Booklist, Sep '02*

"Highly recommended for academic and medical reference collections."
—*Library Bookwatch, Sep '02*

SEE ALSO *Emergency Medical Services Sourcebook, Sports Injuries Sourcebook, 3rd Edition*

Learning Disabilities Sourcebook, 3rd Edition

Basic Consumer Health Information about Dyslexia, Auditory and Visual Processing Disorders, Communication Disorders, Dyscalculia, Dysgraphia, and Other Conditions That Impede Learning, Including Attention Deficit/Hyperactivity Disorder, Autism Spectrum Disorders, Hearing and Visual Impairments, Chromosome-Based Disorders, and Brain Injury

Along with Facts about Brain Function, Assessment, Therapy and Remediation, Accommodations, Assistive Technology, Legal Protections, and Tips about Family Life, School Transitions, and Employment Strategies, a Glossary of Related Terms, and Directories of Additional Resources

Edited by Joyce Brennfleck Shannon. 613 pages. 2009. 978-0-7808-1039-6.

SEE ALSO *Attention Deficit Disorder Sourcebook, Autism and Pervasive Developmental Disorders Sourcebook*

Leukemia Sourcebook

Basic Consumer Health Information about Adult and Childhood Leukemias, Including Acute Lymphocytic Leukemia (ALL), Chronic Lymphocytic Leukemia (CLL), Acute Myelogenous Leukemia (AML), Chronic Myelogenous Leukemia (CML), and Hairy Cell Leukemia, and Treatments Such as Chemotherapy, Radiation Therapy, Peripheral Blood Stem Cell and Marrow Transplantation, and Immunotherapy

Along with Tips for Life During and After Treatment, a Glossary, and Directories of Additional Resources

Edited by Joyce Brennfleck Shannon. 564 pages. 2003. 978-0-7808-0627-6.

"Unlike other medical books for the layperson, . . . the language does not talk down to the reader. . . . This volume is highly recommended for all libraries."
—*American Reference Books Annual, 2004*

"A fine title which ranges from diagnosis to alternative treatments, staging, and tips for life during and after diagnosis."
—*The Bookwatch, Dec '03*

SEE ALSO *Cancer Sourcebook, 5th Edition*

Liver Disorders Sourcebook

Basic Consumer Health Information about the Liver and How It Works; Liver Diseases, Including Cancer, Cirrhosis, Hepatitis, and Toxic and Drug Related Diseases; Tips for Maintaining a Healthy Liver; Laboratory Tests, Radiology Tests, and Facts about Liver Transplantation

Along with a Section on Support Groups, a Glossary, and Resource Listings

Edited by Joyce Brennfleck Shannon. 580 pages. 2000. 978-0-7808-0383-1.

"This title is recommended for health sciences and public libraries with consumer health collections."
—*E-Streams, Oct '00*

"Recommended reference source."
—*Booklist, Jun '00*

SEE ALSO *Gastrointestinal Diseases and Disorders Sourcebook, 2nd Edition, Hepatitis Sourcebook*

Lung Disorders Sourcebook

Basic Consumer Health Information about Emphysema, Pneumonia, Tuberculosis, Asthma, Cystic Fibrosis, and Other Lung Disorders, Including Facts about Diagnostic Procedures, Treatment Strategies, Disease Prevention Efforts, and Such Risk Factors as Smoking, Air Pollution, and Exposure to Asbestos, Radon, and Other Agents

Along with a Glossary and Resources for Additional Help and Information

Edited by Dawn D. Matthews. 657 pages. 2002. 978-0-7808-0339-8.

"Highly recommended for academic and medical reference collections."
—*Library Bookwatch, Sep '02*

SEE ALSO *Respiratory Disorders Sourcebook, 2nd Edition*

Medical Tests Sourcebook, 3rd Edition

Basic Consumer Health Information about X-Rays, Blood Tests, Stool and Urine Tests, Biopsies, Mammography, Endoscopic Procedures, Ultrasound Exams, Computed Tomography, Magnetic Resonance Imaging (MRI), Nuclear Medicine, Genetic Testing, Home-Use Tests, and More

Along with Facts about Preventive Care and Screening Test Guidelines, Screening and Assessment Tests Associated with Such Specific Concerns as Cancer, Heart Disease, Allergies, Diabetes, Thyroid Disfunction, and Infertility, a Glossary of Related Terms, and a Directory of Resources for Additional Help and Information

Edited by Karen Bellenir. 627 pages. 2008. 978-0-7808-1040-2

"This volume has a wide scope that makes it useful . . . Can be a valuable reference guide."
—*ARBAonline, Nov '08*

Men's Health Concerns Sourcebook, 3rd Edition

Basic Consumer Health Information about Wellness in Men and Gender-Related Differences in Health, With Facts about Heart Disease, Cancer, Traumatic Injury, and Other Leading Causes of Death in Men, Reproductive Concerns, Sexual Dysfunction, Disorders of the Prostate, Penis, and Testes, Sex-Linked Genetic Disorders, and Other Medical and Mental Concerns of Men

Along with Statistical Data, a Glossary of Related Terms, and a Directory of Resources for Additional Information

Edited by Sandra J. Judd. 600 pages. 2009. 978-0-7808-1033-4.

SEE ALSO *Prostate and Urological Disorders Sourcebook*

Mental Health Disorders Sourcebook, 4th Edition

Basic Consumer Health Information about the Causes and Symptoms of Mental Health Problems, Including Depression, Bipolar Disorder, Anxiety Disorders, Posttraumatic Stress Disorder, Obsessive-Compulsive Disorder, Eating Disorders, Addictions, and Personality and Psychotic Disorders

Along with Information about Medications and Treatments, Mental Health Concerns in Children, Adolescents, and Adults, Tips on Living with Mental Health Disorders, a Glossary of Related Terms, and a Directory of Resources for Additional Help and Information

Edited by Amy L. Sutton. 600 pages. 2009. 978-0-7808-1041-9.

SEE ALSO *Depression Sourcebook, 2nd Edition, Stress-Related Disorders Sourcebook, 2nd Edition*

Mental Retardation Sourcebook

Basic Consumer Health Information about Mental Retardation and Its Causes, Including

Down Syndrome, Fetal Alcohol Syndrome, Fragile X Syndrome, Genetic Conditions, Injury, and Environmental Sources

Along with Preventive Strategies, Parenting Issues, Educational Implications, Health Care Needs, Employment and Economic Matters, Legal Issues, a Glossary, and a Resource Listing for Additional Help and Information

Edited by Joyce Brennfleck Shannon. 627 pages. 2000. 978-0-7808-0377-0.

"Public libraries will find the book useful for reference and as a beginning research point for students, parents, and caregivers."
—American Reference Books Annual, 2001

"The strength of this work is that it compiles many basic fact sheets and addresses for further information in one volume. It is intended and suitable for the general public."
—E-Streams, Nov '00

"An invaluable overview."
—Reviewer's Bookwatch, Jul '00

Movement Disorders Sourcebook, 2nd Edition

Basic Consumer Health Information about the Symptoms and Causes of Movement Disorders, Including Parkinson Disease, Amyotrophic Lateral Sclerosis, Cerebral Palsy, Muscular Dystrophy, Multiple Sclerosis, Myasthenia, Myoclonus, Spina Bifida, Dystonia, Essential Tremor, Choreatic Disorders, Huntington Disease, Tourette Syndrome, and Other Disorders That Cause Slowed, Absent, or Excessive Movements

Along with Information about Surgical and Nonsurgical Interventions, Physical Therapies, Strategies for Independent Living, a Glossary of Related Terms, and a Directory of Resources for Additional Help and Information

Edited by Amy L. Sutton. 600 pages. 2009. 978-0-7808-1034-1.

SEE ALSO Multiple Sclerosis Sourcebook, Muscular Dystrophy Sourcebook

Multiple Sclerosis Sourcebook

Basic Consumer Health Information about Multiple Sclerosis (MS) and Its Effects on Mobility, Vision, Bladder Function, Speech,

Swallowing, and Cognition, Including Facts about Risk Factors, Causes, Diagnostic Procedures, Pain Management, Drug Treatments, and Physical and Occupational Therapies

Along with Guidelines for Nutrition and Exercise, Tips on Choosing Assistive Equipment, Information about Disability, Work, Financial, and Legal Issues, a Glossary of Related Terms, and a Directory of Additional Resources

Edited by Joyce Brennfleck Shannon. 553 pages. 2007. 978-0-7808-0998-7.

SEE ALSO Movement Disorders Sourcebook, 2nd Edition

Muscular Dystrophy Sourcebook

Basic Consumer Health Information about Congenital, Childhood-Onset, and Adult-Onset Forms of Muscular Dystrophy, Such as Duchenne, Becker, Emery-Dreifuss, Distal, Limb-Girdle, Facioscapulohumeral (FSHD), Myotonic, and Ophthalmoplegic Muscular Dystrophies, Including Facts about Diagnostic Tests, Medical and Physical Therapies, Management of Co-Occurring Conditions, and Parenting Guidelines

Along with Practical Tips for Home Care, a Glossary, and Directories of Additional Resources

Edited by Joyce Brennfleck Shannon. 552 pages. 2004. 978-0-7808-0676-4.

"This book is highly recommended for public and academic libraries as well as health care offices that support the information needs of patients and their families."
—E-Streams, Apr '05

"Excellent reference."
—The Bookwatch, Jan '05

SEE ALSO Movement Disorders Sourcebook, 2nd Edition

Obesity Sourcebook

Basic Consumer Health Information about Diseases and Other Problems Associated with Obesity, and Including Facts about Risk Factors, Prevention Issues, and Management Approaches

Along with Statistical and Demographic Data, Information about Special Populations,

Research Updates, a Glossary, and Source Listings for Further Help and Information

Edited by Wilma Caldwell and Chad T. Kimball. 360 pages. 2001. 978-0-7808-0333-6.

"The book synthesizes the reliable medical literature on obesity into one easy-to-read and useful resource for the general public."
—American Reference Books Annual, 2002

"Well suited for the health reference collection of a public library or an academic health science library that serves the general population."
—E-Streams, Sep '01

Osteoporosis Sourcebook

Basic Consumer Health Information about Primary and Secondary Osteoporosis and Juvenile Osteoporosis and Related Conditions, Including Fibrous Dysplasia, Gaucher Disease, Hyperthyroidism, Hypophosphatasia, Myeloma, Osteopetrosis, Osteogenesis Imperfecta, and Paget's Disease

Along with Information about Risk Factors, Treatments, Traditional and Non-Traditional Pain Management, a Glossary of Related Terms, and a Directory of Resources

Edited by Allan R. Cook. 568 pages. 2001. 978-0-7808-0239-1.

"This resource is recommended as a great reference source for public, health, and academic libraries, and is another triumph for the editors of Omnigraphics."
—American Reference Books Annual, 2002

"Will prove valuable to any library seeking to maintain a current, comprehensive reference collection of health resources. . . . From prevention to treatment and associated conditions, this provides an excellent survey."
—The Bookwatch, Aug '01

SEE ALSO Healthy Aging Sourcebook, Women's Health Concerns Sourcebook, 3rd Edition

Pain Sourcebook, 3rd Edition

Basic Consumer Health Information about Acute and Chronic Pain, Including Nerve Pain, Bone Pain, Muscle Pain, Cancer Pain, and Disorders Characterized by Pain, Such as Arthritis, Temporomandibular Muscle and Joint (TMJ) Disorder, Carpal Tunnel Syndrome,

Headaches, Heartburn, Sciatica, and Shingles, and Facts about Diagnostic Tests and Treatment Options for Pain, Including Over-the-Counter and Prescription Drugs, Physical Rehabilitation, Injection and Infusion Therapies, Implantable Technologies, and Complementary Medicine

Along with Tips for Living with Pain, a Glossary of Related Terms, and a Directory of Additional Resources

Edited by Joyce Brennfleck Shannon. 644 pages. 2008. 978-0-7808-1006-8.

"Excellent for ready-reference users and can be used for beginning students in health fields . . . appropriate for the consumer health collection in both public and academic libraries."
—ARBAonline, Nov '08

Pediatric Cancer Sourcebook

Basic Consumer Health Information about Leukemias, Brain Tumors, Sarcomas, Lymphomas, and Other Cancers in Infants, Children, and Adolescents, Including Descriptions of Cancers, Treatments, and Coping Strategies

Along with Suggestions for Parents, Caregivers, and Concerned Relatives, a Glossary of Cancer Terms, and Resource Listings

Edited by Edward J. Prucha. 575 pages. 1999. 978-0-7808-0245-2.

"An excellent source of information. Recommended for public, hospital, and health science libraries with consumer health collections."
—E-Streams, Jun '00

"A valuable addition to all libraries specializing in health services and many public libraries."
—American Reference Books Annual, 2000

SEE ALSO Childhood Diseases and Disorders Sourcebook, 2nd Edition, Healthy Children Sourcebook

Physical and Mental Issues in Aging Sourcebook

Basic Consumer Health Information on Physical and Mental Disorders Associated with the Aging Process, Including Concerns about Cardiovascular Disease, Pulmonary Disease, Oral Health, Digestive Disorders, Musculoskeletal and Skin Disorders, Metabolic

Changes, Sexual and Reproductive Issues, and Changes in Vision, Hearing, and Other Senses

Along with Data about Longevity and Causes of Death, Information on Acute and Chronic Pain, Descriptions of Mental Concerns, a Glossary of Terms, and Resource Listings for Additional Help

Edited by Jenifer Swanson. 660 pages. 1999. 978-0-7808-0233-9.

"This is a treasure of health information for the layperson."
—CHOICE Health Sciences Supplement, May '00

"Recommended for public libraries."
—American Reference Books Annual, 2000

SEE ALSO Healthy Aging Sourcebook

Podiatry Sourcebook, 2nd Edition

Basic Consumer Health Information about Disorders, Diseases, and Deformities that Affect the Foot and Ankle, Including Sprains, Corns, Calluses, Bunions, Plantar Warts, Plantar Fasciitis, Neuromas, Clubfoot, Flat Feet, Achilles Tendonitis, and Much More

Along with Information about Selecting a Foot Care Specialist, Foot Fitness, Shoes and Socks, Diagnostic Tests and Corrective Procedures, Financial Assistance for Corrective Devices, a Glossary of Related Terms, and a Directory of Resources for Additional Help and Information

Edited by Ivy L. Alexander. 516 pages. 2007. 978-0-7808-0944-4.

"An excellent resource. . . . Although there have been various types of 'foot books' published in the past, none are as comprehensive as this one. 5 Stars (out of 5)!"
—Doody's Review Service, 2007

"Perfect for both health libraries and general-interest lending collections."
—Internet Bookwatch, Jul '07

Pregnancy and Birth Sourcebook, 3rd Edition

Basic Consumer Health Information about Pregnancy and Fetal Development, Including Facts about Fertility and Conception, Physical and Emotional Changes during Pregnancy, Prenatal Care and Diagnostic Tests, High-Risk Pregnancies and Complications, Labor, Delivery, and the Postpartum Period

Along with Tips on Maintaining Health and Wellness during Pregnancy and Caring for Newborn Infants, a Glossary of Related Terms, and Directories of Resources for Additional Help and Information

Edited by Amy L. Sutton. 600 pages. 2009. 978-0-7808-1074-7.

SEE ALSO Breastfeeding Sourcebook, Congenital Disorders Sourcebook, 2nd Edition, Family Planning Sourcebook, Women's Health Concerns Sourcebook, 3rd Edition

Prostate and Urological Disorders Sourcebook

Basic Consumer Health Information about Urogenital and Sexual Disorders in Men, Including Prostate and Other Andrological Cancers, Prostatitis, Benign Prostatic Hyperplasia, Testicular and Penile Trauma, Cryptorchidism, Peyronie Disease, Erectile Dysfunction, and Male Factor Infertility, and Facts about Commonly Used Tests and Procedures, Such as Prostatectomy, Vasectomy, Vasectomy Reversal, Penile Implants, and Semen Analysis

Along with a Glossary of Andrological Terms and a Directory of Resources for Additional Information

Edited by Karen Bellenir. 604 pages. 2006. 978-0-7808-0797-6.

"Certain to be a popular pick among library reference holdings. . . . No prior knowledge is assumed for any of the conditions or terms herein, making it a most accessible general-interest reference."
—California Bookwatch, Apr '06

SEE ALSO Men's Health Concerns Sourcebook, 3rd Edition, Urinary Tract and Kidney Diseases and Disorders Sourcebook, 2nd Edition

Prostate Cancer Sourcebook

Basic Consumer Health Information about Prostate Cancer, Including Information about the Associated Risk Factors, Detection, Diagnosis, and Treatment of Prostate Cancer

Along with Information on Non-Malignant Prostate Conditions, and Featuring a Section

Listing Support and Treatment Centers and a Glossary of Related Terms

Edited by Dawn D. Matthews. 340 pages. 2001. 978-0-7808-0324-4.

"Recommended reference source."
—*Booklist, Jan '02*

"A valuable resource for health care consumers seeking information on the subject. . . . All text is written in a clear, easy-to-understand language that avoids technical jargon. Any library that collects consumer health resources would strengthen their collection with the addition of the *Prostate Cancer Sourcebook*."
—*American Reference Books Annual, 2002*

SEE ALSO *Cancer Sourcebook, 5th Edition, Men's Health Concerns Sourcebook, 3rd Edition*

Rehabilitation Sourcebook

Basic Consumer Health Information about Rehabilitation for People Recovering from Heart Surgery, Spinal Cord Injury, Stroke, Orthopedic Impairments, Amputation, Pulmonary Impairments, Traumatic Injury, and More, Including Physical Therapy, Occupational Therapy, Speech/Language Therapy, Massage Therapy, Dance Therapy, Art Therapy, and Recreational Therapy

Along with Information on Assistive and Adaptive Devices, a Glossary, and Resources for Additional Help and Information

Edited by Dawn D. Matthews. 519 pages. 2000. 978-0-7808-0236-0.

"This is an excellent resource for public library reference and health collections."
—*American Reference Books Annual, 2001*

"Recommended reference source."
—*Booklist, May '00*

Respiratory Disorders Sourcebook, 2nd Edition

Basic Consumer Health Information about Infectious, Inflammatory, and Chronic Conditions Affecting the Lungs and Respiratory System, Including Pneumonia, Bronchitis, Influenza, Tuberculosis, Sarcoidosis, Asthma, Cystic Fibrosis, Chronic Obstructive Pulmonary Disease, Lung Abscesses, Pulmonary Embolism, Occupational Lung Diseases, and Other Bacterial, Viral, and Fungal Infections

Along with Facts about the Structure and Function of the Lungs and Airways, Methods of Diagnosing Respiratory Disorders, and Treatment and Rehabilitation Options, a Glossary of Related Terms, and a Directory of Resources for Additional Help and Information

Edited by Sandra L. Judd. 638 pages. 2008. 978-0-7808-1007-5.

"A great addition for public and school libraries because it provides concise health information . . . readers can start with this reference source and get satisfactory answers before proceeding to other medical reference tools for more in depth information . . . A good guide for health education on lung disorders."
—*ARBAonline, Nov '08*

SEE ALSO *Lung Disorders Sourcebook*

Sexually Transmitted Diseases Sourcebook, 4th Edition

Basic Consumer Health Information about Chlamydial Infections, Gonorrhea, Hepatitis, Herpes, HIV/AIDS, Human Papillomavirus, Pubic Lice, Scabies, Syphilis, Trichomoniasis, Vaginal Infections, and Other Sexually Transmitted Diseases, Including Facts about Risk Factors, Symptoms, Diagnosis, Treatment, and the Prevention of Sexually Transmitted Infections

Along with Updates on Current Research Initiatives, a Glossary of Related Terms, and Resources for Additional Help and Information

Edited by Laura Larsen. 600 pages. 2009. 978-0-7808-1073-0.

SEE ALSO *AIDS Sourcebook, 4th Edition, Contagious Diseases Sourcebook, 2nd Edition, Men's Health Concerns Sourcebook, 3rd Edition, Women's Health Concerns Sourcebook, 3rd Edition*

Sleep Disorders Sourcebook, 2nd Edition

Basic Consumer Health Information about Sleep and Sleep Disorders, Including Insomnia, Sleep Apnea, Restless Legs Syndrome, Narcolepsy, Parasomnias, and Other Health Problems That Affect Sleep, Plus Facts about Diagnostic Procedures, Treatment Strategies,

Sleep Medications, and Tips for Improving Sleep Quality

Along with a Glossary of Related Terms and Resources for Additional Help and Information

Edited by Amy L. Sutton. 567 pages. 2005. 978-0-7808-0743-3.

"This book will be useful for just about everybody, especially the 40 million Americans with sleep disorders."
—*American Reference Books Annual, 2006*

"A welcome addition to public libraries and consumer health libraries."
—*Medical Reference Services Quarterly, Summer '06*

Smoking Concerns Sourcebook

Basic Consumer Health Information about Nicotine Addiction and Smoking Cessation, Featuring Facts about the Health Effects of Tobacco Use, Including Lung and Other Cancers, Heart Disease, Stroke, and Respiratory Disorders, Such as Emphysema and Chronic Bronchitis

Along with Information about Smoking Prevention Programs, Suggestions for Achieving and Maintaining a Smoke-Free Lifestyle, Statistics about Tobacco Use, Reports on Current Research Initiatives, a Glossary of Related Terms, and Directories of Resources for Additional Help and Information

Edited by Karen Bellenir. 595 pages. 2004. 978-0-7808-0323-7.

"Provides everything needed for the student or general reader seeking practical details on the effects of tobacco use."
—*The Bookwatch, Mar '05*

"Public libraries and consumer health care libraries will find this work useful."
—*American Reference Books Annual, 2005*

SEE ALSO *Respiratory Disorders Sourcebook, 2nd Edition*

Sports Injuries Sourcebook, 3rd Edition

Basic Consumer Health Information about Sprains and Strains, Fractures, Growth Plate Injuries, Overtraining Injuries, and Injuries to

the Head, Face, Shoulders, Elbows, Hands, Spinal Column, Knees, Ankles, and Feet, and with Facts about Heat-Related Illness, Steroids and Sport Supplements, Protective Equipment, Diagnostic Procedures, Treatment Options, and Rehabilitation*

Along with a Glossary of Related Terms and a Directory of Resources for Additional Help and Information

Edited by Sandra J. Judd. 623 pages. 2007. 978-0-7808-0949-9.

SEE ALSO *Fitness and Exercise Sourcebook, 3rd Edition*

Stress-Related Disorders Sourcebook, 2nd Edition

Basic Consumer Health Information about Stress and Stress-Related Disorders, Including Types of Stress, Sources of Acute and Chronic Stress, the Impact of Stress on the Body's Systems, and Mental and Emotional Health Problems Associated with Stress, Such as Depression, Anxiety Disorders, Substance Abuse, Posttraumatic Stress Disorder, and Suicide

Along with Advice about Getting Help for Stress-Related Disorders, Information about Stress Management Techniques, a Glossary of Stress-Related Terms, and a Directory of Resources for Additional Help and Information

Edited by Amy L. Sutton. 608 pages. 2007. 978-0-7808-0996-3.

"Accessible to the lay reader. Highly recommended for medical and psychiatric collections."
—*Library Journal, Mar '08*

"Well-written for a general readership, the 2nd Edition of *Stress-Related Disorders Sourcebook* is a useful addition to the health reference literature."
—*American Reference Books Annual, 2008*

SEE ALSO *Mental Health Disorders Sourcebook, 4th Edition*

Stroke Sourcebook, 2nd Edition

Basic Consumer Health Information about Stroke, Including Ischemic, Hemorrhagic, and Mini Strokes, as Well as Risk Factors, Prevention Guidelines, Diagnostic Tests, Medications and

Surgical Treatments, and Complications of Stroke

Along with Rehabilitation Techniques and Innovations, Tips on Staying Healthy and Maintaining Independence after Stroke, a Glossary of Related Terms, and a Directory of Resources for Stroke Survivors and Their Families

Edited by Amy L. Sutton. 626 pages. 2008. 978-0-7808-1035-8.

"An encyclopedic handbook on stroke that is written in a language the layperson can understand. . . . This is one of the most helpful, readable books on stroke. This volume is highly recommended and should be in every medical, hospital and public library; in addition, every family practitioner should have a copy in his or her office."
—ARBAonline Dec '08

SEE ALSO *Hypertension Sourcebook*

Surgery Sourcebook, 2nd Edition

Basic Consumer Health Information about Common Inpatient and Outpatient Surgeries, Including Critical Care and Trauma, Gastrointestinal, Gynecologic and Obstetric, Cardiac and Vascular, Neurologic, Ophthalmologic, Orthopedic, Reconstructive and Cosmetic, and Other Major and Minor Surgeries

Along with Information about Anesthesia and Pain Relief Options, Risks and Complications, Postoperative Recovery Concerns, and Innovative Surgical Techniques and Tools, a Glossary of Related Terms, and a Directory of Additional Resources

Edited by Amy L. Sutton. 645 pages. 2008. 978-0-7808-1004-4.

"Large public libraries and medical libraries would benefit from this material in their reference collections."
—ARBAonline Aug '08

SEE ALSO *Cosmetic and Reconstructive Surgery Sourcebook, 2nd Edition*

Thyroid Disorders Sourcebook

Basic Consumer Health Information about Disorders of the Thyroid and Parathyroid Glands, Including Hypothyroidism, Hyperthyroidism,

Graves Disease, Hashimoto Thyroiditis, Thyroid Cancer, and Parathyroid Disorders, Featuring Facts about Symptoms, Risk Factors, Tests, and Treatments

Along with Information about the Effects of Thyroid Imbalance on Other Body Systems, Environmental Factors That Affect the Thyroid Gland, a Glossary, and a Directory of Additional Resources

Edited by Joyce Brennfleck Shannon. 573 pages. 2005. 978-0-7808-0745-7.

"Recommended for consumer health collections."
—American Reference Books Annual, 2006

"Highly recommended pick for basic consumer health reference holdings at all levels."
—The Bookwatch, Aug '05

SEE ALSO *Endocrine and Metabolic Disorders Sourcebook, 2nd Edition*

Transplantation Sourcebook

Basic Consumer Health Information about Organ and Tissue Transplantation, Including Physical and Financial Preparations, Procedures and Issues Relating to Specific Solid Organ and Tissue Transplants, Rehabilitation, Pediatric Transplant Information, the Future of Transplantation, and Organ and Tissue Donation

Along with a Glossary and Listings of Additional Resources

Edited by Joyce Brennfleck Shannon. 610 pages. 2002. 978-0-7808-0322-0.

"Recommended for libraries with an interest in offering consumer health information."
—E-Streams, Jul '02

"This is a unique and valuable resource for patients facing transplantation and their families."
—Doody's Review Service, Jun '02

Traveler's Health Sourcebook

Basic Consumer Health Information for Travelers, Including Physical and Medical Preparations, Transportation Health and Safety, Essential Information about Food and Water, Sun Exposure, Insect and Snake Bites, Camping and Wilderness Medicine, and Travel with Physical or Medical Disabilities

Along with International Travel Tips, Vaccination Recommendations, Geographical Health Issues, Disease Risks, a Glossary, and a Listing of Additional Resources

Edited by Joyce Brennfleck Shannon. 619 pages. 2000. 978-0-7808-0384-8.

"Recommended reference source."
—*Booklist, Feb '01*

"This book is recommended for any public library, any travel collection, and especially any collection for the physically disabled."
—*American Reference Books Annual, 2001*

SEE ALSO *Worldwide Health Sourcebook*

■

Urinary Tract and Kidney Diseases and Disorders Sourcebook, 2nd Edition

Basic Consumer Health Information about the Urinary System, Including the Bladder, Urethra, Ureters, and Kidneys, with Facts about Urinary Tract Infections, Incontinence, Congenital Disorders, Kidney Stones, Cancers of the Urinary Tract and Kidneys, Kidney Failure, Dialysis, and Kidney Transplantation

Along with Statistical and Demographic Information, Reports on Current Research in Kidney and Urologic Health, a Summary of Commonly Used Diagnostic Tests, a Glossary of Related Terms, and a Directory of Resources for Additional Help and Information

Edited by Ivy L. Alexander. 621 pages. 2005. 978-0-7808-0750-1.

"A good choice for a consumer health information library or for a medical library needing information to refer to their patients."
—*American Reference Books Annual, 2006*

SEE ALSO *Prostate and Urological Disorders Sourcebook*

■

Vegetarian Sourcebook

Basic Consumer Health Information about Vegetarian Diets, Lifestyle, and Philosophy, Including Definitions of Vegetarianism and Veganism, Tips about Adopting Vegetarianism, Creating a Vegetarian Pantry, and Meeting Nutritional Needs of Vegetarians, with Facts Regarding Vegetarianism's Effect on Pregnant and Lactating Women, Children, Athletes, and Senior Citizens

Along with a Glossary of Commonly Used Vegetarian Terms and Resources for Additional Help and Information

Edited by Chad T. Kimball. 337 pages. 2002. 978-0-7808-0439-5.

"Organizes into one concise volume the answers to the most common questions concerning vegetarian diets and lifestyles. This title is recommended for public and secondary school libraries."
—*E-Streams, Apr '03*

"Invaluable reference for public and school library collections alike."
—*Library Bookwatch, Apr '03*

"The articles in this volume are easy to read and come from authoritative sources. The book does not necessarily support the vegetarian diet but instead provides the pros and cons of this important decision. . . . Recommended for public libraries and consumer health libraries."
—*American Reference Books Annual, 2003*

SEE ALSO *Diet and Nutrition Sourcebook, 3rd Edition*

■

Women's Health Concerns Sourcebook, 3rd Edition

Basic Consumer Health Information about Issues and Trends in Women's Health and Health Conditions of Special Concern to Women, Including Endometriosis, Uterine Fibroids, Menstrual Irregularities, Menopause, Sexual Dysfunction, Infertility, Cancer in Women, and Other Such Chronic Disorders as Lupus, Fibromyalgia, and Thyroid Disease

Along with Statistical Data, Tips for Maintaining Wellness, a Glossary, and a Directory of Resources for Further Help and Information

Edited by Sandra J. Judd. 600 pages. 2009. 978-0-7808-1036-5.

SEE ALSO *Breast Cancer Sourcebook, 3rd Edition, Cancer Sourcebook for Women, 3rd Edition, Healthy Heart Sourcebook for Women, Osteoporosis Sourcebook*

■

Workplace Health and Safety Sourcebook

Basic Consumer Health Information about Workplace Health and Safety, Including the Effect of Workplace Hazards on the Lungs,

Skin, Heart, Ears, Eyes, Brain, Reproductive Organs, Musculoskeletal System, and Other Organs and Body Parts

Along with Information about Occupational Cancer, Personal Protective Equipment, Toxic and Hazardous Chemicals, Child Labor, Stress, and Workplace Violence

Edited by Chad T. Kimball. 610 pages. 2000. 978-0-7808-0231-5.

"As a reference for the general public, this would be useful in any library."
—E-Streams, Jun '01

"Provides helpful information for primary care physicians and other caregivers interested in occupational medicine. . . . General readers; professionals."
—CHOICE, May '01

Worldwide Health Sourcebook

Basic Information about Global Health Issues, Including Malnutrition, Reproductive Health, Disease Dispersion and Prevention, Emerging Diseases, Risky Health Behaviors, and the Leading Causes of Death

Along with Global Health Concerns for Children, Women, and the Elderly, Mental Health Issues, Research and Technology Advancements, and Economic, Environmental, and Political Health Implications, a Glossary, and a Resource Listing for Additional Help and Information

Edited by Joyce Brennfleck Shannon. 597 pages. 2001. 978-0-7808-0330-5.

"Named an Outstanding Academic Title."
—CHOICE, Jan '02

"Yet another handy but also unique compilation in the extensive *Health Reference Series*, this is a useful work because many of the international publications reprinted or excerpted are not readily available. Highly recommended."
—CHOICE, Nov '01

SEE ALSO *Traveler's Health Sourcebook*

654

Teen Health Series
Complete Catalog
List price $69 per volume. School and library price $62 per volume.

Abuse and Violence Information for Teens
Health Tips about the Causes and Consequences of Abusive and Violent Behavior
Including Facts about the Types of Abuse and Violence, the Warning Signs of Abusive and Violent Behavior, Health Concerns of Victims, and Getting Help and Staying Safe

Edited by Sandra Augustyn Lawton. 411 pages. 2008. 978-0-7808-1008-2.

"A useful resource for schools and organizations providing services to teens and may also be a starting point in research projects."
—*Reference and Research Book News, Aug '08*

"Violence is a serious problem for teens. . . . This resource gives teens the information they need to face potential threats and get help—either for themselves or for their friends."
—*ARBAonline, Aug '08*

Accident and Safety Information for Teens
Health Tips about Medical Emergencies, Traumatic Injuries, and Disaster Preparedness
Including Facts about Motor Vehicle Accidents, Burns, Poisoning, Firearms, Natural Disasters, National Security Threats, and More

Edited by Karen Bellenir. 420 pages. 2008. 978-0-7808-1046-4.

SEE ALSO Sports Injuries Information for Teens, 2nd Edition

Alcohol Information for Teens, 2nd Edition
Health Tips about Alcohol and Alcoholism
Including Facts about Alcohol's Effects on the Body, Brain, and Behavior, the Consequences of Underage Drinking, Alcohol Abuse Prevention and Treatment, and Coping with Alcoholic Parents

Edited by Lisa Bakewell. 400 pages. 2009. 978-0-7808-1043-3.

SEE ALSO Drug Information for Teens, 2nd Edition

Allergy Information for Teens
Health Tips about Allergic Reactions Such as Anaphylaxis, Respiratory Problems, and Rashes
Including Facts about Identifying and Managing Allergies to Food, Pollen, Mold, Animals, Chemicals, Drugs, and Other Substances

Edited by Karen Bellenir. 410 pages. 2006. 978-0-7808-0799-0.

"This is a comprehensive, readable text on the subject of allergic diseases in teenagers. 5 Stars (out of 5)!"
—*Doody's Review Service, Jun '06*

"This authoritative and useful self-help title is a solid addition to YA collections, whether for personal interest or reports."
—*School Library Journal, Jul '06*

Asthma Information for Teens
Health Tips about Managing Asthma and Related Concerns
Including Facts about Asthma Causes, Triggers, Symptoms, Diagnosis, and Treatment

Edited by Karen Bellenir. 386 pages. 2005. 978-0-7808-0770-9.

"Highly recommended for medical libraries, public school libraries, and public libraries."
—*American Reference Books Annual, 2006*

"Although this volume is nearly 400 pages long, it is so clearly written and well organized that even hesitant readers will be able to find the facts they need, whether for reports or personal information. . . . A succinct but complete resource."
—*School Library Journal, Sep '05*

Body Information for Teens

Health Tips about Maintaining Well-Being for a Lifetime

Including Facts about the Development and Functioning of the Body's Systems, Organs, and Structures and the Health Impact of Lifestyle Choices

Edited by Sandra Augustyn Lawton. 458 pages. 2007. 978-0-7808-0443-2.

Cancer Information for Teens, 2nd Edition

Health Tips about Cancer Awareness, Symptoms, Prevention, Diagnosis, and Treatment

Including Facts about Common Cancers Affecting Teens, Causes, Detection, Coping Strategies, Clinical Trials, Nutrition and Exercise, Cancer in Friends or Family, and More

Edited by Karen Bellenir and Lisa Bakewell. 400 pages. 2009. 978-0-7808-1085-3.

Complementary and Alternative Medicine Information for Teens

Health Tips about Non-Traditional and Non-Western Medical Practices

Including Information about Acupuncture, Chiropractic Medicine, Dietary and Herbal Supplements, Hypnosis, Massage Therapy, Prayer and Spirituality, Reflexology, Yoga, and More

Edited by Sandra Augustyn Lawton. 407 pages. 2007. 978-0-7808-0966-6.

"This volume covers CAM specifically for teenagers but of general use also. It should be a welcome addition to both public and academic libraries."
—*American Reference Books Annual, 2008*

"This volume provides a solid foundation for further investigation of the subject, making it useful for both public and high school libraries."
—*VOYA: Voice of Youth Advocates, Jun '07*

Diabetes Information for Teens

Health Tips about Managing Diabetes and Preventing Related Complications

Including Information about Insulin, Glucose Control, Healthy Eating, Physical Activity, and Learning to Live with Diabetes

Edited by Sandra Augustyn Lawton. 410 pages. 2006. 978-0-7808-0811-9.

"A comprehensive instructional guide for teens. . . . some of the material may also be directed towards parents or teachers. 5 stars (out of 5)!"
—*Doody's Review Service, 2006*

"Students dealing with their own diabetes or that of a friend or family member or those writing reports on the topic will find this a valuable resource."
—*School Library Journal, Aug '06*

"This text is directed to the teen population and would be an excellent library resource for a health class or for the teacher as a reference for class preparation. It can, however, serve a much wider audience. The clinical educator on diabetes may find it valuable to educate the newly diagnosed client regardless of age. It also would be an excellent reference and education tool for a preventive medicine seminar on diabetes."
—*Physical Therapy, Mar '07*

Diet Information for Teens, 2nd Edition

Health Tips about Diet and Nutrition

Including Facts about Dietary Guidelines, Food Groups, Nutrients, Healthy Meals, Snacks, Weight Control, Medical Concerns Related to Diet, and More

Edited by Karen Bellenir. 432 pages. 2006. 978-0-7808-0820-1.

"A very quick and pleasant read in spite of the fact that it is very detailed in the information it gives. . . . A book for anyone concerned about diet and nutrition."
—*American Reference Books Annual, 2007*

SEE ALSO *Eating Disorders Information for Teens, 2nd Edition*

Drug Information for Teens, 2nd Edition

Health Tips about the Physical and Mental Effects of Substance Abuse

Including Information about Marijuana, Inhalants, Club Drugs, Stimulants, Hallucinogens,

Opiates, Prescription and Over-the-Counter Drugs, Herbal Products, Tobacco, Alcohol, and More

Edited by Sandra Augustyn Lawton. 468 pages. 2006. 978-0-7808-0862-1.

"As with earlier installments in Omnigraphics' *Teen Health Series, Drug Information for Teens* is designed specifically to meet the needs and interests of middle and high school students. . . . Strongly recommended for both academic and public libraries."
—*American Reference Books Annual, 2007*

"Solid thoughtful advice is given about how to handle peer pressure, drug-related health concerns, and treatment strategies."
—*School Library Journal, Dec '06*

SEE ALSO *Alcohol Information for Teens, 2nd Edition, Tobacco Information for Teens*

Eating Disorders Information for Teens, 2nd Edition
Health Tips about Anorexia, Bulimia, Binge Eating, And Other Eating Disorders
Including Information about Risk Factors, Diagnosis and Treatment, Prevention, Related Health Concerns, and Other Issues

Edited by Sandra Augustyn Lawton. 377 pages. 2009. 978-0-7808-1044-0.

SEE ALSO *Diet Information for Teens, 2nd Edition*

Fitness Information for Teens, 2nd Edition
Health Tips about Exercise, Physical Well-Being, and Health Maintenance
Including Facts about Conditioning, Stretching, Strength Training, Body Shape and Body Image, Sports Nutrition, and Specific Activities for Athletes and Non-Athletes

Edited by Lisa Bakewell. 432 pages. 2009. 978-0-7808-1045-7.

SEE ALSO *Diet Information for Teens, 2nd Edition, Sports Injuries Information for Teens, 2nd Edition*

Learning Disabilities Information for Teens
Health Tips about Academic Skills Disorders and Other Disabilities That Affect Learning
Including Information about Common Signs of Learning Disabilities, School Issues, Learning to Live with a Learning Disability, and Other Related Issues

Edited by Sandra Augustyn Lawton. 400 pages. 2006. 978-0-7808-0796-9.

"This book provides a wealth of information for any reader interested in the signs, causes, and consequences of learning disabilities, as well as related legal rights and educational interventions. . . . Public and academic libraries should want this title for both students and general readers."
—*American Reference Books Annual, 2006*

Mental Health Information for Teens, 2nd Edition
Health Tips about Mental Wellness and Mental Illness
Including Facts about Mental and Emotional Health, Depression and Other Mood Disorders, Anxiety Disorders, Conduct Disorder, Self-Injury, Psychosis, Schizophrenia, and More

Edited by Karen Bellenir. 424 pages. 2006. 978-0-7808-0863-8.

"This excellent overview of the psychological disorders that affect teens provides clear definitions and descriptions, and discusses resources, therapies, coping mechanisms, and medications."
—*School Library Journal Curriculum Connections, Fall '07*

"A well done reference for a specific, often under-represented group."
—*Doody's Review Service, 2006*

SEE ALSO *Stress Information for Teens*

Pregnancy Information for Teens
Health Tips about Teen Pregnancy and Teen Parenting
Including Facts about Prenatal Care, Pregnancy Complications, Labor and Delivery,

Postpartum Care, Pregnancy-Related Lifestyle Concerns, and More

Edited by Sandra Augustyn Lawton. 434 pages. 2007. 978-0-7808-0984-0.

SEE ALSO Sexual Health Information for Teens, 2nd Edition

Sexual Health Information for Teens, 2nd Edition
Health Tips about Sexual Development, Reproduction, Contraception, and Sexually Transmitted Infections
Including Facts about Puberty, Sexuality, Birth Control, Chlamydia, Gonorrhea, Herpes, Human Papillomavirus, Syphilis, and More

Edited by Sandra Augustyn Lawton. 430 pages. 2008. 978-0-7808-1010-5.

"This offering represents the most up-to-date information available on an array of topics including abstinence-only sexual education and pregnancy-prevention methods. . . . The range of coverage—from puberty and anatomy to sexually transmitted diseases—is thorough and extensive. Each chapter includes a bibliographic citation, and the three back sections containing additional resources, further reading, and the index are all first-rate. . . . This volume will be well used by students in need of the facts, whether for educational or personal reasons."
—*School Library Journal, Nov '08*

SEE ALSO Pregnancy Information for Teens

Skin Health Information for Teens, 2nd Edition
Health Tips about Dermatological Concerns and Skin Cancer Risks
Including Facts about Acne, Warts, Allergies, and Other Conditions and Lifestyle Choices, Such as Tanning, Tattooing, and Piercing, That Affect the Skin, Nails, Scalp, and Hair

Edited by Edited by Kim Wohlenhaus. 400 pages. 2009. 978-0-7808-1042-6.

Sleep Information for Teens
Health Tips about Adolescent Sleep Requirements, Sleep Disorders, and the Effects of Sleep Deprivation

Including Facts about Why People Need Sleep, Sleep Patterns, Circadian Rhythms, Dreaming, Insomnia, Sleep Apnea, Narcolepsy, and More

Edited by Karen Bellenir. 355 pages. 2008. 978-0-7808-1009-9.

SEE ALSO Body Information for Teens

Sports Injuries Information for Teens, 2nd Edition
Health Tips about Acute, Traumatic, and Chronic Injuries in Adolescent Athletes
Including Facts about Sprains, Fractures, and Overuse Injuries, Treatment, Rehabilitation, Sport-Specific Safety Guidelines, Fitness Suggestions, and More

Edited by Karen Bellenir. 429 pages. 2008. 978-0-7808-1011-2.

"An engaging selection of informative articles about the prevention and treatment of sports injuries. . . The value of this book is that the articles have been vetted and are often augmented with inserts of useful facts, definitions of technical terms, and quick tips. Sensitive topics like injuries to genitalia are discussed openly and responsibly. This revised edition contains updated articles and defines sport more broadly than the first edition."
—*School Library Journal, Nov '08*

"This work will be useful in the young adult collections of public libraries as well as high school libraries. . . . A useful resource for student research."
—*ARBAonline, Aug '08*

SEE ALSO Accident and Safety Information for Teens

Stress Information for Teens
Health Tips about the Mental and Physical Consequences of Stress
Including Information about the Different Kinds of Stress, Symptoms of Stress, Frequent Causes of Stress, Stress Management Techniques, and More

Edited by Sandra Augustyn Lawton. 392 pages. 2008. 978-0-7808-1012-9.

"Understanding what stress is, what causes it, how the body and the mind are impacted by it, and what teens can do are the general categories addressed here. . . . The chapters are brief but informative, and the list of community-help organizations is exhaustive. Report writers will find information quickly and easily, as will those who have personal concerns. The print is clear and the format is readable, making this an accessible resource for struggling readers and researchers."

—*School Library Journal, Dec '08*

"The articles selected will specifically appeal to young adults and are designed to answer their most common questions."

—*ARBAonline, Aug '08*

SEE ALSO *Mental Health Information for Teens, 2nd Edition*

Suicide Information for Teens
Health Tips about Suicide Causes and Prevention
Including Facts about Depression, Risk Factors, Getting Help, Survivor Support, and More

Edited by Joyce Brennfleck Shannon. 368 pages. 2005. 978-0-7808-0737-2.

"Highly Recommended for libraries serving teenagers as well as those who work with them."

—*E-Streams, Apr '06*

SEE ALSO *Mental Health Information for Teens, 2nd Edition*

Tobacco Information for Teens
Health Tips about the Hazards of Using Cigarettes, Smokeless Tobacco, and Other Nicotine Products
Including Facts about Nicotine Addiction, Immediate and Long-Term Health Effects of Tobacco Use, Related Cancers, Smoking Cessation, Tobacco Use Prevention, and Tobacco Use Statistics

Edited by Karen Bellenir. 440 pages. 2007. 978-0-7808-0976-5.

"A comprehensive resource. Each chapter is written to stand alone, so students can dip in and use the information in each section for reports or to answer personal questions without having to read the entire book. . . . The book is packed full of statistics, with sources to help students look up more."

—*School Library Journal, Sep '07*

"Pulls together a wide variety of authoritative sources to provide a comprehensive overview of tobacco use for this age group. . . . This reasonably priced reference title should be considered a necessary purchase for all public libraries and school media centers, along with academic libraries supporting teacher education."

—*American Reference Books Annual, 2008*

SEE ALSO *Drug Information for Teens, 2nd Edition*